The Primary Care Clinical Encounter

Field Guide to the Generalist's Craft

The Primary Care Clinical Encounter

Field Guide to the Generalist's Craft

William L. Miller, MD, MA

Illustrations by Su Bin Hahn and Rena Jiang

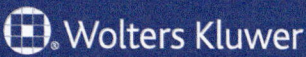

Philadelphia • Baltimore • New York • London
Buenos Aires • Hong Kong • Sydney • Tokyo

Acquisitions Editor: Joe Cho
Development Editor: Cindy Yoo
Editorial Coordinator: Abirami Balakrishnan
Editorial Assistant: Devin Van Gorden
Marketing Manager: Kirsten Watrud
Production Project Manager: Frances Gunning
Manager, Graphic Arts & Design: Stephen Druding
Manufacturing Coordinator: Lisa Bowling
Prepress Vendor: S4Carlisle Publishing Services

Copyright © 2027 Wolters Kluwer.

All rights reserved. This book is protected by copyright. No part of this book may be reproduced or transmitted in any form or by any means, including as photocopies or scanned-in or other electronic copies, or utilized by any information storage and retrieval system without written permission from the copyright owner, except for brief quotations embodied in critical articles and reviews. Materials appearing in this book prepared by individuals as part of their official duties as U.S. government employees are not covered by the above-mentioned copyright. To request permission, please contact Wolters Kluwer at Two Commerce Square, 2001 Market Street, Philadelphia, PA 19703, via email at permissions@lww.com, or via our website at shop.lww.com (products and services).

9 8 7 6 5 4 3 2 1

Printed in United States of America.

Library of Congress Cataloging-in-Publication Data

ISBN-13: 978-1-975267-29-2

Library of Congress Control Number: 2025947283

This work is provided "as is," and the publisher disclaims any and all warranties, express or implied, including any warranties as to accuracy, comprehensiveness, or currency of the content of this work.

This work is no substitute for individual patient assessment based upon healthcare professionals' examination of each patient and consideration of, among other things, age, weight, gender, current or prior medical conditions, medication history, laboratory data and other factors unique to the patient. The publisher does not provide medical advice or guidance and this work is merely a reference tool. Healthcare professionals, and not the publisher, are solely responsible for the use of this work including all medical judgments and for any resulting diagnosis and treatments.

Given continuous, rapid advances in medical science and health information, independent professional verification of medical diagnoses, indications, appropriate pharmaceutical selections and dosages, and treatment options should be made and healthcare professionals should consult a variety of sources. When prescribing medication, healthcare professionals are advised to consult the product information sheet (the manufacturer's package insert) accompanying each drug to verify, among other things, conditions of use, warnings and side effects and identify any changes in dosage schedule or contraindications, particularly if the medication to be administered is new, infrequently used or has a narrow therapeutic range. To the maximum extent permitted under applicable law, no responsibility is assumed by the publisher for any injury and/or damage to persons or property, as a matter of products liability, negligence law or otherwise, or from any reference to or use by any person of this work.

shop.lww.com

Thanks and Dedication

Gratitude for the wonder of life and all the relationships from which it emerges and to all those who practice the generalist craft in primary care and help ensure a healthier life together. Thank you!

Land Acknowledgment

The generalist craft in primary care presented in this *Field Guide* has been learned, taught, and practiced at the Lehigh Valley Family Medicine Residency Program since 1995. We acknowledge and recognize the Lehigh Valley as part of Lënapehòkink, the homelands of the Lenape peoples.

    The Lenape (aka Delaware) are the Indigenous people of the lands we now call Pennsylvania, New Jersey, Delaware, and parts of New York, Connecticut, and Maryland since before any known records. Lenape Chief Tamanend is recognized for establishing a friendship treaty with William Penn when he arrived here in 1682 to found the English colony of Pennsylvania. But following the fraudulent Walking Purchase of 1737, the Lenape were historically removed and forced from their homelands as a result of centuries of settler colonial violence, broken treaties, and dispossession. Today's federally recognized Lenape tribal nations are: Delaware Nation (Anadarko, Oklahoma); Delaware Tribe of Indians (Bartlesville, Oklahoma); the Stockbridge Munsee Community (Bowler, Wisconsin); and the Munsee Delaware Nation and the Eelūnaapèewii Lahkèewiit (Delaware Nation at Moraviantown), both in Ontario Canada. Notice that none of them currently reside near their beloved homeland.

    We strive to understand our place within the legacy of colonization and act as allies to the Lenape today. Land acknowledgments alone are not a solution to the issues facing Indigenous peoples. This statement is a call for establishing meaningful ongoing relationships with the Tribal Nations whose lands we are occupying and which respect tribal sovereignty.

Faculty Reviewers

VERONICA BROHM, DO
Program Director, Family Medicine Residency
Department of Family Medicine
Lehigh Valley Health Network
Jefferson Health
Allentown,
PA, USA

DREW M. KEISTER, MD
Vice Chair of Education
Department of Family Medicine
Lehigh Valley Health Network
Jefferson Health
Allentown,
PA, USA

SUSAN S. MATHIEU, MD
Associate Program Director, Family Medicine Residency
Department of Family Medicine
Lehigh Valley Health Network
Jefferson Health
Allentown,
PA, USA

ERIN SMITH, DO
Associate Program Director, Family Medicine Residency
Department of Family Medicine
Lehigh Valley Health Network
Jefferson Health
Allentown,
PA, USA

Acknowledgments

We are all embedded within the web of wisdom. This project is a manifestation of that web but limited to my experiences, attentions, and understandings within it. So much more wisdom remains to be gleaned. I can only hint at the habitat that nourished, informed, supported, and cared for me over continents and decades as the endeavor to explicate the generalist craft in primary care emerged and evolved.

This *Field Guide* exists, first and foremost, because of my membership in communities of practice and healing that sustained me to thrive through more than 50 years of living the craft. It begins with the patients who I cannot thank enough. It is their hopes, needs, encouragement, gratitude, courage, and many questions that energized my curiosity and seeking to get better at my craft. You are why I do this and do it with love. The craft of making places and situations that generate health does take a village, and I am fortunate for participating in several such villages beginning with the class of 1978 and the Department of Family Medicine at the University of North Carolina School of Medicine. The activist spirit of that class challenged the patriarchal, racist, and sexist underpinnings of clinical medicine while supporting and encouraging each of us, especially those entering primary care disciplines, to reimagine and create a better path forward and to help each other along the way. A special thanks to past friends and mentors Larry Wilson, Sue Snider, Bob Uhren, Tom Mettee, Gregory Strayhorn, Jim Wells, and Robin Blake. The family practice residency community at Harrisburg Hospital ensured my craft would be infused with generalism, community engagement, and attention to the family in family medicine. Special thanks to Joe Cincotta, Geoff James, Bill Keenan, Bev Blaisure, Beth Burns, and Tim Dudley along with so many others. Fellow resident Michael Abgott came with me to South Mountain Family Practice in my hometown in the Lehigh Valley where the craft was informed by our elder colleagues, Dale Grove, and my father, Warren Miller, and patients who had watched me grow up. Thanks to all for being there during these formative times.

The next 10 years found our family nested in central Connecticut and the excitement of innovating, teaching, and learning in the University of Connecticut family medicine department located in downtown Hartford. David Schmidt's vision to build a learning community there was fulfilled. Here I met lifelong friends, Ben Crabtree, Rob Cushman, and Eric Jackson. This is also where being able to articulate and explicitly teach the generalist craft saw its beginnings, nourished and inspired by the remarkable residents, faculty, and staff. Special thanks to Jeri Hepworth, Tina Krause, Pat O'Connor, Sarah Nicklin, and Lu Marchand. They also introduced me to the Society of Teachers of Family Medicine, an incredible collaborative community of scholars, and the North American Primary Care Research Group, an inspiring, innovative, and nurturing community of international researchers. Too many to name and thank, but these connections introduced me to Ian McWhinney, Moira Stewart, and Judith Belle Brown at the University of Western Ontario, and to the small but growing community of family physicians doing qualitative and participatory research, especially Val Gilchrist, Lucy Candib, Paul Thomas, and Tony Kuzel and the special friendships of Kurt Stange and Jeff Borkan. These communities and friends are the hidden sources and inspirations for the tools of the generalist craft.

And then I returned home to the Lehigh Valley where Elliot Sussman, Bob Laskowski, and Headley White offered me the opportunity to develop a family medicine department and residency program at Lehigh Valley Health Network. This community of practice and healing is the family and village that raised the tools of turtle craft, the tools of the generalist craft, from infancy to maturity and into this *Field Guide*. Every member of this community, over the past 30 years, contributed to the development. They exemplify our core practice of hospitality using the disciplines of fidelity, thought, and community through celebrating abundance, mystery, and grace. I love and thank them all with extra hugs to Julie Dostal, Joanne Cohen-Katz, Drew Keister, Lou Lukas, Jeff Sternlieb, Holly Binnig, Abby Letcher, Eamon Armstrong, and Brian Stello and the first pioneer class of residents, Paul Branch, Aaron Katz, Jeff and Sue Mathieu, Bindi Patel, and Andrew McLaren.

Communicating the craft through illustrations to younger generations learning the generalist craft became possible through the creative magic of Rena Jiang and Su Bin Hahn who were third year medical students when they began working with me. They were and continue to be sources of inspiration and motivation along with keeping me up-to-date on the latest memes for which I am grateful. I am thankful for Joseph Cho, acquisitions editor for the publisher, who wisely guided and coached me through the publishing adventure, and his colleague, Cindy Yoo, development editor, as we explored how to make this a living text that honors the living craft.

Converting a dynamic craft without losing its energy was a daunting challenge. Fortunately, I am blessed with an editor, Angel Batts, and seven intrepid friends who spent hours and days reading every word and critiquing a great many of them. Thank you Kurt Stange, Stefan Topolski, and David Loxtercamp and the faculty reviewers, Veronica Brohm, Drew Keister,

Sue Mathieu, and Erin Smith. I have tried to honor your recommendations and insights, but what resulted is my responsibility.

My family and the Delaware River watershed are the deep well from which I draw my love for self and others. My life partner and best friend, Deb, has always been there with her patience, insight, support, wise challenges, and reassuring smile. Our children, Lindsay and Ethan, and their partners, Bill and Kate, my parents and grandparents, nine generations of ancestors living in the greater Lehigh Valley, and the source of that extra bright sparkle in my eye, my grandson Loren—they create a love in my heart greater than the sum of its parts. Thank you!

Contents

Dedication   v
Faculty Reviewers   vii
Acknowledgments   ix
Contents   xiii
List of Tables   xix
List of Figures   xxiii

PRELUDE   1

- Welcome   1
- Purpose   4
- The Origins of Craft   5
- Developing the Clinical Hand Tool of the Generalist's Craft   6
- Lehigh Valley Health Network and the Tools of Turtle Craft   8
- How the Tools of the Generalist's Craft Were Selected   10
- Language   11
- Overview of the *Field Guide*   12
- Reflections   14

PART I: Getting Ready   17

MODULE 1   Thriving Skills   19

- Overview   19
- The Importance of Wellness and Care of the Self   19
- Thriving Skill 1: Mindfulness and Attending   23
  Introduction   23
  Emotional and Social Intelligence   24
  Mindful Practice and Mindfulness Meditation   26
  Clinical Tools for Mindfulness and Attending   27
- Thriving Skill 2: Eye Juggling   29
- Thriving Skill 3: The BATHE Technique   30
- Thriving Skill 4: Ritual   33

MODULE 2   Metaphors and Tools Overview   39

- Introduction   39
- Four Guiding Metaphors of the Generalist's Craft   39
  River of Health   40
  Spiral of Healing   41
  Windmill Sails of Generalism   42
  The Elephant and the Rider of Changing Behavior   44

- Reflective Pause — 46
- The Clinical Hand and Supporting Tools of the Generalist's Craft — 47
  - Clinical Hand Tool — 48
  - Ecological Clinical Map Tool — 51
  - Relationship-Centered Clinical Method Tool — 54
  - Round Table of Evidence Tool — 56
- How the Tools Fit Together — 59

PART II: Embodying the Craft — 65

MODULE 3 Heart of the Craft—Journey of the Clinical Encounter — 67

- Introduction — 67
- The Fingers of Direction—The Ritual Structure of the Five Guideposts — 69

UNIT ONE: Journey to Connect — 71

- Orientation — 71
- Achieving Situational Awareness Using the Ecological Clinical Map — 71
- Prepare and Open the Hand — 72
- Attending and the Grip of Power — 74
- Getting to the Connect Guidepost — 75

UNIT TWO: The Journey to Set Agenda — 80

- Orientation — 80
- The Wrist Lines of Guidance: Three Goals and Encounter Types — 81
  - Guiding Wrist—Goals of Encounter — 81
  - Guiding Pulses—Encounter Types — 84
- Getting to the Set Agenda Guidepost — 92

UNIT THREE: The Journey to Hand Over: Exploring the Patient's Stories — 98

- Moving Toward the Hand Over Guidepost — 98
- Observation and Listening Skills — 100
- Exploring the Patient's Stories — 103
- Understanding the Whole Person in Context — 107
  - Reflective Pause — 109

UNIT FOUR: The Journey to Hand Over: Clinical Discovery and Evaluation — 119

- Clinical Discovery and Evaluation — 119
  - Touching Skills — 119
  - Clinical Discovery — 121

Contents   **XV**

- The Palm of Hope and Swinging on the Tree   127
- Reflective Pause   137

UNIT FIVE: The Journey to Hand Over: Sensemaking   140

- The Round Table of Evidence and Information Mastery   140
  The Round Table of Evidence   140
  Information Mastery   147
- Sensemaking   149

UNIT SIX: The Journey to Hand Over: Finding Common Ground   158

- Finding Common Ground and Making Shared Decisions   158
  Conceptual Strategies for Finding Common Ground   158
  Concerns: Problems and Priorities   161
  Goals: Goal-Oriented Care and Personalizing   161
  Roles   164
- Getting to the Hand Over Guidepost   167

UNIT SEVEN: The Journeys to Safety Net and Housekeep   169

- The Safety Net Guidepost   169
- The Housekeep Guidepost   171

MODULE 4   Doing the Encounter Types   175

- Introduction   175
- Routines   179
- Maintenance Ceremonies   182
- Dramas   185
- Transition Ceremonies   191

MODULE 5   Deepening Practical Wisdom   195

- Overview   195
- Ecological Clinical Map Add-Ons   196
  Patient   196
  Clinic, Community, and Healing Landscapes   199
- Clinical Hand Add-Ons   204
  The Swinging Cultural Ape   204
- Relationship-Centered Clinical Method Add-Ons   210
  Understanding the Whole Person   210
  Discovering Clinical Evidence: Heuristics, Clues, and Biases   212
  Organizing the Health Story   212
  Patient (and Clinician) Denial—or Is It?   218
- Round Table of Evidence Add-Ons   220
  Sensemaking and Mindlines   220

POSTLUDE — 225

- Our Partners in Health — 225
- Aphorisms and Wisdom — 225
- More Than a Craft — 226

PART III: Supplements — 227

SUPPLEMENT 1 Empirical and Theoretical Foundations of the Generalist's Craft — 229

- Overview — 229
- Primary Medical Care — 230
  Primary Health Care — 230
  Primary Medical Care: Functions, Facilitators, and Principles — 231
- Patients Who Seek Primary Medical Care — 233
  The Ecology of Medical Care — 233
  Health, Symptoms, and Illness Behavior — 234
  Frequent Attenders and Power Laws — 238
  Developmental Trauma and Trauma-Informed Care — 238
- Health and Healing — 241
  Introduction — 241
  Health as Concept — 242
  Health in Complexity Theory — 243
  Health as Membership — 245
  River of Health — 247
  Drivers of Health — 247
  How Healing Happens — 249
  Healing Relationships — 250
  Spiral of Healing — 252
- Changing Human Behavior — 252
- Generalism — 254
  Generalist Ways — 254
  Generalist as Jack-of-All-Trades, Polymath, Eclectic, and *Phronimos* — 256
  Principles of Generalism — 257
  Montreal Statement on Generalist Practice — 260
- High-Value Primary Medical Care and Generalism — 262
- Summary — 265

SUPPLEMENT 2 Educational Resources — 271

- Introduction — 271
- GEMs: Generalist Enhancement Methods — 272
  Camera Walk — 272
  Fox Walking — 274
  Sculpting Health — 275

- Teaching Strategies for Generalist's Craft 276
  Continuity Case Conference 277
  Mega Clinic 279
  Paired Precepting 280
- Assessment Tools 281
- Clinical Hand Direct Observation Tool 284
  Ground Rules and Goals 284

GLOSSARY OF MNEMONICS 289

- General Mnemonics 289
- Diagnostic Mnemonics 291

Index 293

List of Tables

Table P.1	Examples of Current Tensions and Pressures Facing General Practitioners	3
Table P.2	Outcomes of Good Generalist Craft	10
Table P.3	Principles Informing Design and Selection of Tools of the Generalist's Craft	11
Table 1.1	Whole Person Self-Care Activities	20
Table 1.2	Tools of the Creative Hero(ine)	23
Table 1.3	Tool for Self-Evaluating Emotional and Social Intelligence	25
Table 1.4	Simple Steps for Mindfulness Meditation	26
Table 1.5	Features of Mindful Practice	27
Table 1.6	Implementing the Attending Imagery Technique	28
Table 1.7	The Three Eyes of Eye Juggling	31
Table 1.8	Features of BATHE	32
Table 1.9	Ritual or Habit?	33
Table 1.10	Components of Ritual	35
Table 1.11	Functions of Ritual	36
Table 2.1	Four Guiding Metaphors of the Generalist Craft	40
Table 2.2	Simple Rules of Specialists	43
Table 2.3	The Clinical Hand and Supporting Tools of the Generalist's Craft	47
Table 2.4	Clinical Hand Highlights	49
Table 2.5	Ecological Clinical Map Highlights	52
Table 2.6	Relationship-Centered Clinical Method Highlights	57
Table 2.7	Round Table of Evidence Highlights	59
Table 2.8	Features of Clinical Jazz Improvisation	60
Table 3.1	Preparation for the Encounter	73
Table 3.2	Managing Power in the Encounter	76
Table 3.3	The Path to Connect	77
Table 3.4	POISED Mnemonic for Using the Electronic Health Record	78
Table 3.5	Actual Reason for Connecting	83
Table 3.6	Overview of Encounter Types	85
Table 3.7	Features of Routines	86
Table 3.8	Features of Dramas	88

List of Tables

Table 3.9	Features of Transition Ceremonies	89
Table 3.10	Types of Transition Ceremonies	90
Table 3.11	Features of Maintenance Ceremonies	91
Table 3.12	Types of Maintenance Ceremonies	92
Table 3.13	Eliciting and Prioritizing the Agenda	94
Table 3.14	Patient Requests	95
Table 3.15	Indicators of Completing Set Agenda	96
Table 3.16	Enhancing Observation	100
Table 3.17	Enhancing Active Listening	101
Table 3.18	Meta-Models as Speech Cues	103
Table 3.19	Components of FIFE	105
Table 3.20	Eliciting an Explanatory Model	106
Table 3.21	Eliciting Illness Prototypes	106
Table 3.22	Eliciting Sickness Story Features	107
Table 3.23	Story and the Generalist Craft	108
Table 3.24	Understanding the Whole Person: Examples of Contexts	110
Table 3.25	Family as Process	111
Table 3.26	Features of the Family APGAR Measurement of Capacity	113
Table 3.27	Eliciting Livelihoods Identity	114
Table 3.28	Highlights of the Whole Person's Life Story	115
Table 3.29	The Six Stages of Change	116
Table 3.30	Preparation for Touching (Examining) the Patient	120
Table 3.31	How to Touch (Exam) the Patient	120
Table 3.32	Clinical Discovery Recognition Processes	125
Table 3.33	Physical Naming and Caring	130
Table 3.34	Emotional Naming and Caring	131
Table 3.35	Cognitive Naming and Caring	132
Table 3.36	Social Naming and Caring	132
Table 3.37	The SCREEM Resources	133
Table 3.38	Spiritual Naming and Caring	134
Table 3.39	Habitat Naming and Caring	135
Table 3.40	Additional Evidence Questions for Generalists	143
Table 3.41	Types and Sources of Evidence	144
Table 3.42	The Four Questions for Information Evaluation	145
Table 3.43	Questions for Evaluating Quantitative Studies	146

List of Tables

Table 3.44	Questions for Evaluating Qualitative Studies	146
Table 3.45	POEMs Versus DOEs	147
Table 3.46	Questions to Identify Useful Information	148
Table 3.47	STEPS for Evaluating Pharmacotherapeutics	148
Table 3.48	The Sensemaking Process in the Clinical Encounter	151
Table 3.49	The Sensemaking Process for Pedro's Clinical Encounter	154
Table 3.50	Tips for Principled Negotiation and Positive Criticism	160
Table 3.51	Goal Types	162
Table 3.52	Values History	162
Table 3.53	Questions to Guide Tailoring the Care Plan	163
Table 3.54	Roles	164
Table 3.55	Pedro's Explanatory Story and Engaging Plan	165
Table 3.56	Indicators of Completing Hand Over	167
Table 3.57	Indicators of Completing Safety Net	170
Table 3.58	Tools for Housekeeping	172
Table 3.59	Indicators of Completing Housekeeping	173
Table 4.1	Domains of the Cynefin Framework Within Primary Medical Care	176
Table 4.2	Remembering the Family in Routines	180
Table 4.3	Precise Treatment	181
Table 4.4	Mastering Routines	181
Table 4.5	Remembering the Family in Maintenance Ceremonies	183
Table 4.6	Mastering Maintenance Ceremonies	184
Table 4.7	Facilitators of Effective Dramas	186
Table 4.8	Mastering Dramas	188
Table 4.9	Family Questions in Dramas	189
Table 4.10	Breakthrough Tactics for Dramas	190
Table 4.11	Aims for Transition Ceremonies	192
Table 4.12	LATE—Mastering Transition Ceremonies	193
Table 5.1	Model of Reflective Practice	196
Table 5.2	Characteristics of Four Patient Faces	198
Table 5.3	Optimal Healing Environments	201
Table 5.4	Features of the Community-Oriented Primary Care Process	202
Table 5.5	Features of Bioregion	203

Table 5.6	Ecological Identity	203
Table 5.7	Mechanisms of Heritable Change and Variation	206
Table 5.8	Why Bioculture and Evolution Matter to Clinicians	207
Table 5.9	Behavior Rules of Thumb From Evolutionary Psychology	209
Table 5.10	When to Convene the Family	211
Table 5.11	Heuristics, Clues, and Biases	213
Table 5.12	Story Tools	216
Table 5.13	MENCH: The Multiple Stories of the Generalist Craft	217
Table 5.14	Faces of Safeguarding and Denial	219
Table 5.15	Mindlines of General Practice	220
Table S1.1	The Four Functions of Primary Medical Care	232
Table S1.2	The Four Cs and the Shared Principles of Primary Medical Care	233
Table S1.3	Symptom Formation Process	236
Table S1.4	Who Connects With Primary Medical Care	239
Table S1.5	Key Principles of Trauma-Informed Approach	240
Table S1.6	Trauma-Informed Primary Medical Care at the Practice Level	241
Table S1.7	Properties of Complex Adaptive Systems	243
Table S1.8	Definitional Features of Health	246
Table S1.9	Drivers of Health (Longevity and Quality of Life)	248
Table S1.10	Three Ways for Healing	249
Table S1.11	Three Common Factors Inducing Healing	251
Table S1.12	Significant Aspects of Healing Relationships	251
Table S1.13	The Generalist Ways	255
Table S1.14	Principles of the Generalist's Craft in Primary Care	258
Table S1.15	Montreal Statement on Generalist Practice	260
Table S1.16	High-Value Primary Medical Care	262
Table S1.17	Features of High-Value Primary Medical Care	263
Table S1.18	Person-Centered Primary Care Measure	264
Table S2.1	Q-List for General Medical Practice	282

List of Figures

Figure P.1	The Four-Circle Curriculum for Lehigh Valley Health Network Family Medicine Residency	9
Figure 1.1	Attending Imagery Technique	29
Figure 1.2	Eye Juggling	30
Figure 1.3	BATHE on Fingernails	32
Figure 2.1	River of Health	41
Figure 2.2	Spiral of Healing	42
Figure 2.3	Windmill Sails of Generalism	43
Figure 2.4	The Elephant and the Rider of Changing Behavior	45
Figure 2.5	Clinical Hand Tool	48
Figure 2.6	Ecological Clinical Map Tool	52
Figure 2.7	Relationship-Centered Clinical Method Tool	55
Figure 2.8	Round Table of Evidence Tool	58
Figure 2.9	Using All the Tools in a Clinical Encounter	60
Figure 3.1	Clinical Hand Tool	68
Figure 3.2	Journey of the Clinical Encounter	68
Figure 3.3	The Fingers of Direction—The Five Required Guideposts of Ritual Structure	70
Figure 3.4	The Connect Finger	71
Figure 3.5	Achieving Situational Awareness Using the Ecological Clinical Map	72
Figure 3.6	Opening the Hand of Intention	74
Figure 3.7	The Grip of Power	75
Figure 3.8	The Set Agenda Finger	80
Figure 3.9	Clinical Hand Tool	81
Figure 3.10	Guiding Wrist	82
Figure 3.11	Guiding Pulses	84
Figure 3.12	A LOT (High-Yield Information) Moments	95
Figure 3.13	The Hand Over Finger	98
Figure 3.14	Expressive Eyes	102
Figure 3.15	Weaving Among the Stories	103
Figure 3.16	Understanding the Whole Person	109
Figure 3.17	Family Life Cycle	112

List of Figures

Figure 3.18	The Wheel of Readiness to Change	117
Figure 3.19	The Dance of Clinical Discovery and Sensemaking	121
Figure 3.20	The Expanding Field of Shared Understanding from the Point of View of the Clinician	122
Figure 3.21	Clinical Discovery Strategies and Related Tactics	123
Figure 3.22	The Palm of Hope and the Naming and Caring Tree	128
Figure 3.23	The Round Table of Evidence	140
Figure 3.24	The Generalist Wheel of Inquiry	141
Figure 3.25	Sensible Scales for Generalists	150
Figure 3.26	Finding Common Ground	158
Figure 3.27	Continuum of Decision-Making	160
Figure 3.28	The Safety Net Finger	169
Figure 3.29	The Housekeep Finger	171
Figure 4.1	Cynefin Framework: Making Sense of Situations	176
Figure 4.2	Drama Illness Trajectory	187
Figure 5.1	Four Faces of Patient	197
Figure 5.2	The Swinging Cultural Ape	204
Figure 5.3	Drivers of Life Story	205
Figure S1.1	Domains and Context of Primary Health Care	231
Figure S1.2	The Health-Seeking Process	234
Figure S1.3	Symptom Awareness Process	235
Figure S1.4	River of Health	247
Figure S1.5	Spiral of Healing	252
Figure S1.6	The Elephant and the Rider of Changing Behavior	253
Figure S1.7	The Generalist Wheel of Inquiry	259
Figure S1.8	Windmill Sails of Generalism	259
Figure S2.1	The Experiential Learning Cycle	272

Prelude

Welcome

The Primary Care Clinical Encounter: Field Guide to the Generalist's Craft is a gateway to the wonder, joy, and humility of general practice and family medicine and mastering its *craft*. The range of skills needed to master the generalist craft in primary care is as diverse as its patients. A practitioner might wonder: *How do I make and maintain a safe space for vulnerable patients to optimize their willingness to share and ability to listen? How do I know where to pay attention and what to notice? How do I prioritize and personalize? How do I know what the high-value questions are and when to explore other bodies of evidence not dependent on randomized controlled trials or expert opinion? How can I calm an emotional moment? How will I know when to keep an encounter brief and routine and when to dive deeper? How can I more fully engage patients in their own care?*

 By Learning and Mastering the Craft

Generalist practice is rife with surprises and challenges, but for those who persist in the adventure and the learning, it is a celebration of life's abundance, mystery, and grace. We discover in our patients and ourselves the many ways of being alive and healthy. As a wise family doc and friend recently wrote, "Our job is to help acutely ill patients recover, chronically ill patients maintain control, and people who are making self-destructive choices make better ones. It is a human enterprise: people helping people."[1] The *Field Guide* offers a way to excel in doing the work of clinical healing encounters, of making better health for ourselves and our patients, and in performing the clinical jazz of the generalist's craft in relational primary care.

Medicine advances and adapts and advances again at an ever-accelerating rate. Over the course of my career, it seems a vast amount of medical knowledge has changed. Fortunately, technological advances and the availability of up-to-date evidence databases allow us unprecedented access to medical content at the point of care, helping us maintain our bearings in an ever-evolving landscape. No matter how quickly the content of medicine changes, however, the craft of applying that knowledge in each clinical encounter and within each patient relationship in the primary medical care setting remains consistent. My experience in doing and teaching the craft allows this *Field Guide* to honor and integrate 60 years of innovations in the teaching and doing of primary medical care.

A trained general practitioner will come to this *Field Guide* pre-armed with communication skills, knowledge of their local community, and access to virtually unlimited medical content. Trainees arrive learning the same. Both will leave this *Field Guide* mastering the craft of their generalist primary care practice.

But what exactly is this generalist's craft? The craft is how we weave all our skills, all our knowledge, all our intuitions together to make better health with our patients. Excelling in the generalist's craft won't increase your wRVUs (work relative value units), tick your boxes, or follow protocols better, nor will it necessarily improve your prevention-and-disease quality metrics. But it will facilitate managing your time more effectively, increase your patient experience scores, significantly improve your patients' health, and help you rediscover the joy and fulfillment of clinical practice and your love of being with patients.

Whether you have been doing clinical primary care for several years or are just starting, you may be scratching your head wondering, *What part of what I am already doing is "the craft"?* and, importantly, *How will this* Field Guide *help me through my busy day?*

Let's begin by considering what one of those busy days might look like from a clinical perspective. At the start of each new patient encounter, a portal opens—an exam room door, the threshold into a patient's home, a virtual-visit window on a computer screen. Almost anything a body can experience may be waiting for you on the other side. A parent with a crying infant, a pregnant woman with spotting, an adolescent with urethral discharge. A young man in a wheelchair hoping to get a driver's license, or an overweight adult with diabetes and hypertension wanting to start a new exercise and diet program. Perhaps you find a recently retired person with palpitations or an older woman with multiple problems and now a new cough and low-grade fever. The list stretches on and on.

As if that weren't daunting enough, in addition, the primary care healer must manage any external pressures weighing on the encounter. These stem from a variety of contemporary pressures and expectations (see Table P.1), including changes to clinical reality; practice and health system expectations; patient and personal expectations; and social, ecological, and political issues. These tensions require the generalist's craft, now more than ever before, to help prioritize clinical attention and action.[2]

How can anyone be prepared to respond effectively to so much? This question, or a version of it, is likely to arise in the mind of any medical student contemplating a career in family medicine or any other generalist field.

But pause for a moment and reflect on the history of healing. Since the appearance of *Homo sapiens* 200,000 to 300,000 years ago, in every known

TABLE P.1 Examples of Current Tensions and Pressures Facing General Practitioners

Sources of Tensions and Pressures	Examples
Clinical Reality	• Multiple complicated and complex problems • Multiple care options
Practice/Health System Expectations	• High volume • Limited time • Revenue generation • Electronic medical records • Quality metrics • Resource management • Administrative requirements • Big data and artificial intelligence (algorithms) • Employee status challenging professionalism
Patient Expectations	• Availability and action • Quick response to email
Personal Expectations	• Self-care • Time for family and friends (work/life balance)
Social/Ecological/Political Issues	• Social media • Information overload • Consumerism and public rating systems • Cultural and language diversity • Wealth and income inequality • Climate change and habitat destruction

human culture, people have performed this work of primary care healing.[3] From the first midwives[4] and shamans,[5] through Asklepios[6] and Hildegard of Bingen,[7] to the general practitioners of the mid-20th century and the family physicians of today, generalist primary care healers have developed and honed the healing craft.

At the heart of this craft is a body of tacit knowledge, mostly learned through observed apprenticeships, aphorisms, stories, and ritualized routines, that serves as a critical ingredient enabling the effectiveness of primary care healers. Because of this enigmatic and tacit nature, the craft can seem hidden and magical. No more. This *Field Guide* explicitly guides you in the generalist's craft of primary care healing, so you can learn how the magic works, and how you can make it work for your patients.

Though the generalist's craft originally developed among small, mostly kin-based groups working with a very limited set of treatment options,[8] that early context has changed dramatically. Fortunately, the craft has proven highly adaptable. While it may not be able to solve all the dilemmas that arise in a day of general practice, it does offer a way to remain actively aware and sensitive to them. It will help you prioritize competing, sometimes daunting demands while staying focused on the source of joy and fulfillment that called you to this amazing and foundational sacred vocation—the person waiting for you on the other side of the portal.

Purpose

The *Field Guide for the Generalist's Craft* integrates 60 years of innovations in the teaching and doing of primary medical care in service of one predominant aim:

> **To provide practical, easy-to-recall tools and models for doing the craft of generalist primary medical care and to guide you in how to apply them in daily clinical practice.**

By illuminating this long-obscured dimension of the generalist's practice, I hope to restore the heart, soul, and integrity of the profession by raising awareness and understanding of what primary medical care can be—for active clinicians, residents, and students as well as patients. Everyone and every community deserves personal primary care from clinicians who are skilled in the generalist's craft of healing.

Who you are influences how you will most benefit from using this *Field Guide*. Students and residents, begin using the *Field Guide* when training starts, either in residency or advanced nursing education. Like most starting clinicians, you may be tempted to put most of your energy into learning clinical content in search of a sense of competence, but don't wait to begin learning the craft. The craft sets the habits that make the clinical content useful and helpful. Learn the craft, the content, and the communication skills together.

Experienced clinicians, I see your eyes rolling, and I hear your voices. "I'm running behind; my inbox is overflowing; I need to get home to my family; I just need quick clinical content answers. No time for the craft." You just identified your primary reasons for using this *Field Guide*. I recognize the moral distress. You once loved this work, and you can again. Do I notice a smile? I encourage finding one or two colleagues with whom to explore the *Field Guide* together. Even consider observing each other to discover the many variations on how the craft is performed.

Patients, while the *Field Guide* is primarily written for clinicians, you can also benefit. It can teach you what to look for in your personal clinician, what to expect, and how to better engage in the healing relationship. The thriving skills discussed in Module 1 are beneficial for anyone living in the 21st century, so begin there.

The Origins of Craft

The word *craft* derives from the Old English, *cræft*, and the Old High German, *kraft*, which both refer to the skill involved in doing, making, or executing some object or process. Sociologist Richard Sennett adds that *craft* specifically refers to doing a job well for its own sake or to a "joined skill in community."[9] Alexander Langlands, an archeologist, views craft as "a form of intelligence, an ingenuity, that can shift in accordance with a changing world."[10]

I use *craft* in all these forms: as a set of skills, developed within communities of healers, that creatively work the hands of practitioners as they interact with patients. In that sense, craft is not the same as *art*, which is committed to self-expression. Craft commits to the medium, the healing relationship. The generalist's craft of healing involves resourcefulness, the skill "to use as little as possible in relation to the job that needs undertaking."[10] It also involves power in the form of adeptness and fitness; knowledge and understanding of the materials used; the knack to make decisions about the approaches to the work; and the ability to factor in the wider capacities and time constraints impacting the work.[10]

The Clinical Hand and its supporting tools in the *Field Guide for the Generalist's Craft* are designed to help you master the *craft* of primary care medicine. They use, but are not about, the clinical content of family medicine and primary medical care: the pathologies and diseases, the diagnostic tools and treatments. A myriad of textbooks and other resources are available on these topics. Similarly, the tools in this guide are intended to draw upon, not to develop, your communication and relationship skills; community engagement strategies; and skills and approaches for ensuring better self-awareness, self-understanding, or mindfulness. Again, there are many texts and resources about these, and the *Field Guide* assumes you are mastering them. Instead, the *Field Guide*'s focus on craft will present you with tools and strategies for how to bring the clinical content, communications, community engagement, and self-awareness together in a healing relationship to skillfully cocreate and make health.

Developing the Clinical Hand Tool of the Generalist's Craft

The attribution of single authorship for the *Field Guide* profoundly misrepresents the material. The content of the *Field Guide* is gathered from the community of primary care healers. The author's contribution is to make selections from that content and organize it into the Clinical Hand and its supporting tools to aid generalist clinicians as they practice their craft. I also organized it as a coherent curriculum for family medicine residency education. Even those actions involved multiple collaborations. As a user of this *Field Guide*, you may find the following brief overview of the influences and sources of the content helpful.

I am thankful I answered the call to general practice. I love doing family medicine! I discovered the magic of general practice from observing my father, a general practitioner for more than 50 years in the small town where I grew up. I learned the importance of place and relationships and the difference general practice made in people's lives. I also experienced the emotional and developmental consequences of being the child of a solo practice general practitioner with poor self-care and neglect of his family life. No surprise that my first career wasn't in family medicine.

I began my vocational life in 1971 as a medical anthropologist fascinated by shamanism, divination, the cultural traditions and diversity of healing practices, human evolution, midwifery and birthing practice through time, and the perspective of generalism. Shamans introduced me to the concept of understanding the whole person within their community and ecological context and to intimacy with the larger living world. Midwives taught me about attending and the importance of presence and the personal. Evolution reminded me of our deep ancestral roots in the story of life, and the healing traditions revealed the significance of stories, meaning, and rituals in how our bodies work and make sense. Anthropology also connected me to international public health and the broad and exciting understandings of primary health care developed at Alma Ata in 1978.[11] But it was only after I discovered self-care skills and learned that being a good healer, partner, friend, and parent was possible that I was ready to hear the call to general practice.

Life as a family physician started in 1978 when I began residency. I experienced the thrill of full-scope (ambulatory, hospital, and birthing) care for 30 years, an additional 5 years doing both ambulatory and hospital care, and another 5 years focusing only on ambulatory care. Across those decades, I remained deeply immersed in the wonder and joy of doing the generalist's craft. And I still am! My love for family medicine will be unapologetically evident throughout.

Being present in clinical practice for so many of the most poignant and memorable moments in people's lives, discovering the hidden strengths and heroism in others and in yourself, and making sense of an endless stream of puzzles and questions all foster a lifetime of adventure. What an amazing service and vocation! The generalist's craft presented here lies at the heart of doing this work well and experiencing the accompanying sense of purpose and mastery.

I've been a family medicine educator for more than 45 years, an administrator for 35 years, and a researcher for more than 50 years. The tools of the generalist's craft have been gathered and organized across these roles and experiences and were informed by all of them. My first full-time faculty role was at the University of Connecticut from 1984 to 1993. It was there that the Clinical Encounter Series was developed as a formal curriculum on the craft of family medicine. Since early on, fellow faculty and many residents have been included in its yearly revisions. When I moved to Lehigh Valley Health Network (LVHN) in 1994 and began its family medicine residency, that curriculum followed me and became the Tools of Turtle Craft, which are outlined in this guide and remain the keystone of that residency curriculum. It was also at LVHN that we developed the Clinical Hand and its three supporting tools of the generalist's craft. Again, that work involved fellow faculty and a number of residents. Most of the tools and content come from the primary care and family medicine literature.

The Clinical Hand is the centerpiece tool for the generalist craft. Roger Neighbour, a British general practitioner and educator and brilliantly insightful describer of the generalist primary care craft, inspired the principal Clinical Hand tool and the ritual structure of the five checkpoints or guideposts.[12] I strongly encourage exploring his text in depth. Two additional sources serve as stimulators and anchors for two of the three supporting tools. The Relationship-Centered Clinical Method tool is a direct adaptation of the remarkable patient-centered clinical method developed and evaluated over a 40-year span by a core group of faculty, educators, and researchers in the

Department of Family Medicine at Western University, London, Ontario.[13] This is one of the few clinical methods demonstrated to improve primary medical care clinical outcomes. The many publications and workshops on information mastery by David Slawson and Allen Shaughnessy[14] significantly shaped our understanding and approach to evidence-informed care and inspired the Round Table of Evidence supporting tool.

As you will discover, each of the tools is filled with additional craft wisdom. Faculty, residents, and I frequently discovered these gems at the Society of Teachers of Family Medicine meetings. We also shared our tools and curriculum at those meetings, which often led to revisions and additions.

The tools and approaches presented here build upon many existing consultation and patient interviewing models and are compatible with them. These include Byrne and Long's Six Phases model,[15] Stott and Davis' Four Areas framework,[16] the Calgary-Cambridge model,[17] Helman's Folk Model,[18] Pendleton's Model of the Consultation,[19] the Three Function model,[20] Robert Smith's Patient-Centered Interviewing approach,[21] the REDE (Relationship: Establishment, Development, Engagement) model,[22] the CARE approach,[23] the Four Habits model,[24] and the Collaborative Deliberation framework.[25]

Lehigh Valley Health Network and the Tools of Turtle Craft

The tools and curriculum presented in this *Field Guide* have been a centerpiece of the curriculum for the family medicine residents at LVHN since 1996. Large posters of the Clinical Hand and its three supporting tools hang in the learning center of the residency, and a smaller version of the Clinical Hand tool is posted in many exam rooms where the residents practice. How we position the tools within a larger four-circle curriculum for the residency is depicted in Figure P.1. In the figure, three small circles nest within a larger circle, and all of them rest on the shell of a large freshwater common snapping turtle. The turtle is the symbol for our residency, and we use the term *turtle craft* to signify our relationship-centered, evidence-informed curriculum that emphasizes the unity of science and sensibility in the practice of the generalist's craft of healing.

Why use the enigmatic and formidable snapping turtle as our foundation? Because it is a place-based animal that is watchful, patient, and represents wisdom in many cultural folklores. It is an enduring creature with a lifespan of over 100 years that is at home navigating the muddy space between land and water, reflecting our skills at helping our patients traverse their journey through the daunting, enigmatic, and mucky terrain of bodily affliction.

The turtle also features prominently in the creation story of the Lenape people native to eastern Pennsylvania and the Lehigh Valley bioregion prior to European colonization. In that story, when the future of life seems bleak, a turtle offers its back as a foundation upon which new life can rise, just as we are there for patients when they fall into the mud of ill health and help them rise again. Oral tradition holds many versions of this story, with some referring to a tortoise and others mentioning a domed turtle.[26-28] I chose the common snapping turtle for the model because it is the largest and most domed turtle in our region.

The term *turtle craft* also refers to the culture of inquiry and open dialogue that is the foundation for our interactions within the residency.[29,30] That culture is founded upon the values of our residency—what we call the *Footsteps of the Turtle Path*: the *practice of hospitality*, the *engagement of the disciplines of thought, fidelity, and community*, and the *celebration of mystery, abundance, and grace*.

We at LVHN visualize the curriculum on the back of a turtle as a reminder of the importance of turtle craft and its values within our program. The large circle covering the top of the turtle's shell represents the core content of clinical knowledge and evidence that informs our medical practice. That clinical content springs to life through the mediation of the three intersecting circles of self-understanding, relationship skills, and community and system activation. The body of the turtle signifies the craft of healing, the tools of generalist turtle craft that activate and integrate the four circles.

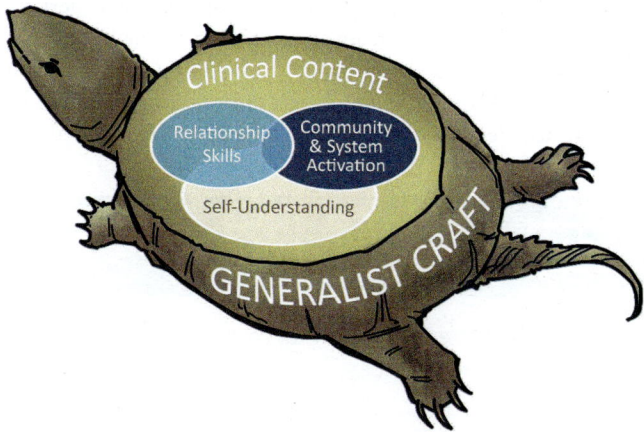

FIGURE P.1. The Four-Circle Curriculum for Lehigh Valley Health Network Family Medicine Residency.

We believe that best practice in generalist primary care occurs at the intersection between the three smaller circles and clinical content. The generalist turtle craft makes that integrated delivery possible. In this way, LVHN's residency curriculum design empowers residents with competence in both the content of the four circles *and the craft*.

The *Field Guide for the Generalist's Craft* is the first-ever full-length comprehensive guide to the content of LVHN's curriculum based on turtle craft. In it, I will walk you through the Clinical Hand of the generalist's craft and its supporting tools and explain how to integrate them in the service of making health with your patients.

How the Tools of the Generalist's Craft Were Selected

Our goal is health. Our approach is generalist. Our setting is primary medical care. Our care needs to recognize the human condition in our living ecology as well as its limits and possibilities, including the impact of developmental trauma on human health and the challenges of changing human behavior. When the generalist's craft is done well, healing is activated and behavior changes, and the result is better health (see Table P.2).

The *Tools of the Generalist's Craft* are intended to facilitate these outcomes. These tools need to support the implementation of the generalist's craft. All of the tools and strategies presented in this *Field Guide* are designed and selected accordingly (see Table P.3).

The tools also need to promote the development of expertise in the craft. A healer takes the voyage from apprentice to journeyman to expert as they learn to master and embody the craft. That begins with learning and practicing the tools of the generalist's craft until playing them out becomes second nature, like learning the scales, cadences, chords, and arpeggios of

TABLE P.2 — Outcomes of Good Generalist Craft

Activate Healing: Offer a meaningful response, communal support, targeted treatment

Change Behavior: Alter perception and increase adherence/self-management

Better Health: Guide patients back into life

TABLE P.3	Principles Informing Design and Selection of Tools of the Generalist's Craft

The tool must...
Help to generate healing and health.
Promote generalism.
Be personal.
Promote relationships.
Facilitate trauma-centered care.
Be goal-oriented.
Activate behavior change.
Be realistic.

the piano and then progressing, with even more practice, to be able to reliably perform the great concertos. In other words, by mastering *clinical jazz*. An expert knows how to improvise in the face of uncertainties and how to create communities of practice so that they might improvise with other people, recover from the unexpected, and work safely and confidently when guidelines don't apply.[31]

Language

I am excited to finally share this lifetime of learning from my world of amazing collaborators and colleagues. The generalist's craft of healing in the primary medical care setting, like most crafts, is best learned as a *hands-on oral tradition in established apprentice–master relationships*. I say this with two important caveats. First, the word *master* as used here refers to skill level rather than to a hierarchy of dominance. I use an adult learning approach that embraces apprentices' knowledge and expertise and emphasizes self-directed learning and transformation while remaining sensitive to cultural and gender differences.[32,33] This approach models and parallels the healing relationships being developed through the craft, particularly, though not exclusively, through residencies and preceptorships. The success of these relationships, as we learned early and frequently at Lehigh Valley, depends on a well-prepared faculty developing a safe learning culture and habitat.

Second, I would like to take a moment to reflect on the phrase *hands-on oral tradition*. Oral traditions are dynamic, immediately responsive to the present moment and its audiences. There are always subtle changes, sometimes in the words, often in the rhythm and voice inflections, and even occasionally in the plot and action. That all stops when an oral tradition gets frozen by an alphabet in the written word. I do not intend for this *Field Guide* to be such an enterprise, and I hope it won't. The generalist's craft of healing is never done in the same way. I have taught the tools of the generalist's craft for over 30 years, and no two learning sessions and their presentations were ever the same. What is in the *Field Guide* are guides and principles, not rules. Other than the Guideposts of the Clinical Hand, the content you will find here consists of sensitizing concepts designed to alert you to pay special attention. How the suggestions, guides, and principles get applied in each specific clinical encounter is up to you. Improvisation and personal expression are strongly encouraged. Make the craft yours, add your art to the craft. One of the many beauties of the generalist's craft is how easily it adapts to change. It fits comfortably with new innovations in technology and artificial intelligence and with the rapidly changing platforms and modes of clinical care.

These caveats are important because words matter. They communicate to others, to ourselves, and to our integrity, as individuals and as a community.[34,35] I try to honor that in the *Field Guide*. I will not be using the word *provider* when referring to physicians, nurse practitioners, and other professionals serving as primary medical care professionals. Provider is a transactional word, and the work of primary care healing is relational. Instead, I'll interchange the words *clinician*, *healer*, and *practitioner*. Additionally, I use the phrases *electronic health record* and *electronic medical record* interchangeably—mostly the former because that is what I hope these documents will become.

Finally, I intend to do my best to discuss this craft in a way that is accessible to all in the generalist practices of primary care, whether you are a family doctor, general practitioner, family nurse practitioner or related advanced practice clinician, general internist, pediatrician, midwife, or chiropractor.

Overview of the *Field Guide*

The *Field Guide for the Generalist's Craft* offers a concise, user-friendly format with tools, selected information, tips, and recommendations for orienting and assisting you in performing the generalist's craft. It is devised for use on your smart phone or other handheld device, on the clinic computer with your electronic health record, and as a convenient, portable hand-size text. Use it in the clinical field at the point of care when seeking to improve your craft. Use it when you want to reflect and make better sense about particularly surprising or challenging moments that arise. Use it during group learning activities.

But most of all, use it to restore and refresh your love for generalist relational primary care and to renew your sense of joy and fulfillment at the end of a long day shared with your patients.

Part 1 prepares you for learning and mastering the generalist's craft. In Module 1, I present the prerequisite tools and skills needed to thrive in this endeavor. It serves as a prompt and review for those who learned these tools and skills in medical school or other professional training setting or as a primer for those who may be new to them. Module 2 introduces and highlights the four guiding metaphors for the generalist's craft: the River of Health, the Spiral of Healing, the Windmill Sails of Generalism, and the Elephant and Rider of Changing Behavior. This is followed by an overview of the Clinical Hand and its three supporting tools: the Ecological Clinical Map, the Relationship-Centered Clinical Method, and the Round Table of Evidence. The module ends with a summary of how these tools fit together for use in a clinical encounter.

In Part 2, you will learn how to embody the generalist's craft in practice. In Modules 3 and 4, the heart of the *Field Guide*, I will guide you through the details of the integrated use and application of the Clinical Hand and its supporting tools. Across the seven units of Module 3, you will learn, in detail, how to move through a clinical encounter using these tools, and Module 4 describes how to apply the skills from Module 3 across various encounter types: routines, ceremonies, and dramas. Module 5 offers advanced postgraduate competencies, including supplementary skills and tools for further mastering and deepening your practical wisdom within the generalist's craft in primary care.

The Postlude shares summary reflections about the generalist's craft, the importance of patients as our partners, and some aphorisms and tips from masters of the craft.

Part 3 includes a contextual supplement and supportive resource. Supplement 1 uncovers the empirical and theoretical foundations of the generalist's craft—the context and the why. We will briefly explore the meaning of health and healing, how they happen, and what promotes them. Supplement 2 contains educational resources for teaching the generalist's craft, including methods and strategies, and an observation tool for assessing the use of the Clinical Hand tool in a clinical encounter. I have included descriptions of GEMs, or generalist enhancement methods, used in the LVHN family medicine residency to engage learners—apprentices of the craft—in enhancing the use of their senses and enriching their integrative clinical use of the tools of turtle craft. This supplement is followed by a Glossary of the many mnemonics presented in the *Field Guide*.

Reflections

Hopefully, you've noticed this *Field Guide* does not read like a standard medical text or journal article. The latter are intentionally stylized to be formal, rational, scientific, objective, and laden with specialized language. The craft represented in the *Field Guide* is none of those. It flows like improvisational jazz, with emotional empirical subjectivity, both cool and warm, in whatever language is understood by the players—the clinician and patient. Clinical care is where their two worlds meet, and I have tried to write in a language that respects both.

The concept of generalist relational clinical jazz was beautifully described by Paul Haidet in a 2007 *Annals of Family Medicine* article that included illustrative jazz excerpts.[36] (In that same tradition, I highly recommend the Paul Winter Consort and their earth jazz as excellent accompaniment for your exploration of this *Field Guide*.) Build space that is multidimensional within the fertile span between the notes. Develop your voice, your curiosity and self-reflection, and your sense of purpose, embodied by the unique clinician you are becoming. Cultivate ensemble in a way that is considerate of how all your practice colleagues both solo with and support each other. Make this *Field Guide* your own, tuned in to your local place and particular relationships.

REFERENCES

1. Loxterkamp D. What humans need. *Ann Fam Med.* 2023;21(5):465-467.
2. Korownyk C, McCormack J, Kolber MR, et al. Competing demands and opportunities in primary care. *Can Fam Physician.* 2017;63(9):664-668.
3. Hardy K. Paleomedicine and the evolutionary context of medicinal plant use. *Rev Bras Farmacogn.* 2021;31(1):1-15.
4. Mitteroecker P, Fischer B. Evolution of the human birth canal. *Am J Obstet Gynecol.* 2024;230(3 suppl):S841-S855.
5. Winkelman M. *Shamanism: A Biopsychosocial Paradigm of Consciousness and Healing.* 2nd ed. Praeger; 2010.
6. Bailey JE. Asklepios: ancient hero of medical caring. *Ann Intern Med.* 1996;124(2):257-263.
7. Sweet V. *Rooted in the Earth, Rooted in the Sky: Hildegard of Bingen and Premodern Medicine.* Routledge; 2006.
8. Kessler SE, Aunger R. The evolution of the human healthcare system and implications for understanding our responses to COVID-19. *Evol Med Public Health.* 2022;10(1):87-107.
9. Sennett R. *The Craftsman.* Yale University Press; 2008.

10. Langlands A. *Craeft: An Inquiry into the Origins and True Meaning of Traditional Crafts*. W. W. Norton & Company; 2017.
11. World Health Organization. *Primary Health Care: Report of the International Conference on Primary Health Care, Alma Ata, USSR, 6-12 September 1978*. World Health Organization; 1978.
12. Neighbour R. *The Inner Consultation: How to Develop an Effective and Intuitive Consulting Style*. 2nd ed. CRC Press; 2005.
13. Stewart M, Brown JB, Weston WW, et al. *Patient-Centered Medicine: Transforming the Clinical Method*. 4th ed. CRC Press; 2024.
14. Slawson DC, Shaughnessy AF, Bennett JH. Becoming a medical information master: feeling good about not knowing everything. *J Fam Pract*. 1994;38:505-513.
15. Byrne PS, Long BE. *Doctors Talking to Patients: A Study of the Verbal Behavior of General Practitioners Consulting in Their Surgeries*. Her Majesty's Stationery Office; 1976.
16. Stott NCH, Davis RH. The exceptional potential in each primary care consultation. *J R Coll Gen Pract*. 1979;29(201):201-205.
17. Kurtz S, Silverman J, Benson J, et al. Marrying content and process in clinical method teaching: enhancing the Calgary-Cambridge guides. *Acad Med*. 2003;78(8):802-809.
18. Helman CG. Disease versus illness in general practice. *J R Coll Gen Pract*. 1981;31(230):548-552.
19. Pendleton D, Schofield T, Tate P, et al. *The New Consultation: Developing Doctor-Patient Communication*. Oxford University Press; 2003.
20. Cole SA, Bird J. *The Medical Interview: The Three Function Approach*. 3rd ed. Elsevier Saunders; 2014.
21. Fortin AH VI, Dwamena FC, Frankel RM, et al. *Smith's Patient-Centered Interviewing: An Evidence-Based Method*. 4th ed. McGraw-Hill Education; 2019.
22. Windover AK, Boissy A, Rice TW, et al. The REDE model of healthcare communication: optimizing relationship as a therapeutic agent. *J Patient Exp*. 2014;1(1):8-13.
23. Bikker AP, Cotton P, Mercer SW. *Embracing Empathy in Healthcare: A Universal Approach to Person-Centred, Empathic Healthcare Encounters*. Radcliffe Publishing; 2014.
24. Frankel RM, Stein T. Getting the most out of the clinical encounter: the four habits model. *J Med Pract Manage*. 2001;16(4):184-191.
25. Elwyn G, Lloyd A, May C, et al. Collaborative deliberation: a model for patient care. *Patient Educ Couns*. 2014;97(2):158-164.
26. Hitakonanu'laxk (Tree Beard). *The Grandfathers Speak: Native American Folk Tales of the Lenape People*. Interlink Books; 1994.
27. Bierhorst J, ed. *Mythology of the Lenape: Guide and Texts*. University of Arizona Press; 1995.
28. Townsend C, Michael NK. *On the Turtle's Back: Stories the Lenape Told Their Grandchildren*. Rutgers University Press; 2023.

29. Cohen-Katz JL, Miller WL, Borkan JM. Building a culture of resident well-being: creating self-reflection, community, and positive identity in family practice residency education. *Fam Syst Health*. 2003;21(3):293-304.
30. Cohen-Katz J, Miller WL, Dostal JA. Growing relationships on the turtle's back: family medicine at Lehigh Valley Health Network. In: Suchman A, Sluyter D, Williamson P, eds. *Leading Change in Healthcare: Transforming Organizations Using Complexity, Positive Psychology, and Relationship-Centered Care*. Radcliffe Publishing; 2011:83-119.
31. Kneebone R. *Expert*. Viking; 2020.
32. Knowles MA. *Andragogy in Action: Applying Modern Principles of Adult Learning*. Jossey-Bass; 1984.
33. Freire P. *Pedagogy of the Oppressed*. Rev 30th Anniversary ed. Continuum; 2000.
34. Le Guin UK. *Words Are My Matter: Writings About Life and Books, 2000-2016*. Small Beer Press; 2016.
35. Berry W. *Standing by Words: Essays*. Counterpoint; 2011.
36. Haidet P. Jazz and the "art" of medicine: improvisation in the medical encounter. *Ann Fam Med*. 2007;5(2):164-169.

PART 1

Getting Ready

MODULE 1

Thriving Skills

Overview

The generalist's craft in primary care begins with you! Well-done craft work requires a thriving craftsperson. This first module shares an approach to wellness and care of the self that corresponds to some of the tools of the generalist's craft. I review four skills that help you thrive while performing the craft: mindfulness and attending, eye juggling, the BATHE technique, and ritual. Mindfulness and attending prepares you to optimize your presence with patients, while eye juggling awakens your generalist awareness and ability to appropriately multitask. The BATHE technique teaches you questions to ask when trouble arises during any clinical encounter to deepen understanding and relationships. Finally, you will discover how to utilize ritual to shift time and create a protective, safe healing space. Since these skills are ideally learned in medical or nursing school, what follows is a review and reminder to keep these thriving skills active. They are how you find joy in the midst of fear and uncertainty as you immerse yourself in the lives of others struggling with life's afflictions and support them as they find their way back to health. It all starts with self-care.

The Importance of Wellness and Care of the Self

Imagine yourself as a tree with five large limbs. Those limbs represent your physical, emotional, cognitive, social, and spiritual lives. Envision how the limbs integrate to ensure the whole tree's livelihood. Reflect on how to care for that tree so it thrives, even in times of rapid climate change. Now, apply those lessons to yourself. Table 1.1 lists several strategies for the self-care of these five limbs, its livelihood, within the habitat of your life. Be selective. What would you recommend to a patient seeking advice for promoting their health? Not everything in Table 1.1. You recognize the information in the table as what's possible, but you would prioritize and personalize the advice based on who the patient is and what they need at the time.

Care for your physical limb with stretching, strengthening, aerobics, getting outside, and healthy eating. For the latter, I relish Michael Pollan's guidance. "Eat food. Not too much. Mostly plants."[1] The secret in that advice

TABLE 1.1 Whole Person Self-Care Activities

Self-Care Feature	Activities
Physical	Daily physical activity (mix of stretching, strengthening, aerobics) Daily time outside Maintain healthy eating patterns. Avoid drug, tobacco, and alcohol misuse.
Emotional	Experience your emotions without judgment; let go. Learn to say, "No." Get enough sleep. Regularly schedule time for yoga, tai chi, forest walking, etc. Make music, pottery, knitting, woodworking, poetry, etc.
Cognitive	Do the work to squash stinking thinking. Do puzzles (crossword, sudoku, jigsaw, etc.). Read multiple genres. Learn a new language. Practice journaling.
Social	Nurture a circle of friends and gather with them regularly. Practice self-disclosure. Join a group (choir, theater, sports team, etc.). Engage in hobbies with others.
Spiritual	Practice gratitude every day. Reserve silent time. Connect with a faith community. Engage with spiritual mystery, e.g., prayer.
Livelihood	Maintain a sense of purpose and mastery. Share gifts and skills. Achieve adequate financial health. Ensure proportionality among personal, social, and professional. Compose a life; avoid creating silos.
Habitat	Connect with your place. Decrease your carbon footprint. Minimize plastic use. Advocate for parks, trails, and more public commons. Advocate for more public transportation.

resides in the definition of food. This could simply be fresh, mostly unprocessed food. Again, I am fond of Pollan's guidance to avoid eating "anything your great grandmother wouldn't recognize as food"[1]; products with unfamiliar, unpronounceable names, or more than five ingredients (refers to chemically related words, not cultural names of whole foods); and products that make health claims, as well as to avoid the middle of supermarkets.[1]

Care for your emotional limb by noticing your emotions, paying attention and owning them, neither suppressing nor attaching. Get enough sleep and direct emotional energy into an artistic endeavor such as music, knitting, pottery, woodworking, or poetry. Actively practice emotional self-management.

Care for your cognitive limb by doing the work to squash stinking thinking, those negative intrusive thoughts that shrink your sense of self. Recognize and challenge those thoughts; be your own friend. Bring the inside out and share your thoughts with others. Stimulate, expand, stretch, and discipline.

Care for your social limb by developing an intimate friend network, managing family relationships, and expanding your network of engagement. Ensure diversity.

Care for your spiritual limb with a daily practice of gratitude and the use of prayer or whatever form of engagement relates you with spiritual mystery. Connect with a faith community and spend time in the presence of silence.

Put all five limbs together and care for your livelihood, your whole self, by composing your life over time in a way that allows all of your parts and desires to grow. Insist on proportionality across the personal, social, and professional, not as silos but as a whole of interdependences. Budget and plan to build adequate financial security.

Care for your habitat and all that lives there. Care for your roots that connect you with habitat; the land desperately needs our help to heal and vice versa. Robin Wall Kimmerer posits, "Our relationship with land cannot heal until we hear its stories. But who will tell them?"[2] Go outside, listen, and share the stories that emerge. Let them inform your generalist's craft.

For generalist healers, a common source of self-torment, and an inadvertent basis for poor performance of the craft, is our inner chatter. Two voices compete for attention in our inner chatter: the voice of scarcity and the voice of abundance. When we neglect aspects of our self-care, the voice of scarcity booms loudly. When we take good care, the voice of abundance speaks confidently. Listen for both voices in this excerpt from one of my journal entries from my first years in family practice. It's early April, I'm tired, I haven't been taking care of myself, and I've taken on more than I can handle.

> *8:30 PM. The phone rings. I turn from the 1040 tax form on my desk with clenched fist and answer. It's a mother worried about her 8-year-old son's 3-week dry cough; she sounds frightened. My inner chatter:* Nuts, I don't have time for this; I've got to get this stupid tax stuff done. It's not adding up and I owe money. It's only a cough. What's her problem[?] *"I'm just, like, really scared. Josh was getting better, but I got home from work …" My inner chatter:* Oh no, another guilt-ridden working mom […] Why won't these figures work out? Yikes, I must also get ready for my friend's visit tomorrow. I can get rid of this phone call quickly. **I explain, "Some coughs persist after a bad cold. I'll be happy to see you and Josh in the morning at the office." She interrupts, "But I'm really not sure. I think I hear wheezing." More inner chatter:** […] I'm not up for this. She's not hearing me. Gosh I'm tired. **And so goes the conversation and mental chatter. Eventually, Josh gets seen in the emergency room at 2 AM for status asthmaticus. Another story not heard.** Aaargh! What's happened to me?

Not my finest moment, but I used it to motivate significant changes in my self-care and in how I managed my inner chatter and ability to listen to others. The voice of scarcity has fear at its core, is filled with lists of "to dos" and prejudgments, and takes everything personally. It wants to stay in control and impose its story on others—and for us, "others" is our patients. The voice of abundance is one of awareness, curiosity, and insight. It wants to learn, to listen, to discover what's happening and to stay with the seeking. The voice of abundance has no investment in the answers it receives. Peace nestles at its core, confident that answers are everywhere and solutions will appear.

Both voices are always present. One intensifies the storm that's brewing; the other finds attentive presence in the midst of the storm. What to do when the voice of scarcity predominates, as in the above example? From a longer-term perspective, better daily self-care calms the voice of scarcity. Yet, it still occasionally breaks through. What then?

Listen and acknowledge. Recognize that the voice of scarcity is reminding you of the current tempestuous situation of your life. Pay heed and make note; say thank you and let the voice know you will get back to it shortly. Put it aside, laugh, and take a deep breath. Invite the voice of abundance to come forth and be present as you direct your attention to the person before you. Get comfortable, even consider changing locations; lighten up. Use the tools of attending and mindfulness to be discussed in the next section. Now, with a more open attitude and learning stance, concentrate and focus on who is inviting you into their dilemma. Be assured that you and the patient are where

TABLE 1.2	Tools of the Creative Hero(ine)

Have faith in your creativity.
Suspend negative judgment.
Practice precise observation.
Ask penetrating questions.
Deepen relationships.

you are supposed to be and doing what you are supposed to be doing. And as the challenging situation unfolds, and the voice of scarcity starts to get restless, remember the wisdom of the tools of the creative hero(ine) (see Table 1.2).[3] These tools help you to stay calm in the storm without losing your own wholeness and integrity. I keep these five statements in my cell phone so I can see them when my voice of scarcity troubles the waters.

As generalist primary care healers, we experience a lot of weather. Without help, we can easily end each day with a laundry bag full of wet and muddied clothes. If we aren't diligent, all that laundry comes home with us and gets emptied onto those awaiting us. But with good self-care, management of our inner chatter, the tools of the creative hero(ine), and application of the four thriving skills in this section, we keep our laundry bag at least much lighter, if not empty.

Thriving Skill 1: Mindfulness and Attending

Introduction

Effective performance of the generalist's craft rests on a foundation of mindfulness and attending. Mindfulness refers to the experience of full awareness of the present moment without interpretation or judgment, of coming to attention. Attending denotes what's being noticed when mindful. I am most alive in deep snow on skis or snowshoes in temperatures many degrees below zero; that is where I am fully mindful and attending. I purposefully seek that experience with a group of friends every winter. It reinforces my neural pathways for when I am with patients the rest of the year. Two winters in Yellowstone National Park are especially memorable. It was just us, the wilderness, the weather, and the area's natural inhabitants: wolf packs, coyotes, bison, elk, birds. After a few days, all of my senses tingled with intense awareness.

When I'm in that environment, I know the temperature of every body part, my state of hydration, fatigue, hunger, soreness. I know what animals are near, which are paying attention to me and which not. I know where I am relative to home base and possible routes back, and I know how to quickly find refuge. The air, sky, and light all glow brighter, even when cloudy, and I know the present weather and what is coming. The glittering crystals of snow dazzle. I know all of this at the same time without thinking. Not magic, although it is magical. I am experiencing mindfulness. My inner chatter is as quiet as the enveloping white silence of the winter landscape. Subconsciously, I am attending to all of it; it is all there awaiting recognition. But at any given moment, I have prioritized what gets fuller attention and, usually, that relates to the unique personal circumstances. I am applying the simple rules of generalism to my attending.[4] I recognize, prioritize, and personalize. I am ready and prepared for whatever comes next.

Imagine being that awake when doing the generalist's craft in primary care! As noted by Ron Epstein, "Attending to each patient's concerns means being prepared to greet whatever concerns patients bring with curiosity and resolve."[5] That means enhancing your ability to enact mindfulness and attending. I begin this section with an overview of emotional and social intelligence, which builds capacity for mindfulness and attending. Then, I will briefly explore mindfulness meditation and mindful practice in clinical situations. I will end by sharing some techniques for recentering mindfulness and boosting self-awareness in situations where you feel stuck or frustrated while caring for patients.

Emotional and Social Intelligence

Mindfulness and attending come easier with higher levels of emotional and social intelligence. Emotional intelligence is the ability to notice, express, and control your emotions and understand, interpret, and respond to the emotions of others.[6,7] Social intelligence is the ability to understand and manage interpersonal and social relationships.[8,9] Table 1.3 identifies the components of both emotional and social intelligence, but more importantly, it lists some questions for self-reflection to aid you in identifying aspects of these intelligences that may need additional attention. I recommend checking in several times a year, especially when you've experienced some stormy times. Ask friends and mentors to offer feedback on the indicator questions. They often notice the blind spots in our mirrors.

TABLE 1.3 — Tool for Self-Evaluating Emotional and Social Intelligence

Intelligence Type	Components	Indicator Questions

Emotional Intelligence	High Self-Awareness	• Do you have accurate understanding of:
		  ◦ How you behave?
		  ◦ How others perceive you?
		  ◦ How you respond to others?
		  ◦ Your own attitudes, feelings, intents?

	Mood Regulation	• Are you able to:
		  ◦ Soothe yourself?
		  ◦ Shake off anxiety, gloom, irritability?
		  ◦ Maintain emotional perspective?
		  ◦ Put yourself in a good mood?

	Self-Motivation	• Are you able to:
		  ◦ Channel emotions to achieve a goal?
		  ◦ Postpone immediate gratification?
		  ◦ Persist in the face of frustration?
		  ◦ Self-generate initiative?

Social Intelligence	High Social Awareness	• Are you able to:
		  ◦ Feel with others; attune to a person?
		  ◦ Understand another person?
		  ◦ Interpret the social world around you?

	Social Facility	• Are you able to:
		  ◦ Interact smoothly at the non-verbal level?
		  ◦ Present yourself effectively?
		  ◦ Shape the outcome of interactions?
		  ◦ Care about others' needs and respond?

Mindful Practice and Mindfulness Meditation

Mindfulness meditation is a technique that is relatively simple to learn, yet remarkably difficult to sustain.[10,11] When practiced, we discover the stickiness of our inner chatter, and, with persistence, we develop the ability to listen, acknowledge, and let go. We learn how not to attach, which makes us more available to what else is in our presence. Table 1.4 offers instructions on how to get started with mindfulness meditation. Developing your emotional and social intelligence and the regular practice of mindfulness meditation prepare you for mindful practice.

The four features or "habits of mind" shown in Table 1.5 characterize mindful practice.[12-15]

Engaging *beginner's mind* means seeing each situation as new and fresh. You suspend preconceptions and expectations and presume naivete. This is how anthropologists are trained to enter and explore cultures new to them: observe, listen, don't assume, and delay trying to explain. Seek with the surprise and wonder of a child. With beginner's mind active, bring yourself into *presence*, the experience of undistracted attention on the patient, task, and moment. This is where your mindfulness meditation enters to help. You have come into attention, the place of sacred silence where intuition resides. Now you are ready to practice attentive observation and critical curiosity. *Attentive observation* refers to looking for the unexpected. Move back and forth between your central and peripheral vision and keep shifting what is in the foreground and what is in the background. At times, hold the patient in the foreground, and at other times, focus on the concerns being addressed. *Critical curiosity* welcomes doubt and uncertainty and invites self-questioning.

TABLE 1.4 Simple Steps for Mindfulness Meditation

Action	Description
Settle In	Get comfortable, preferably in a sitting position.
Breathe	Take slow, relaxed breaths, in and out, for 5 or more minutes.
Focus	Stay focused on the movement and sound of your breathing.

Variation: Put a raisin in your mouth and focus on it as you breathe.

TABLE 1.5　Features of Mindful Practice

Beginner's mind
Presence
Attentive observation
Critical curiosity

Data from Epstein RM. Mindful practice in action (I): technical competence, evidence-based medicine, and relationship-centered care. *Fam Syst Health*. 2003;21(1):1-9.

These four habits of mindful practice prepare you for masterful performance of the generalist's craft in primary care.

A day in the vocational life of a generalist healer vibrates with the sounds and chords of multiple relationships coming and going with all the diverse emotions and thoughts that accompany them. We've learned that the sequencing of relationships influences what happens next.[16] The music of each encounter enters into the ones that follow. Practice mindfully and learn to quiet those sounds, diminish the amplitude of the vibrations, and become more fully present and fresh for each. Ronald Epstein, a family doc and leader of workshops on mindful practice, offers this advice:

 Over the years I have developed a habit of pausing momentarily before entering any patient's room. With my hand on the doorknob, I quietly take a breath to help me become more present in preparation for the visit—I mentally set aside everything that has happened with the patient I have just finished seeing and other events of the day so that I can be fresh and available. I let go of expectations.[5]

You will meet this habit again in Module 3.

Clinical Tools for Mindfulness and Attending

There are many moments in primary care clinical practice where achieving beginner's mind and presence seems nearly impossible. The sound of a pager beeping in the middle of the night still causes my body to react with vigilance and a surge of fight-or-flight hormones. The Attending Imagery Technique helps dampen the hormone storm and make space for beginner's mind and presence. This technique combines established work on the relaxation

TABLE 1.6 — Implementing the Attending Imagery Technique

Practice	Duration
Inhale for 5 s, then exhale for 10 s. Repeat this breathing pattern for 5 min. (It will be helpful to use a timepiece at first.)	Twice per day until the practice comes naturally and a timepiece is no longer needed.
Add imagery to the breathing exercise. Focus on an image you associate with calm and presence.	Twice per day for 3 wk, and once per day thereafter.

response, guided imagery, and progressive muscle relaxation to help you achieve presence at any time.[17-19]

Table 1.6 describes the steps for learning the attending imagery technique. Focus for the first week on breathing and triggering the relaxation response—the sense of calm evidenced by your pulse slowing, inner chatter diminishing, and presence emerging.

When you are able to practice the breathing comfortably and without a timepiece, add imagery. Choose a place, sound, color, and/or image that you most associate with calm and presence. For me, it's Moore Cove Falls in Pisgah National Forest, North Carolina, near the Shining Rock Wilderness (see Figure 1.1).

Once you've conditioned the image, you will be able to trigger the attending response by just bringing the image to mind. Of course, daily reinforcement is required to keep this response active. I try to practice this technique at lunchtime, which helps me reset for the next part of the day.

A second tool for supporting mindfulness and attending is a Balint group.[20-22] Though they were initially developed to enhance understanding of the doctor–patient relationship, especially in the generalist primary medical care setting, they turned out to do much more, including enhance mindful practice. Balint group is the place you take "cases" where you feel frustrated, stuck, and/or confused. In the group, you discover, in the facilitated safe presence of colleagues, how "stuckness" happened, including what role you inadvertently played and why. Balint groups have become common in family medicine residencies in the United States and for general practitioners

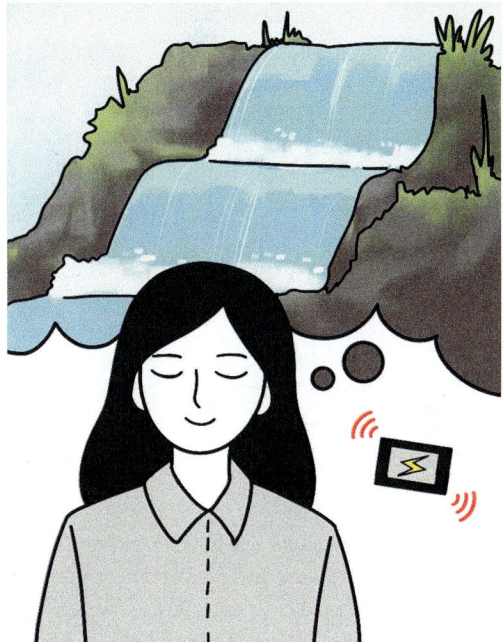

FIGURE 1.1. Attending Imagery Technique.

throughout Europe. If there aren't any in your residency or in your community, please contact the American Balint Society for next steps in getting one started. Your patients, family, and you will be grateful.

Thriving Skill 2: Eye Juggling

Eye juggling is a form of attentive observation and an important tool for the sensemaking of the generalist's craft. The metaphor of eye juggling is rooted in a Cheyenne story about a shaman who could sing his eyes to the top of a tree and look in all four directions—and a coyote who learned the song but lacked discipline and got into all sorts of trouble.[23] For our purposes, eye juggling refers to the ability to juggle three different fields of awareness at the same time (see Figure 1.2). One of those fields is the *eye of self*, which sees you as you are present with a patient. A second field is the *eye on the patient*, which is focused on what's happening with the person in front of you. The third field of awareness is the *eye of context*, which seeks to understand the unique situational contexts, past and present, of the moment, as well as the

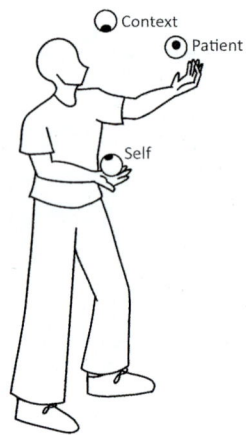

FIGURE 1.2. Eye Juggling.

concerns being explored. The context eye looks near and far as well as back in time. I often ask patients to show me pictures of where they live and of family members and important places to help my context eye see more clearly.

When juggling three objects, one is being held, ready for tossing; one is being caught; and one is in the air—and so it is for eye juggling. At any given moment, one field of awareness, the one in the air, is foregrounding your attention: it's focused on learning. Another field of awareness, the one being caught, is now in the background: it's what you now know. The third is waiting, ready to win your attention: it's what you don't know yet.

Eye juggling recognizes that doing the generalist's craft requires the seemingly contradictory need to multitask, focus, and manage inner chatter at the same time. Like juggling, it takes practice to do this. Table 1.7 highlights some questions to consider when each of the three eyes, or fields of awareness, is attending.

These questions are just starters; many others will arise. For exercises to help learn to eye juggle and translate the practice to the clinical setting, see the work of Donald Krill.[24] And for help learning to juggle, which I encourage you to do, see John Cassidy, who also happens to hold several Guinness World Records in balloon sculpting.[25]

Thriving Skill 3: The BATHE Technique

When in trouble—BATHE! Imagine the letters BATHE on your fingernails so you will notice them when, in a clinical encounter, you begin to clench

TABLE 1.7	The Three Eyes of Eye Juggling
The Eye	**Questions to Ask**
Self	What past experiences have I had like this one?
	What are my expectations?
	Where are my blind spots?
	What am I feeling?
	What else?
Patient	Who is this person?
	What are they feeling?
	What are they thinking?
	What am I observing? Eyes? Posture? Facial expressions? Dress?
	What else?
Context	Where did the patient come from?
	What's happening back at their home? At work?
	What's happening in the clinic?
	How did the patient get here?
	What else?

your fist or feel as if you're hanging by your nails (see Figure 1.3). These are often moments of emotional tension, tears, anger, feeling stuck. Pause and begin BATHEing the patient. BATHE is a remarkable technique to help you through these nail-biting moments during a clinical encounter.[26]

You will also find the BATHE letters on the nails of the Clinical Hand tool described in Module 2 (see Figure 2.5).

Table 1.8 describes the features and key questions for using this tool.[26] Begin to BATHE by exploring the background for the current situation. What was happening just before the patient started crying? If that isn't clear, have the patient sit up and take a deep breath, and ask them what they were thinking, what memory was triggered, what they heard just before they got upset. Inquire: Has this happened before? Gently invite them to share their feelings, and then expand and ask what most troubles them about it. Give the patient time to reflect and answer. End your questioning by having the patient share ways they've handled situations like this before. When the patient has finished speaking, summarize what you heard in a way that conveys empathy.

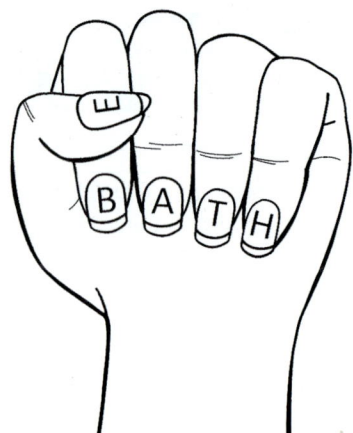

FIGURE 1.3. BATHE on Fingernails.

The BATHE technique works in dealings with family and friends as well as in clinical encounters. For example, I once visited a close friend but found him more irritable and distant than usual. I sat back in my chair, made eye contact, and, in a subdued and serious voice, asked him what was really happening right now. He choked up.

"I can't concentrate," he explained. "I just learned that my wife's best friend has terminal cancer."
"How do you feel about that?" I inquired.
"I feel lost, uncertain about my own future."

TABLE 1.8	Features of BATHE	
Letter	Feature	Question
B	Background	*What's been happening?*
A	Affect	*How does it make you feel?*
T	Troubles	*What troubles you the most about it?*
H	Handle	*How have you been handling it?*
E	Empathy	*Give empathic response.*

After a few cleansing breaths, I asked, "What troubles you the most about this situation?"

"She was helping my wife find us a smaller, single-floor home so we could eventually move there closer to my wife's family after I retire."

Calmly, I replied, "How are you handling it so far?"

"Not well. Worries keep flooding into my head, worries about my own mortality."

Leaning closer to him, I responded, "This sounds like quite a distressing situation for you. Let's pause and take a walk and brainstorm some future options."

"Great idea. Thanks! Let's get our coats," he said with greater assurance in his voice.

You will have many opportunities to BATHE.

Thriving Skill 4: Ritual

When is coffee drinking a habit, and when is it a ritual? I often ask this question of family medicine residents when I'm introducing them to the importance of ritual when doing the generalist's craft. They are usually sipping coffee at the time.

Table 1.9 explores the differences between habit and ritual. People drinking coffee as a habit are barely aware of the coffee and focused more on other activities—their cell phone, lecture, whatever. They are often in a hurry, the coffee being transported from place to place without playing a significant part in the day's drama unless it accidentally spills. Coffee-as-ritual looks entirely different. The intent is to savor, the person's full attention on not only drinking the coffee, but its careful preparation. In that way, coffee-as-ritual is

TABLE 1.9 Ritual or Habit?

Feature	Ritual	Habit
Intentionality	Conscious	Unconscious
Attention	Fully Present	Scattered
Time	Kairos	Chronos
Performance	Excellent	Variable

similar to a Japanese tea ceremony.[27] The ritualist is meticulous in the details, appearing lost in time—*kairos time*. Kairos time is deep time, unlike *chronos* or "clock" time. Kairos, in Greek, means "the right or critical moment." Kairos time feels as if time has stopped. When you spend 15 minutes with a patient and do the generalist's craft with excellence, the patient will comment that you "took all the time in the world." They experienced kairos time, a ritual done well. Excellence in ritual performance matters.

Ritual is "a patterned, repetitive, and symbolic enactment of cultural (or individual) beliefs and values."[28] Let's unpack these words. *Patterned* indicates that rituals have a discernible structure and form that is *repeated* with each enactment. Each performance includes *symbols* rich with *cultural and personal meaning* related to the intention(s) underlying the ritual. Ritual has also been defined as "acts of display through which one or more participants transmit information concerning their physiological, psychological, or sociological states either to themselves or to one or more of their participants."[29] This definition highlights how ritual communicates whole-body information to the participants in the ritual; ritual moves us. It moves us physically, emotionally, and relationally. When used in the primary medical care setting, ritual enables healing. As William Howells noted, affliction is "like a tangled head of hair, and ritual is the comb."[30]

Ritual works through activating and integrating the left and right hemispheres of the brain and its three evolutionary layers: the triune forebrain, limbic system, and neocortex. This happens through the framing of ritual performance in the clinic itself—its common smells, appearance, stylized and patterned processes of checking-in and rooming—an order and formality that separates clinical space from everyday life. The framing is followed by the use of multilayered symbols of healing that generate an edge of fear but, even more, of hopefulness, creating a liminal state of heightened suggestibility. All of this happens within a cognitive matrix of cultural beliefs surrounding health, malady, and healing. Done well, the ritual engenders a sense of safety, of inviolability and inevitability driven by an expected rhythm, repetition, and redundancy performed, stylized, and staged using techniques and technologies.[28] For us as generalist healers and our clinical ensemble, the cabinets of gauze, tongue blades, syringes and needles, and suture kits; the electronic scale, point-of-care ultrasound device, computer screens, microscope, and centrifuge; our stethoscopes and otoscopes are the stuff of our daily work. For patients, they impart a bit of anticipation, a sense of magic, a glimmer of hope. Ritual creates the safe harbor where those perspectives meet and where the start of healing begins.

Table 1.10 highlights the critical components of ritual with examples from the primary medical care setting. We begin the healing ritual by creating

TABLE 1.10 Components of Ritual

Component	Example(s)
Sacred Space	The exam room
Ritual Intention	Agency and belonging through clinician–patient relationship
Ritual Gestures	Rhythm and sequence of touch; handwashing; procedures; positioning
Ritual Words	Voice of medicine (but presented in a manner accessible to the patient)
Ritual Objects	Stethoscope, prescription, gloves, medical record, anatomic displays

sacred space, moving the patient from the everyday world of the waiting room into the ritual space of an exam or consultation room. Within this room (or virtual screen), we divide the space into listening and examination spaces, the latter being the exam table, the inner chamber for physical contact. We set ritual intention as we enter this space and then use ritual gestures, words, and objects as we do the healing craft work.

Ritual serves us by fulfilling several functions. These are named and elaborated in Table 1.11.[31-33] Ritual helps take the edge off the fear patients frequently feel as they enter clinical space. It's reassuring. This feeling of security and sense of control results from the "stereotyped sequence of activities including gestures, words, and objects, performed in a sequestered place designed to influence forces on behalf of the actor's (physician's) goals and interests."[34] This reassurance is enhanced by respecting the patient's cultural expectations.

Good ritual stimulates the parasympathetic nervous system, helping to reduce stress and relieve tension. Ritual also functions to enhance a sense of safety where one can risk more vulnerability, making any external intrusion more quickly noticeable.[35] We recognize symptoms and life circumstances previously overlooked. Reinforcing status quo values represents the conservative function of ritual, one usually invoked within religious ceremonies. This can be a powerful help when patients present with simple concerns needing a fix and a return to life as it was, a restitution narrative.[36]

But that's often not the case. Patients with unexplained symptoms, complex chronic disease, or a new diagnosis of metastatic cancer will not be able

TABLE 1.11 Functions of Ritual

Function	Description
Provide Reassurance	Generates a feeling of security, sense of control
Relieve Tension	Activates parasympathetics, reduces stress
Enhance Sense of Safety	Creates spatial and psychological order
Reinforce/Validate Values	Preserves status quo values (the conservative function of ritual)
Transformation	Opens space for something new
Facilitate Status Change	Smooths transition from "sick role" to "healthy"

to return to their earlier life. A greater change is in order, a more fundamental type of transformation to move on to a new life chapter or story. Fortunately, ritual can perform this function as well. Whether preserving status quo or transforming, ritual usually facilitates status change from the sick role toward a healthy one, stabilizing and reestablishing important relationships and patterns of interaction. Ritual serves especially well in situations of multi-morbidity[37] and in creating some reassuring order among the multiple competing demands and opportunities of primary medical care.[38]

Ritual can be the comb that untangles the knotted strands of malady's hair, but to do so, it must be performed well and with lots of room for improvisation. Use ritual to create structure and a safe space, but remain flexible enough to ensure openings for creativity and respect for the uniqueness of each person who enters into it. Rituals can easily turn into habits or become too rigid and restrict our vision and imagination.

Now that you've taken the time to learn some techniques to help you thrive as a healer, you are ready to learn and discover the joy of the generalist's craft of healing. In the modules that follow, I will introduce the Clinical Hand, the primary tool that provides the ritual structure of the craft. Its five fingers will guide you through all the components required for its mastery. How the rest of the craft manifests is up to you, to be danced and sung into life.

REFERENCES

1. Pollan M. *In Defense of Food: An Eater's Manifesto*. The Penguin Press; 2008.
2. Kimmerer RW. *Braiding Sweetgrass: Indigenous Wisdom, Scientific Knowledge, and the Teachings of Plants*. Milkweed Editions; 2013.
3. Catford L, Ray M. *The Path of the Everyday Hero: Drawing on the Power of Myth to Meet Life's Most Important Challenges*. Jeremy P. Tarcher, Inc; 1991.
4. Etz R, Miller WL, Stange KC. Simple rules that guide generalist and specialist care. *Fam Med*. 2021;53(8):697-700.
5. Epstein R. *Attending: Medicine, Mindfulness, and Humanity*. Scribner; 2017.
6. Goleman D. *Emotional Intelligence: Why It Can Matter More Than IQ*. 25th Anniversary ed. Bantam Books; 2020.
7. Dott C, Mamarelis G, Karam E, et al. Emotional intelligence and good medical practice: is there a relationship? *Cureus*. 2022;14(3):e23126.
8. Albrecht K. *Social Intelligence: The New Science of Success*. Jossey-Bass; 2006.
9. Goleman D. *Social Intelligence: The New Science of Human Relationships*. Bantom Books; 2006.
10. Kabat-Zinn J. *Wherever You Go, There You Are: Mindfulness Meditation in Everyday Life*. 30th Anniversary ed. Hachette Book Group; 2023.
11. Kabat-Zinn J. *Mindfulness for Beginners: Reclaiming the Present Moment—And Your Life*. Sounds True, Inc; 2012.
12. Epstein RM. Mindful practice in action (I): technical competence, evidence-based medicine, and relationship-centered care. *Fam Syst Health*. 2003;21(1):1-9.
13. Epstein RM. Mindful practice in action (II): cultivating habits of mind. *Fam Syst Health*. 2003;21(1):11-17.
14. Epstein RM. Mindful practice. *JAMA*. 1999;282(9):833-839.
15. Schon DA. *The Reflective Practitioner*. Basic Books; 1983.
16. Seaburn DB, Harp J. Sequencing: the patient caseload as an interactive system. *Fam Syst Med*. 1988;6(1):107-111.
17. Benson H, Klipper MZ. *The Relaxation Response*. Avon; 1975.
18. Rossman ML. *Guided Imagery for Self-Healing*. HJ Kramer, Inc; 2000.
19. Jacobson E. *Progressive Relaxation*. The University of Chicago Press; 1938.
20. Balint M. *The Doctor, His Patient, and the Illness*. International Universities Press, Inc; 1957.
21. Otten H. *The Theory and Practice of Balint Group Work: Analyzing Professional Relationships*. Routledge; 2018.
22. Milberg L, Knowlton K. *Restoring the Core of Clinical Practice: What Is a Balint Group and How Does It Help?* Independently Published; 2019.
23. Frey R. *Eye Juggling: Seeing the World Through a Looking Glass and a Glass Pane*. University Press of America; 1995.
24. Krill DF. *Practice Wisdom: A Guide for Helping Professionals*. Sage Publications, Inc; 1990.
25. Cassidy J, Rimbeaux BC. *Juggling for the Complete Klutz*. Klutz Press; 1988.
26. Stuart MR, Lieberman JA III. *The Fifteen Minute Hour: Efficient and Effective Patient-Centered Consultation Skills*. 6th ed. CRC Press; 2019.

27. Sadler AL. *The Japanese Tea Ceremony: Cha-No-Yu*. Tuttle Publishing; 2008.
28. Davis-Floyd R, Laughlin CD. *Ritual: What It Is, How It Works, and Why*. Berghahn Books; 2022.
29. Rappaport RA. The sacred in human evolution. *Annu Rev Ecol Evol Syst*. 1971;2:23-44.
30. Howells W. *The Heathens*. Doubleday; 1962.
31. Achterberg J, Dossey B, Kolkmeier L. *Rituals of Healing: Using Imagery for Health and Wellness*. Bantam Books; 1994.
32. Imber-Black E, Roberts J, Whiting R, eds. *Rituals in Families and Family Therapy*. W. W. Norton & Company; 1988.
33. Turner V. *The Ritual Process: Structure and Anti-Structure*. Aldine; 1969.
34. Turner VW. Symbols in African ritual. *Science*. 1973;179(4078):1100-1105.
35. Boyer P, Liénard P. Why ritualized behavior? Precaution systems and action parsing in developmental, pathological and cultural rituals. *Behav Brain Sci*. 2006;29(6):595-613; discussion 613-650.
36. Frank AW. *The Wounded Storyteller: Body, Illness, and Ethics*. 2nd ed. The University of Chicago Press; 1997.
37. Grumbach K. Chronic illness, comorbidities, and the need for medical generalism. *Ann Fam Med*. 2003;1(1):4-7.
38. Jaén CR, Stange KC, Nutting PA. Competing demands of primary care: a model for the delivery of clinical preventive services. *J Fam Pract*. 1994;38(2):166-171.

MODULE 2

Metaphors and Tools Overview

Introduction

The generalist's craft in primary care resides in the community where it is practiced and thrives when time, place, and relationships find appreciation. Generalist primary care healers live in the woven tapestry connecting the neighborhood with the house of medicine and the land of the healthy with the domain of the afflicted. In these in-between worlds, we use our generalist's craft to make health for the individuals we encounter and for the families and communities in which we all live. What a gift and privilege!

Module 2 introduces four guiding metaphors, the Clinical Hand and its three supporting tools to guide your mastery of this healing craft. I conclude the module with an overview of how the three supporting tools fit together with the Clinical Hand to craft clinical jazz and make health.

Four Guiding Metaphors of the Generalist's Craft

The generalist's craft of primary care requires you to mobilize your whole body and person in pursuit of engaging and understanding the whole body and personhood of your patient so that, together, you can make better health. Rational, scientific speech, by itself, interferes with this craft work by unconsciously suppressing the personal and emotional.[1] We need a language that speaks to all of our parts: the physical, emotional, cognitive, social, and spiritual. That is the work of metaphor.[2,3] Metaphor and symbols evoke memorable images for better understanding and seeing from a new perspective by combining the literal, objective, and subjective. The four guiding metaphors in this section will help you, the generalist clinician, recall the overall intention and vision that bind together the Clinical Hand and its supporting tools of the generalist's craft in primary care (see Table 2.1).

The *River of Health* evokes the geography of health and malady and the purpose of our craft. The *Spiral of Healing* reminds us of the necessary steps that facilitate the restoration of health. The *Windmill Sails of Generalism* illustrate three concurrent activities—recognize, prioritize, and personalize—that

TABLE 2.1	Four Guiding Metaphors of the Generalist Craft
Guiding Metaphor	**Description**
River of Health	Geography of health and malady
	Illustration of purpose of the generalist's craft
Spiral of Healing	Iterative steps toward restoring health
Windmill Sails of Generalism	Simple rules of generalist practice from which health emerges
	Recognize, prioritize, personalize
The Elephant and the Rider of Changing Behavior	Fast and slow thinking
	Steps for changing behavior

drive an effective generalist's craft in primary care. The *Elephant and the Rider of Changing Behavior* conjures an image for how to help patients change their behavior in the direction of health. Let's explore each of the guiding metaphors.

River of Health

When teaching the generalist's craft of healing, I begin with the River of Health as a guiding metaphor (see Figure 2.1). The River of Health metaphor is grounded in concepts originally developed from complexity theory as the Stacey matrix.[4] Healthy people thrive and live together within the River of Health, their place of membership, a zone of complexity flowing through time. While in the river, people feel well, experience meaningful agency, and feel a sense of purpose and communion with others, observing a "horizon of significance" up ahead.[5] When maladies (disease, illness, sickness) afflict us, we leave the River of Health and are washed up on its banks as patients who, hopefully, seek and find help so that we may return to the waters of health. On the left bank of the river in Figure 2.1, the physiologic systems of our bodies and their responsiveness to each other and their surroundings become more rigid, as occurs in aging with its loss of complexity and reduction in heart rate variability. Chronic stress and malnutrition can also move us further up this side of the river, making us feel stuck.[6]

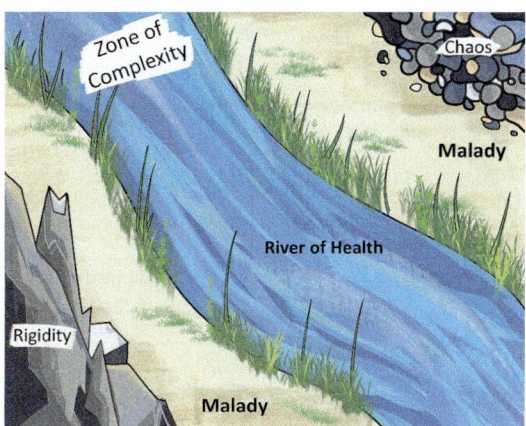

FIGURE 2.1. River of Health.

On the right slope of the river in Figure 2.1, our bodies move closer to chaos and catastrophe such that the dynamics of our life and bodies begin to break apart. These are moments when we benefit from intensive hospital care and powerful allopathic treatments. The medical specialties build their facilities on the land above the river. Primary care healers enact their generalist's craft along the shoreline; we are the "turtles" of health, edge-walkers along the shores at the boundary of health and malady. We swim in the river, helping to promote and maintain the health of those entrusted to our care. We help those who have been washed up on the riverbank by restoring agency and belonging and returning them to the water. We help love grow through healing and enhance our lives together. We craft health through healing the brokenness in life one person at a time.

Spiral of Healing

Our explorations of health, healing, and healing relationships as the purpose, ways, and means for enacting the generalist's craft in primary care come together in the Spiral of Healing (see Figure 2.2). Healing involves a repeated four-step cycle, a spiral over time.[7] The spiral begins with a person experiencing suffering and/or disability of some kind; they are now a patient who has left the River of Health. The spiral ends, after one or more iterations, with that patient feeling better and/or with less disability; they have returned, or at least moved closer, to the River of Health.

The first step of the spiral requires the clinician to engage with the person and *accept and validate* their experience of malady. This does not mean

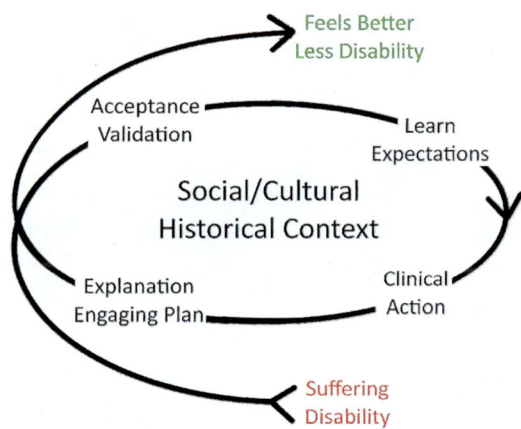

FIGURE 2.2. Spiral of Healing.

agreeing with their explanations for that experience; it's respecting and appreciating the truth of their embodied experience, which is essential to establishing trust. The second step involves *learning the patient's expectations* for care. What are their hopes and goals? What is the actual reason they connected with you today? These first two steps primarily comprise active listening and summarizing what is learned. The third step generates *clinical action* and the use of hands; the suffering and affliction are touched. The primary care clinician creatively and competently intervenes physically to further uncover and alter the current malady. If the encounter is virtual, the clinician can guide the patient in how to examine or manipulate their own body. The fourth step asks the clinician to *explain* what is happening in a way that addresses the patient's expectations and to present an *engaging plan* that moves the patient back toward health. You name their suffering and answer the question, "What is going on?" You activate the patient's agency with caring or a treatment plan that encourages a return to belonging or membership and answers the question, "Now what?" While you both move through the Spiral of Healing, you pay special attention to the particular *social, cultural, and historical contexts* of the encounter and the patient's situation. The Spiral of Healing acts as the cauldron for the magic of the generalist's craft in which you cocreate a relationship oriented toward making a right and good healing action for each particular patient in their particular circumstances.[8]

Windmill Sails of Generalism

Just as some birds, such as geese, use simple rules for flocking behavior, specialists and generalists use their own unique sets of simple rules when

TABLE 2.2	**Simple Rules of Specialists**
Identify	Identify and classify disease for management through filter of defined expertise.
Interpret	Interpret through specialized knowledge tuned to idiosyncrasies of unique person and case.
Manage	Manage using specialty expertise to generate and carry out treatment/management plan.

doing their work.[9] Specialists, in a fairly linear fashion, identify, interpret, and manage (see Table 2.2). When a specialist first sees a patient, they carefully scan for evidence that the patient has a problem that fits within their defined specialty; they identify and classify through the filter of their special expertise. If such a diagnosis is not present, the patient is referred elsewhere. If an appropriate diagnosis is identified, then the specialist interprets the patient's diagnosis, unique characteristics, and situation through their particular knowledge base and proceeds to manage the care using their focused expertise. These simple rules are part of the hidden curriculum of medical school and become part of the tacit knowledge of specialists.

Generalists have a distinctly different set of simple rules, namely: recognize, prioritize, and personalize (see Figure 2.3). These are performed not

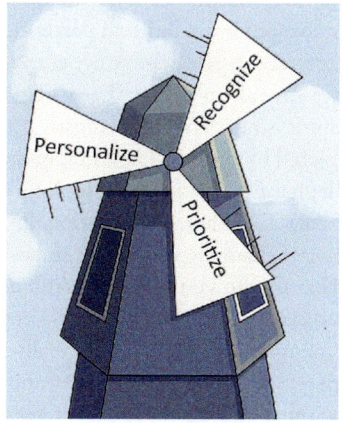

FIGURE 2.3. Windmill Sails of Generalism.

linearly but concurrently, like the sails or blades of a windmill, always moving to generate an engaging plan for better health. This occurs in a continuous exchange of give-and-take between sufferer and healer, as they negotiate a shared path among their worlds. All problems are welcome.

Whereas specialists screen and identify as if sifting through a sieve for gold, generalists search the beach at low tide, recognizing and gathering the broken shells of evidence. We search for cues and hunches, for insights into who the patient is and what they are experiencing, exploring all the aspects of what is going on—the emotional, physical, cognitive, social, spiritual, and habitat related. While working to recognize, we are prioritizing among what we find. Why is the patient here today? What is most worrisome among what I'm recognizing? At the same time, we, as generalist healers, personalize and tailor the information as we make sense. We hold science, art, and humanities together in our healing hands and gaze upon them at once. Whereas specialists foreground disease, we foreground the whole person in context with emphasis on health and malady and on interdependences over time. The Clinical Hand of the generalist's craft presented in this *Field Guide* explicitly operationalizes these Windmill Sails, these simple rules of generalism.

The Elephant and the Rider of Changing Behavior

For the Spiral of Healing to help your patient return to the River of Health, they need to change a health behavior, develop a new behavior, and/or change a belief. As healers, we seek to facilitate that change. Never easy! Quite helpful in this challenge is the analogy of the Elephant and the Rider, drawn from the research of Jonathan Haidt.[10,11] Figure 2.4 illustrates a path toward change.[11,12] The Elephant represents the ancient, fast thinking, usually subconscious, emotionally charged brain built on perception and heuristics. The Rider signifies our more recent, slow thinking, cortical, rational brain that analyzes mostly what we have already done. The Rider, although rather small, thinks it is in charge, but it is not. The Rider mostly rationalizes the actions/decisions already completed by the very large Elephant.

Notice that the Elephant in the figure is looking out at you. Make eye contact with your patient's Elephant, the emotionally charged part of their brain. The first step toward changing resistant human behavior entails motivating the Elephant. That is who you connect with and who you communicate with. Learning to connect with the Elephant compels you to appreciate any history of developmental trauma. To be culturally sensitive, we learn the patient's story and experiences, their expectations and the actual reason for connecting (ARC). You must address those expectations. This work not only enhances safety and gains trust but also helps you uncover their hidden fears

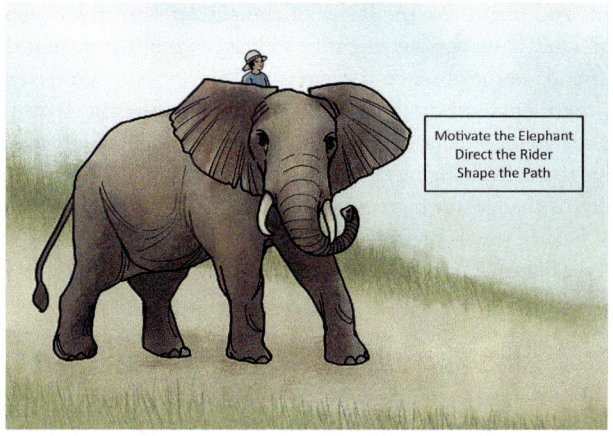

FIGURE 2.4. The Elephant and the Rider of Changing Behavior.

and desires. A key to behavior change is helping your patient convert their fear into a motivating desire they value.

For example, when a patient seemingly trapped in the addiction of smoking presents with an aggravating upper respiratory infection, disruptive coughing, and concerns about lung cancer, do not dwell on the lung cancer. Most smokers know that cigarettes cause cancer and would like to stop. Remember that activating desire is better than fear. People smoke because it fulfills some desire; it helps them handle problems, feel better, and resolve boredom, and it even serves as a surrogate buddy.[13] Do not frighten them out of smoking; find a better way to address the desires.

The stories we hear and those we tell ourselves speak directly to the Elephant[14] and influence what we perceive. Perceptual control theory informs us that our brains don't preplan behavior in a predictive, rational manner; rather, we behave in order to manage what we perceive. In other words, behavior is the control of perception.[15,16] Change the stories, and perception shifts, and behavior changes. Much of our work as generalist healers in primary care is motivating the Elephant, helping patients reveal, revisit, and revise their stories.

Step 2 for changing human behavior directs the Rider, gives them the reins, and helps them support the Elephant. This is where all that medical content and rational analysis you learned in professional training come into play. Notice how the Rider in Figure 2.4 is looking out and away from you, lost in past memories and old stories or worries about the future. For this second step, you speak directly to the Rider, so they can provide the Elephant with a sense of satisfaction with the decisions the patient and you have already motivated. You might ask the Rider of the patient with the cough to help figure out what some options might be to help with boredom and the desire for new friends in the absence of cigarettes. This not only reinforces and encourages the Elephant but also begins to shift what the Elephant perceives, boosting self-management capabilities and providing new information and knowledge to begin changing the patient's story.

Finally, to change our human behavior, we shape the path toward the direction of health, which keeps the Rider and the Elephant aligned. You assist the Rider in Figure 2.4 in shaping the desires now motivating the Elephant into goals with plans. You provide the Rider with explanations and knowledge that support the Elephant's awakened aspiration to shift its attention from the grass and begin moving toward the River of Health. The patient with the upper respiratory infection leaves the encounter with new goals and an immediate plan to join a hiking club in the next week. The field of marketing has known all about the Elephant and the Rider for decades.[14]

Reflective Pause

When teaching the generalist's craft to family medicine residents, this is usually the moment when I pause to address two questions reflected in the eyes of the residents. Do we really need to learn the metaphors? When do we finally get to the actual generalist's craft? Yes, and you are already learning the craft. I follow with a story based on a poem by the Taoist Chuang Tzu and translated by Thomas Merton.[17] Khing, a master woodcarver, was ordered by a prince to craft a bell stand "of precious wood" that "astounded" all who saw it. When asked for the secret of his work, Khing replied, "I have no secret," and proceeded to describe how he found the tree and crafted the bell stand. He prepared himself using the disciplines reviewed in Module 1 and centered himself with guiding metaphors, went to the forest, and began. The master carver concluded, "What happened? My own collected thought encountered the hidden potential in the wood; from this live encounter came the work which you ascribe to the spirits."[17]

The thriving skills in Module 1 and the four guiding metaphors are part of the generalist's craft. They prepare you for using the Clinical Hand and associated tools in the next section more wisely, prudently, and effectively with your patients to make healing. Print them out; add them as photos on your handheld device or cellphone. Frequently glance at them. They help you re-center your healing intentions and frame the implementation of your craft tools.

Now that you've been introduced to the four guiding metaphors, begin processing them by focusing on the one that speaks most to you. Apply this same approach as you become acquainted with the Clinical Hand and its supporting tools of the generalist's craft in the next section of this module. Then practice, keep practicing, prioritize, persist, and let the joy and wonder of the generalist's craft emerge.

The Clinical Hand and Supporting Tools of the Generalist's Craft

The generalist's craft inhabits the Clinical Hand and associated tools to be used in every clinical encounter. Each of these tools contains multiple alerts, guides, tactics, and minitools designed to trigger our engagement with the Rider and the Elephant and the other metaphors so central to the effective practice of the generalist's craft. Table 2.3 provides a brief look at each of the tools. The *Clinical Hand* represents the primary tool of the generalist's craft and provides an overall ritual structure for the clinical encounter. The *Ecological Clinical Map*, a supporting tool, helps us know where we are when using the *Clinical Hand* and what contexts may be important. The next two supporting tools provide more detail on how to navigate between the second and third fingers of the *Clinical Hand*. The *Relationship-Centered Clinical Method* offers guidance on getting the clinical work done once you know the agenda for the visit. The *Round Table of Evidence* displays the information and knowledge you will need for clinical decision-making.

TABLE 2.3 — The Clinical Hand and Supporting Tools of the Generalist's Craft

Core Tool	Brief Description
Clinical Hand	Guide Tool 　Ritual guideposts 　Multipurpose pocketknife
Ecological Clinical Map	Mapping Tool 　Where are we? 　What contexts are important?
Relationship-Centered Clinical Method	Process Tool 　How to do the clinical work
Round Table of Evidence	Information Tool 　What information and evidence are needed?

Clinical Hand Tool

Open your left hand and examine it. Transcribe the details of the Clinical Hand tool from Figure 2.5 onto its surface. You are now gazing at the guide tool for the primary care craft; you have embodied it and will take it with you to every clinical encounter. You will touch patients with it. The Clinical Hand provides a framework for comprehensively approaching and managing the clinical encounter. This comprehensive approach is a vital part of the generalist skillset and is responsible for much of the benefits that primary medical care generates for person and population health.

The most prominent features of the Clinical Hand—your five fingers—reveal the ritual structure of the clinical encounter and give it direction. These are the *Five Fingers of Direction*, revealing the guideposts or way stations to be reached as the patient and you proceed through the clinical encounter. The journey begins with both of you seeking to *Connect* at the index finger and moves on to the middle finger, where you *Set Agenda*. The craft work of clinical discovery and sensemaking occurs after the agenda is set and ends

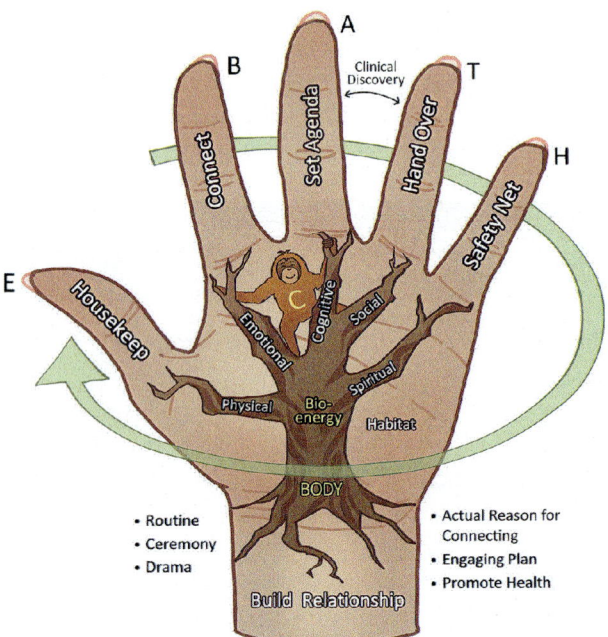

FIGURE 2.5. Clinical Hand Tool. (Adapted from Miller WL. The clinical hand: a curricular map for relationship-centered care. *Fem Med*. 2004;36(5):330-335.)

when you move to the next finger and *Hand Over* what you've discovered and have to offer. Next you reach the little finger, the *Safety Net*, where you make sure nothing important is neglected or missed. As the encounter ends, you cross over the palm to the thumb to *Housekeep* and check-in about how you and your colleagues are doing. Now you are ready to begin the next clinical encounter.

The *Wrist Lines of Guidance* direct your attention to the important what and why of your work. The radial side wrist lines highlight the three kinds of clinical encounters—routines, ceremonies, and dramas—and the ulnar side of the wrist reminds you of the three goals of every visit—to address the ARC, to cocreate an engaging plan for identified concerns, and to promote health. The wrist itself prompts you to always look for ways to build the relationship between yourself and the patient (see Table 2.4 for a highlight summary of the Clinical Hand tool).

In the palm of your hand, the *Palm of Hope*, dwells the *Naming and Caring Tree* within its habitat. This tree and its limbs and roots hold all the possible names or diagnoses of malady and the many possible treatments or means of care for those afflictions. The tree represents a person's body and its bioenergies.[18,19] The tree in its habitat represents the whole person. Its five

TABLE 2.4 Clinical Hand Highlights

Highlight	Description
Fingers of Direction	Ritual structure of clinical encounter: the five guideposts

Wrist Lines of Guidance	• Radial side
	  ○ Three kinds of clinical encounters
	• Ulnar side
	  ○ Three goals for each clinical encounter
	• Reminder to build relationship

Palm of Hope	Naming and caring tree Habitat
Swinging Cultural Ape	Culture and evolutionary heritage "Keep swinging"
Trouble Tool	Don't bite your nails—BATHE

limbs embody different manifestations of our biocultural being—the emotional, physical, cognitive, social, and spiritual—each one a potential source of trouble, and each offering a means back to health. Imagining the body this way helps you, the primary care healer, overcome the fallacy of mind–body dualism, creates a space for multiple healing traditions and approaches, and assures an expansive differential diagnosis and many pathways to healing. There is always something you can do to help. The *Cultural Ape* hangs out in this tree, usually swinging from limb to limb and occasionally exploring the habitat. The ape prompts us to recognize the importance of culture and of our evolutionary heritage, reminds us to acknowledge how they both influence health and malady, and nudges us to "keep swinging."

The Clinical Hand offers us a guide for getting out of trouble when, in a clinical encounter, we feel stuck, upset, spinning, or just hanging on to the cliff edge by our nails. Fittingly, then, you will find the initials BATHE etched onto its fingernails.[20] As you may recall from Module 1, BATHE stands for Background, Affect, Troubles, Handle, and Empathy, words that refer to questions or actions that help to relieve tensions that may arise during the clinical encounter and to create an opening for moving forward as in the following example:

Luisa, a 52-year-old divorced woman with two high-school-age daughters and limited financial resources despite full-time work as a housekeeper, has been a patient in my practice for 6 years and is being monitored for chronic hypertension. She presents for a follow-up visit and also has a mild headache. The visit is going okay, except she seems quieter and more easily distracted than usual. I comment on that observation, and Luisa begins crying. I offer her tissues, turn away from the computer screen, and pause for half a minute before I inquire, "What's happening in your life right now?" (**B**ackground question)

> "I found out that Maribel, my youngest daughter, is using drugs with some of her friends. Drugs! I can't believe it!"
>
> I take a breath and ask, "How do you feel about that?"
> (**A**ffect question)
>
> "I'm angry and ashamed. And I'm so worried. I don't know what to do."
>
> "What troubles you the most about this?" I respond.
> (**T**roubles question)
>
> She sinks in her chair and shakes her head, then looks up toward me. "Maribel had finally found some friends after years of bullying and feeling like she didn't belong. How do I tell her she can't be with these friends anymore?"

I nod my head and query, "How are you handling this?" (**H**andle question)

"Not very well. I'm avoiding my daughters. I think Maribel knows. It's affecting my work."

I lean in a bit closer to Luisa and comment, "That sounds like quite a disturbing and messy situation. Thank you for sharing. That must have been hard." (**E**mpathic response)

Luisa, finally looking more relaxed, adds, "Feels good to finally tell someone. Any suggestions?"

With this new information and both of us now more comfortable and hopeful, the encounter proceeds through the Spiral of Healing.

See Stuart and Lieberman[20] for even more examples and ways to use BATHE in the clinical encounter.

Ecological Clinical Map Tool

The Clinical Hand resides in the world depicted by the Ecological Clinical Map that provides a view of the geography of importance for generalist primary medical care clinicians (see Figure 2.6 and Table 2.5). Here we see how each part of the ecology of our craft nests within the context of the whole, an essential generalist skill. It shows us the circles of our clinical lives—where we and our patients live and do our craft work of mending and healing, where we grow our gardens of health.

At the center of the map breathes the clinical encounter, the meeting of person and healer, the heart of the generalist's healing craft. The encounter generally takes place in a clinic. The word *clinic* derives from the Greek words *klinikos*, or "of the bed," and *klinike*, or "practice at sickbed." The word *patient* derives from the Latin word, *patiens*: "one who suffers, who is reclined." Combining these translations brings us a definition of patients as individuals who have been flattened by life, brought to bed, who have come to our practice to be restored to uprightness and meaningful life. The clinic, for the primary care healer in the 21st century, is much more than a building, office, or home. It is a safe space, whether physical or virtual, that we create in which a patient and their family and friends can connect over time with a healer and their ensemble or team to cocreate a path back toward health. Clinics nest within their community and bioregion with health care services with which they seek to ensure horizontal and vertical integration.

Both healer and patient arrive at the encounter in the midst of separate journeys through a myriad of life choices and fortunes. The set of circumstances that brings them together has the potential to profoundly influence

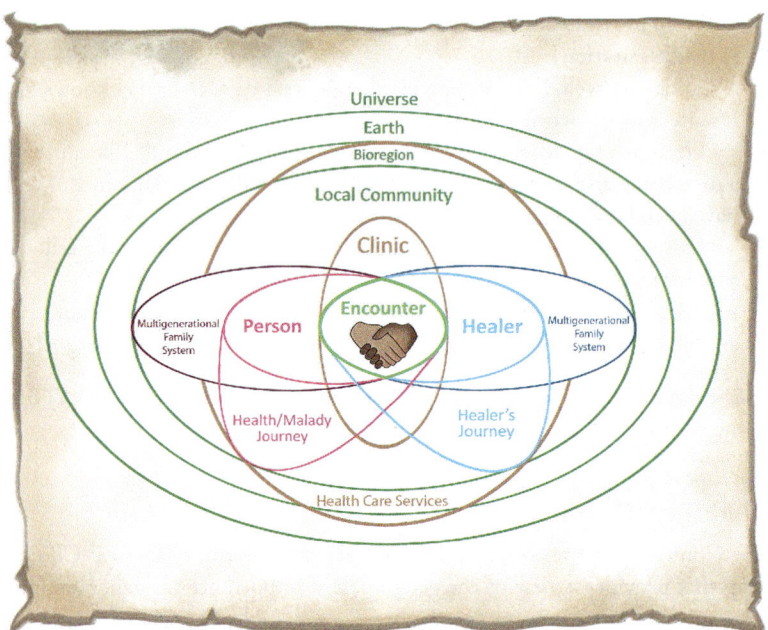

FIGURE 2.6. Ecological Clinical Map Tool. (Adapted from Crabtree BF, Miller WL. *Doing Qualitative Research*. 3rd ed. Sage Publications, Inc; 2023.)

TABLE 2.5	Ecological Clinical Map Highlights
Highlight	**Description**
Encounter	Clinician and person/patient
	Center of attention
Clinic	Safe space where encounter happens
	Ensemble/team with clinician
Person	Becomes a patient when afflicted with malady
	Culture and friendships
	Life plans and developmental perspective
	Multigenerational family system

TABLE 2.5	*Continued*
Health/Malady Journey	Pathway and experience of affliction and efforts to heal
Healer	A generalist with supporting ensemble/team
	Culture and friendships
	Life plans and developmental perspective
	Multigenerational family system
Healer's Journey	Pathway to becoming healer and ongoing learning
	Professional socialization
Local Community	Local people, places, and things
Bioregion	Larger region and habitat (often watershed)
Health Care Services	Primary, secondary, and tertiary services
Earth/Universe	Our planetary home
Grip of Power	Power flows through all of map
	Remember to share the power

what happens between them during the encounter. Patients come as part of their journey through the land of affliction. They could be early or later along that journey, which, as you recall, began when they realized they had left the River of Health and began struggling in a maze and muck of malady. For healers, each encounter represents another step on a vocational trek that began in medical or nursing school or even earlier. The Ecological Clinical Map reminds us, the healers, to pay attention to where both the patient and we are on our respective journeys.

Like all travelers, we journey with baggage. For good and bad, both healer and patient carry with them into every encounter a multigenerational family system, culture, network of friends, set of life plans, and position on the developmental life cycle like a hidden suitcase full of the influences that inform what is said and how it is heard. The Ecological Clinical Map reminds us to pay attention to these variations because the challenges we face in coming together with our patients to make health may intensify as the cultural, class, and other contextual distances separating us on the map grow wider.

The welcoming handshake at the center of the Ecological Clinical Map signifies a coming together while prompting us to recognize the flow and importance of power in our lives and places. Patients arrive at the encounter having experienced a loss of personal power and agency, of the ability to fully enact their lives; healers possess the powers of knowledge, skills, and prestige. This imbalance of power meets in the clinical encounter with the hope for transfer and sharing. Pay attention to that dynamic.

Use the Ecological Clinical Map to survey what's in your suitcase, the contexts that may matter, and what to notice or look for among the bags your patient brings with them to the encounter. And remember: the map suggests where to look, but it doesn't predict what you'll see.

Relationship-Centered Clinical Method Tool

The Relationship-Centered Clinical Method is a process tool; it depicts the clinical method utilized after the clinical encounter's agenda is set. It is applied in the process of clinical discovery and sensemaking, the diagnostic and treatment planning phase of the clinical encounter that appears between the second and third fingers of the Clinical Hand. We use this tool to discover the sweet spot between the patient's agenda and the clinician's knowledge.

The Relationship-Centered Clinical Method represented in Figure 2.7, which is directly adapted from the patient-centered clinical method developed at Western University in London, Canada,[21] is the generalist primary care substitute for the traditional history and physical examination, diagnostic reasoning, and treatment planning taught in medical school.

The Relationship-Centered Clinical Method highlights the importance of exploring not only the disease story in search of a diagnosis but also the other malady stories: those of illness and sickness.

Let me explain.

Malady is the more global word for bodily affliction. Any given malady may be associated with a particular *disease*, a pathophysiologic condition defined by scientific medicine. It may also be associated with the patient's experience of *illness*, whereas *sickness* refers to societal expectations, understandings, and responses. The *health story* also needs to rise to the surface since our goal is to return to our home in that story. These stories and their relationships are depicted on the left side of the figure.

The primary care healer weaves back and forth between the patient's stories and developing a deeper understanding of the whole person, including their pertinent *proximal and distal contexts*. This exploration is represented by the wavy line.

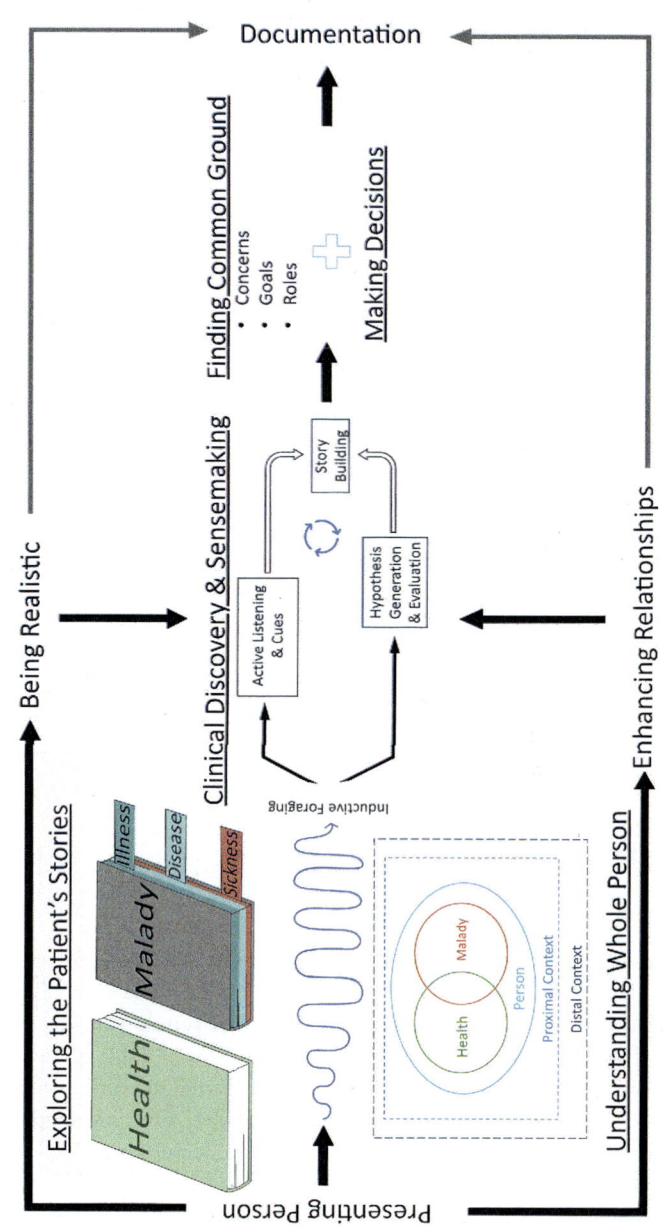

FIGURE 2.7. Relationship-Centered Clinical Method Tool.

As the exploration and understanding of the patient's stories proceed, you, the clinician, slide into more active clinical discovery and sensemaking, beginning with open-ended *inductive foraging* using questions, observations, and active listening. Thus begins the cycle depicted at the center of the figure. Expanding on what's being learned, you search for possible leads and then pursue them based on emergent *cues*. This is the Windmill Sail recognition work drawn from the simple rules of generalism. Some of those cues become *hypotheses*, which you evaluate with new questions and physical examination. All the while, you *build an explanatory story*, with the help of your patient, to frame what's going on and how to address it.

Once sensemaking is completed, you are ready to move on to the right side of the figure, where you hand the story over to the patient. Here is where you *find common ground* within the current context and *make shared decisions* on the identified *concerns*, *goals* of care, and *roles* for each of the participants; take time for the Windmill Sails of prioritization and personalization; and follow the simple rules of generalism. At the end of the process, the Relationship-Centered Clinical Method even reminds you to *document* the care and complete any associated forms.

Table 2.6 provides a highlight summary of the Relationship-Centered Clinical Method.

Throughout the use of the Relationship-Centered Clinical Method, you are to *be realistic* and *enhance the relationship* with your patient. Being realistic is especially important in the primary medical care setting, given its associated high demand and limited time. Here, it helps to remember the Clinical Hand tool and its guidance to set the agenda early, prioritize, recognize the encounter type, and develop your clinic ensemble, all of which support being realistic. Cultural sensitivity and practicing the principles of trauma-informed care help enhance the relationship.

Round Table of Evidence Tool

The Round Table of Evidence tool supplements the Relationship-Centered Clinical Method (see Figure 2.8). It is designed to help you recognize and assess what information and knowledge you need as you do your diagnostic work of clinical discovery and sensemaking. The Round Table of Evidence depicts who is involved in gathering the evidence during the clinical encounter, what evidence is needed, and how to assess the relevant information on the way toward common ground and collaborative decision-making. In this way, the work at the Round Table of Evidence is collaborative, with the goal to reach shared understanding.

At the table, we find the *patient* and the primary care *healer*. We are also likely to notice a *computer* with its many internet search capabilities and,

TABLE 2.6 Relationship-Centered Clinical Method Highlights

Highlight	Description
Exploring the Patient's Stories	Health stories Malady stories—illness, disease, and sickness Explore FIFE (feelings, ideas, effect on function, expectations)

Understanding Whole Person	Weaving patient's stories with whole-person understanding
	Proximal context:
	  Family and friends, livelihood, leisure, etc.
	Distal context:
	  Community, media, economy, habitat, etc.

Clinical Discovery and Sensemaking	Inductive foraging Active listening and cues Hypothesis generation and evaluation Story building
Finding Common Ground and Making Decisions	Concerns, goals, and roles in context Shared decision-making
Being Realistic	Set agenda and prioritize Know what kind of encounter Develop effective clinic ensemble
Enhancing Relationships	Trauma-informed care Culturally sensitive and responsive
Documentation	Medical records Pertinent forms, etc.

when needed, any number of *others* who may include additional family and friends of the patient, a specialist via a virtual link, or colleagues from the clinic ensemble.

There are usually multiple forms of information and evidence on the table that stem from the four ways of knowing identified at its center. The *"I" perspective* offers insights to the question, "What are the words?" and

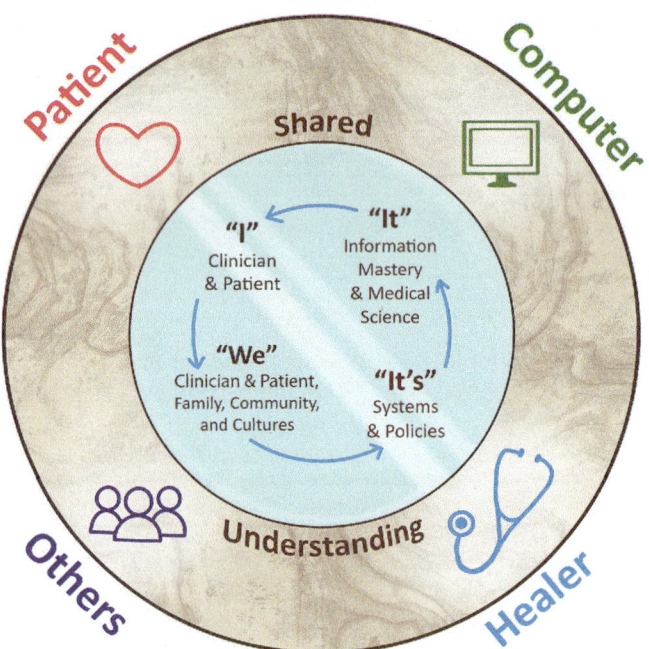

FIGURE 2.8. Round Table of Evidence Tool.

derives from qualitative and self-reflective methods for understanding. The *"It" perspective* answers the question, "What are the numbers?" This is the territory of biomedicine, epidemiology, and most clinical research using quantitative methods. This evidence is assessed using information mastery. The question, "Who benefits?" is addressed by the *"It's" perspective* and uses mixed methods and multiple voices to generate knowledge about systems, organizations, and policy. Finally, the *"We" perspective* answers the question, "What else?" This section requires qualitative, mixed methods, and many voices as it witnesses the knowledge of family and community and clinical team experiences. The generalist's craft integrates these many ways of knowing in service of health. It all matters!

Some of this information can be assessed using the minitools of information mastery, which include differentiating and evaluating POEM (**P**atient-**O**riented **E**vidence that **M**atters) from DOE (**D**isease-**O**riented **E**vidence) and using a STEPS (**S**afety, **T**olerance, **E**fficacy, **P**rice, **S**implicity) approach when considering pharmaceutical options for treatment.[22,23]

Table 2.7 provides a highlight summary of the Round Table of Evidence tool.

TABLE 2.7 Round Table of Evidence Highlights

Highlight	Description
Who Is at the Table?	Patient, healer, computer, others
What Is on the Table?	Four different ways of knowing: The Generalist Wheel of Inquiry/Knowledge
Information Mastery	POEM—Patient-Oriented Evidence that Matters
	DOE—Disease-Oriented Evidence
	STEPS—Safety, Tolerance, Efficacy, Price, Simplicity
Shared Understanding	Feedback, disclosure, exploration

How the Tools Fit Together

The Clinical Hand of the primary care craft neatly fits all the tools together for use in all clinical encounters. It provides overall guidance throughout the encounter and is located and informed by the Ecological Clinical Map, which maps the situation and context for care. The Relationship-Centered Clinical Method gets used between the second- and third-finger guideposts and is supported by the Round Table of Evidence, which stipulates the necessary information and evidence (see Figure 2.9). Combined, they enact the principles of the generalist's craft in primary care by assuring whole-person scope, relational process, integrative practical wisdom, a healing orientation, and a sense of safety.[24]

We're almost ready to do the generalist's craft! But first, another reminder that this is a living craft, always changing and adjusting to each unique time, place, and relationship. Only the ritual structure of the five fingers of direction is set. The rest of the tools are all cues and guides. The generalist's craft in primary care resembles improvisational jazz in its performance. Jazz, like the generalist's craft, is a mongrel, an urban music with deep rural roots, springing from the meeting of Africa and Europe in the Mississippi River Valley, the stockyards of Chicago and Kansas City, and the skyscrapers of Manhattan Island. Global in its reach, local in its performance, jazz is a music of exile, voicing our nomadic urges as well as our longings for home, rooted in the blues of yearning, anger, and dashed hopes.[25] The generalist's craft in primary

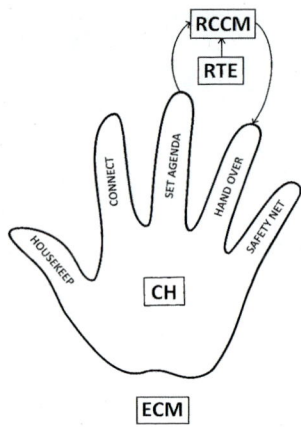

FIGURE 2.9. Using All the Tools in a Clinical Encounter. CH, Clinical Hand; ECM, Ecological Clinical Map; RCCM, Relationship-Centered Clinical Method; RTE, Round Table of Evidence.

care listens for those same voices as it invites patients to leave their exile in the land of affliction and return home to the River of Health. The generalist's craft, like jazz, combines technical mastery with focused personal improvisation,[26] and every encounter becomes a "jam."[27] Table 2.8 notes crucial features of jazz improvisation that pertain to doing the generalist's craft in primary care.[28,29]

TABLE 2.8 Features of Clinical Jazz Improvisation

Feature	Description
Turn-Taking	Alternating between soloing and supporting roles; engaging in call and response
	Requires diversity of tunes and skills, including the following:
	Soloing: Offering both melody and improvisation
	Passing off: Transitioning to other soloists
	Supporting: Carrying rhythmic and harmonic background; creating space for other soloists to develop their ideas
	Cueing: Indicating the occurrence of or need for changes in rhythm, speed, pitch, volume; hesitation or turbulence; silence; gesture

TABLE 2.8	Continued
Building	Adding your voice to what others are doing
Empathic Listening	Paying mindful regard to what others are trying to do while also monitoring yourself and what you want to play
Continual Negotiation	Valuing the distribution of tasks in the interest of working toward synchronization
Facilitative Leadership	Offering guidance that: Is unobtrusive, open Initiates and ends Distributes power and decision-making Facilitates sensemaking Raises questions
Hanging Out	Creating a community of practice Creating folklore, stories, and tricks of the trade Building collective memory
Here and Now	Carrying out the work in a way that is local, performative, in the moment, and immediately responsive to the setting and audience
In the Groove	Performing beyond capacity because of latent capacities the ensemble draws out through its support and joint efforts

Learning these features is key to becoming an expert in the generalist's craft of primary medical care. Remember them as you explore Modules 3 and 4. Let's start jamming!

REFERENCES

1. Miller WL, Yanoshik MK, Crabtree BF, et al. Patients, family physicians, and pain: visions from interview narratives. *Fam Med.* 1994;26(3):179-184.
2. Lakoff G, Johnson M. *Metaphors We Live By.* New ed. University of Chicago Press; 2003.
3. Ortony A, ed. *Metaphor and Thought.* 2nd ed. Cambridge University Press; 1993.
4. Stacey RD. *Complexity and Creativity in Organizations.* Berrett-Koehler Publishers; 1996.

5. Taylor C. *The Ethics of Authenticity*. Harvard University Press; 1991.
6. Topolski S. Understanding health from a complex systems perspective. *J Eval Clin Pract*. 2009;15(4):749-754.
7. Coulehan JL. Chiropractic and the clinical art. *Soc Sci Med*. 1985;21(4):383-390.
8. Pellegrino ED. Toward a reconstruction of medical morality. *Am J Bioeth*. 2006;6(2):65-71.
9. Etz R, Miller WL, Stange KC. Simple rules that guide generalist and specialist care. *Fam Med*. 2021;53(8):697-700.
10. Haidt J. *The Happiness Hypothesis*. Basic Books; 2006.
11. Haidt J. *The Righteous Mind: Why Good People Are Divided by Politics and Religion*. Pantheon Books; 2012.
12. Heath C, Heath D. *Switch: How to Change Things When Change Is Hard*. Broadway Books; 2010.
13. Willms D. A new stage, a new life: individual success in quitting smoking. *Soc Sci Med*. 1991;33(12):1365-1371.
14. Akerlof GA, Shiller RJ. *Animal Spirits: How Human Psychology Drives the Economy, and Why It Matters for Global Capitalism*. Princeton University Press; 2009.
15. Mansell W. The perceptual control model of psychopathology. *Curr Opin Psychol*. 2021;41:15-20.
16. Powers WT. *Behavior: The Control of Perception*. 2nd Expanded ed. Benchmark; 2005.
17. Merton T. *The Way of Chuang Tzu*. New Directions; 1969.
18. Valenti D, Atlante A. Mitochondrial bioenergetics in different pathophysiological conditions 2.0. *Int J Mol Sci*. 2022;23(10):5552.
19. Belal M, Vijayakumar V, Prasad KN, et al. Perception of subtle energy "prana," and its effects during biofield practices: a qualitative meta-synthesis. *Glob Adv Integr Med Health*. 2023;12:27536130231200477.
20. Stuart MR, Lieberman JA III. *The Fifteen Minute Hour: Efficient and Effective Patient-Centered Consultation Skills*. 6th ed. CRC Press; 2019.
21. Stewart M, Brown JB, Weston WW, et al. *Patient-Centered Medicine: Transforming the Clinical Method*. 4th ed. CRC Press; 2024.
22. Slawson DC, Shaughnessy AF. Becoming an information master: using POEMs to change practice with confidence. Patient-oriented evidence that matters. *J Fam Pract*. 2000;49(1):63-67.
23. Shaughnessy AF. STEPS drug updates. *Am Fam Physician*. 2003;68(12):2342-2348.
24. Lynch JM. *A Whole Person Approach to Wellbeing: Building Sense of Safety*. Routledge; 2020.
25. Eisenberg E. *The Ecology of Eden*. Alfred A. Knopf; 1998.

26. Shaughnessy AF, Slawson DC, Becker L. Clinical jazz: harmonizing clinical experience and evidence-based medicine. *J Fam Pract*. 1998;47(6):425-428.
27. Begel A. The family conference: a jazz jam. *Fam Syst Health*. 1998;16(4):437-441.
28. McDaniel RR Jr. Management strategies for complex adaptive systems sensemaking, learning, and improvisation. *Perform Improv Q*. 2007;20(2):21-41.
29. Berliner P. *Thinking in Jazz*. University of Chicago Press; 1994.

PART II

Embodying the Craft

MODULE 3

Heart of the Craft—Journey of the Clinical Encounter

Introduction

Welcome to Module 3, where you will explore how to enact the essentials of the generalist's craft of healing in primary care. This is the heart of the craft and the crux of this *Field Guide*. You will discover how the Clinical Hand and its supporting tools (Ecological Clinical Map, Relationship-Centered Clinical Method, and Round Table of Evidence) combine and integrate to ensure optimal performance of the generalist's craft in all clinical encounters.

The journey of the clinical encounter begins with your open hand. This is the foundational Clinical Hand, always with you. Recall the illustration of the Clinical Hand tool from Module 2, shown here in Figure 3.1 for reference.

View the volar surface, its palm, fingers, and wrist. Visualize the wrist lines of guidance with their goals for each visit and the different kinds of encounters. Picture the palm of hope and the five-limbed tree of naming and caring. Imagine seeing the Fingers of Direction inscribed there. Then recall the graphic shown in Figure 3.2 and notice how the other supporting tools of the generalist's craft (Ecological Clinical Map, Relationship-Centered Clinical Method, and Round Table of Evidence) fit together with the Clinical Hand, mapping the adventure of the clinical encounter.

Within the Clinical Hand tool, trace the movement as you journey through the five guideposts, represented by your five fingers, marking the way.

Module 3 is organized around these five guideposts or checkpoints, which create the ritual structure for the clinical encounter. I describe, in detail, how to journey, finger-by-finger, from the beginning to the end of any visit whether in person or virtual.

The recommendations, tips, guidance, and approaches packed into Module 3 are summarized in tables and figures to help you on the way to the essential goal of reaching each of the five guideposts. The ritual structure—Connect, Set Agenda, Hand Over, Safety Net, and Housekeep—does not change, but which of the many strategies you use at any given moment

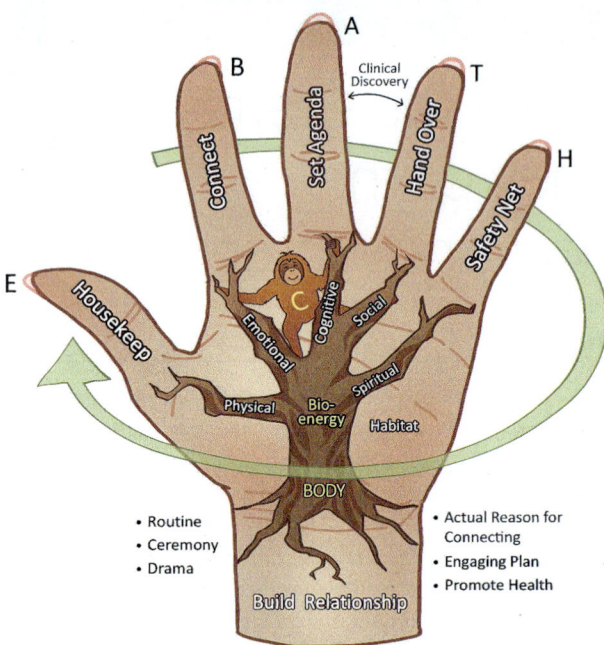

FIGURE 3.1. Clinical Hand Tool.

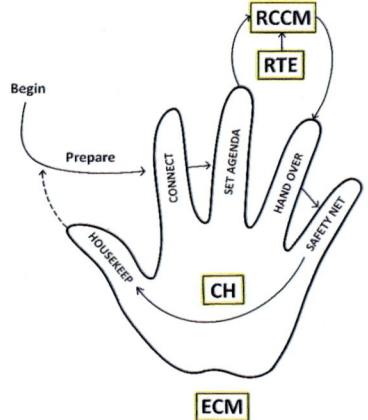

FIGURE 3.2. Journey of the Clinical Encounter. CH, Clinical Hand; ECM, Ecological Clinical Map; RCCM, Relationship-Centered Clinical Method, RTE, Round Table of Evidence.

depends on the particulars of the specific clinical encounter. The strategies are a starting point for improvisation. Welcome to clinical jazz.

This material can feel a bit overwhelming. That is expected. No one can learn the whole craft in just a few sessions or readings. Mastering a craft is developmental. Be patient. Take it slowly. Find the strategies that fit you, your setting, and patients. I'll remind you of this several times and offer reflective and summative pauses along the way. Do the same for yourself.

To help, this module is divided into seven units that follow the ritual structure of the Fingers of Direction. Unit 1 focuses on getting to the Connect guidepost. Unit 2 journeys on to the Set Agenda guidepost. Units 3 through 6 cover the work of Clinical Discovery, Sensemaking, and Finding Common Ground, then on to the Hand Over checkpoint. Unit 7 walks you through the Safety Net and Housekeep guideposts.

May doing the generalist's craft remind you of the joy and gift of being with patients. Before we start, a quick review about the ritual structure of the clinical encounter, the Fingers of Direction.

The Fingers of Direction—The Ritual Structure of the Five Guideposts

"Give me five!" Your fingers that is, beginning with the index finger and ending with the thumb. Before you initiate your next clinical encounter, learn the Fingers of Direction. They are your guideposts for every encounter in the office, at home, or on the phone, video screen, or email. They constitute the ritual structure of the clinical encounter and are the ONLY required part of the generalist's craft. In the discipline of ritual, you must get to each guidepost or checkpoint before moving on to the next (see Figure 3.3). This discipline ensures your travel through the Spiral of Healing detailed in Module 2 (see Figure 2.2). The directional movement transfers from patient-directed at Connect and Set Agenda to clinician-directed on the way to Hand Over followed by shared decision-making as you approach Safety Net. The movement returns to clinician-focused at Housekeep. Learn and memorize this required ritual structure, these five guideposts, for every clinical encounter. Consider writing the guidepost words on your fingers with a washable marker for a few days to help you imprint the ritual flow.

Since every patient and every situation is unique, you will need to improvise on the strategies in this *Field Guide*. You and your clinical ensemble will practice a beautiful clinical jazz, part of the wonder and exhilaration of human life and the generalist's craft. The ritual structure of the five-finger guideposts provides the theater for optimizing the healing music. Let's begin!

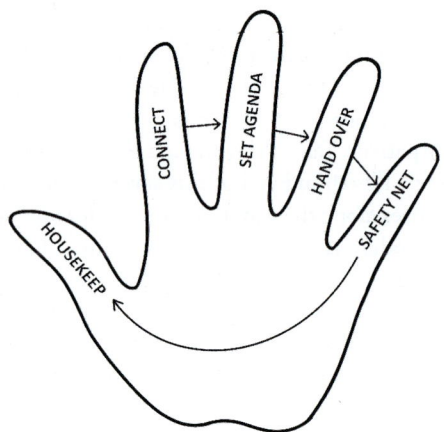

FIGURE 3.3. The Fingers of Direction—The Five Required Guideposts of Ritual Structure.

Part II • Embodying the Craft

Unit One: Journey to Connect

Orientation

The adventure of the clinical encounter commences with the journey to the first guidepost: Connect (see Figure 3.4). The journey to connect begins before you meet the patient and starts with a map.

Achieving Situational Awareness Using the Ecological Clinical Map

Every clinical encounter starts with the question, "Where are we?" The "we" encompasses all the people, institutions, places, and others present on the Ecological Clinical Map detailed in Module 2. Answering this question begins with a self-check-in—by asking the question, "Where am I?" The next questions ask you to also locate your patient and those who accompany them, then your immediate supporting clinical staff or ensemble (see Figure 3.5).

The Ecological Clinical Map is both a map and a story tool. It presents where you are in relation to what else potentially matters for the current clinical situation. Each of the identified sections of the map also serves as a source for stories that inform and promote the healing process. Stories arise from the patient's health and malady journey, the healer's journey, their families, and the local community. The map is a snapshot reminder of the healing landscape and of the many relationships and interdependences that potentially matter.

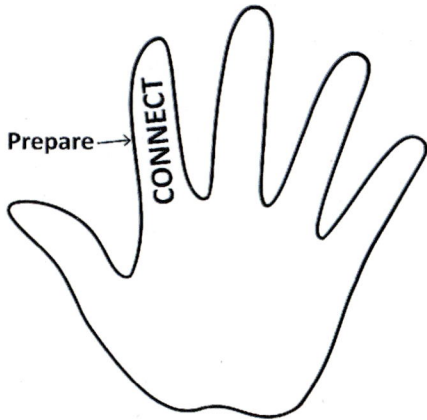

FIGURE 3.4. The Connect Finger.

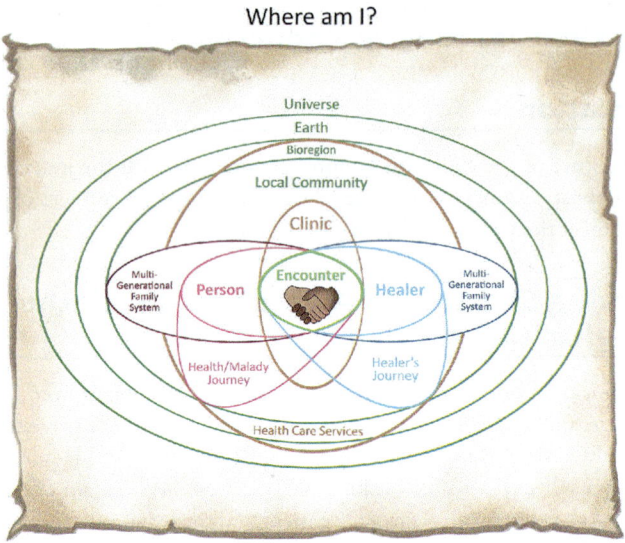

FIGURE 3.5. Achieving Situational Awareness Using the Ecological Clinical Map.

Prepare and Open the Hand

Now that we know where we are, it is time to prepare for the clinical encounter. In most practices today, that usually means opening the electronic health record (EHR) and reviewing the patient's chart before entering the encounter (see Table 3.1). This prompts making a personalizing reference to prior contacts, especially the most recent one. Use the chart review to begin forming a "story" of this person in your imagination. Reviewing the prior three or four visits along with the patient's past medical history can be helpful in creating the story framework. Note of caution! This initial storybuilding is intended to activate your narrative creativity and construct a personalized memory of critical moments in the person's past. Recognize that this story could be wildly incorrect and full of bias. Be ready to build a new one with the patient after you meet.

Next, mentally note what modality is being used for the upcoming encounter. Is it in person at the clinic? At the patient's home? In a skilled nursing facility? Is it virtual, and if so, with video, phone, or email? Your approach and how you engage your clinical ensemble changes with the modality.

TABLE 3.1	Preparation for the Encounter

Ecological Clinical Map Awareness

Review Chart
- Who is this person?
- Note most recent contact(s)/visit(s).
- Take an overview of past medical history.
- Look for personalizing reference(s).

Summarize "Story"
- Create an initial "story" framework.
- What happened in the last visit? 3-4 visits ago?

Center on Modality (e.g., office, virtual, email)

Ensemble Check (mental or in huddle)
- Initial contact
- Arrival
- "Room" entry
- Memories of past encounters
- Did ensemble use patient's name? Greet warmly?

Now you are ready to prepare yourself and your ensemble or clinic team for the meeting. If your clinic has team huddles before the day or half-day begins, there are additional questions and reminders to consider. Who made initial contact with the patient when they requested an appointment? How was that interaction? Who will greet the patient when they arrive, and who will facilitate entry into the "room," whether in space or virtually? How were those interactions? Remind each other to use the patient's name and greet them warmly. What memories of past encounters with this patient do members of the ensemble have? Sometimes, such exchanges are not possible. No worries. In those situations, do what you can in advance, prioritizing a personalizing reference and entering the encounter in the way that encourages the patient to fill in what is missing from your preparation.

Preparation is now almost complete. You have reviewed the chart, summarized what you already know, and spoken with ensemble members. But do not open the portal to the encounter yet. In order to turn the knob on the door or touch the keyboard, you must open your hand (see Figure 3.6). This is your invitation to set healing intention. Ask yourself, "Am I ready to 'attend,'

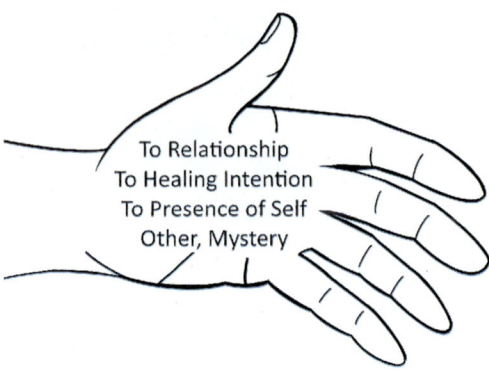

FIGURE 3.6. Opening the Hand of Intention.

to be there; am I situationally aware and willing to go wherever the encounter leads? How do I feel, right now? Am I, and my hand, open so that I am ready to listen, learn, and discover?"

If you can answer these questions in the affirmative and are open to compassion, relationship, and presence to self, other, and mystery, then recall and set healing intention in your mind. Our purpose is to seek health as membership through healing relationships enacting agency and belonging. Note what is not in that intention, specifically wRVUs (work relative value units), performance metrics, dollars. They matter but are secondary concerns. Attend to the prize—health—and help it grow!

Attending and the Grip of Power

As your hand opens the portal to the patient, the ritual begins, and you initiate connection. We are on our way to the Connect guidepost. The introduction to the patient starts with our greeting, whether typed, spoken virtually, or in person. An in-person greeting may be accompanied by eye contact, a smile, and a culturally appropriate physical exchange of respect such as a handshake, nod, or bow. Given rising concerns about hygiene, the handshake has become less common in health care settings and elsewhere. But the smile remains germ-free.[1]

The power imbalance that is often present at the start of a clinical encounter charges the space with the moral imperative for the healer to wield that power wisely and to minimize harm. The Grip of Power (see Figure 3.7)

Remember the importance of power!

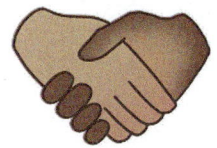

Power-over to Power-with

FIGURE 3.7. The Grip of Power.

reminds us of the importance and role of power in this and all relationships. As you greet the patient, mentally share a metaphorical handshake. Most clinical encounters begin with your hand being stronger and more assured than the hand of the patient: a situation of power-over. Relatively equal pressure between the grips in the handshake at the end of the visit is an indicator of a successful clinical encounter. You have transferred power-over to power-with.

Your professional and moral duty is to locate where the power is and is not, own your part of it, aim your power toward the patient and community's best interest, and share the power available (see Table 3.2).[2] Locating the power includes you, the patient, their family, the community, the clinic, and the health neighborhood.

The Ecological Clinical Map tool discussed in Module 2 (see also Figure 3.5) will help you locate power in the clinical encounter. Recognize power in its many dimensions and in its sociocultural context[3] and approach with humility.[4] Be wary; the potential for abuse of power is omnipresent.

Getting to the Connect Guidepost

Finally, it is time to embark on the Path to Connect (see Table 3.3).

The Path to Connect begins by welcoming the patient. Use names and give personal attention. Determine the patient's preferred language and gender pronouns. Find out if anyone has accompanied them. Welcome them with confidence. Next, help the patient get as comfortable as possible, paying special attention to light, warmth, position, and hydration. Do not forget to make yourself comfortable as well. Ensure the space is safe. If you find the patient

TABLE 3.2	Managing Power in the Encounter

Locate
   Where is the power?
   Where is power lacking?
Own
   Recognize your power.
   Take responsibility for your power.
Aim
   Direct your power toward the patient's interest.
   Direct your power toward the community's interest.
   Do not target the financial bottom line.
Share
   Move and redistribute the power.
   Convert power-over to power-with.

sitting on the exam table, suggest they sit down in a chair for the first part of the visit. I have found that limiting the use of the exam table for the more vulnerable moments where the patient needs to remove clothing and/or experience physical contact for examination helps maintain safety during the encounter and predictability for the patient. Agree to how cell phones are managed. Many patients are uncomfortable turning them off but are amenable to entering silent mode and agreeing to not take calls. Begin in a listening mode.

Commence developing rapport during the first few moments of the encounter with some connecting "small talk." Ask about the patient's experience getting to the office and into the room or what they recently had to eat—or, yes, about the weather. Even better is to ask about something personal you know about them that isn't uncomfortable. Consider using EHR aids such as Post-it Notes® to remind yourself if the patient told you something they were looking forward to such as an upcoming trip or becoming grandparents. If the encounter is a video visit, use this time to adjust the screen and confirm the equipment is all working well. If you are not the regular personal clinician for this patient, name and share a few respectful comments about their personal clinician and note that you will communicate with that clinician concerning what happens during the encounter. Sit near the patient where you can maintain easy eye contact and comport yourself as if you had all the time in the world.

TABLE 3.3	The Path to Connect

Welcome
　Use names.
　Give personal attention.
　Check on preferred language and pronouns.
　Welcome with confidence and warmth.

Comfort
　Check on patient's comfort.
　Help patient get as comfortable as possible.
　Negotiate cell phone management, suggesting off or silent mode.

Develop Rapport
　Connect using "small talk" (traffic, weather, video connection, etc.).
　Mention something personal.

Relational Connection
　Sit down or otherwise place yourself at eye level with the patient as if you have all the time in the world.
　If Return Visit: Connect to prior visits. ("What's happened since last time?")
　If Not Regular Clinician: Name and comment on regular clinician and assure the patient that information about the encounter will be relayed to them.

Orient to Computer

Connect
　"Ready to start..."
　"Let's begin..."

The final step in getting to the Connect guidepost is to orient the patient to the computer you will use to keep track of the information referenced and gathered during the encounter. Table 3.4 unveils a mnemonic, POISED, specifically designed for this purpose.[5] Start with P or Prepare. Peruse the EHR for information concerning the person you are about to see. Orient them (the O in POISED) to the EHR and how it will be used during the visit. Address any questions or concerns they have about the EHR.

TABLE 3.4 POISED Mnemonic for Using the Electronic Health Record

P Prepare
   Review the electronic health record before seeing the patient.

O Orient
   Explain how the computer will be used during the encounter.

I Information Gather
   Enter data to demonstrate that the patient's concerns are being taken seriously.

S Share
   Show the computer screen so patient can see information.

E Educate
   Display graphs of information such as weight or blood pressure, etc.

D Debrief
   Make sure the patient understands what is being said.

Data from Frankel RM. Computers in the examination room. *JAMA Intern Med*. 2016;176(1):128-129.

This mnemonic is consistent with the Clinical Hand tool. Information Gather, Share, and Educate happen on the way to both Set Agenda and Hand Over, and Debrief occurs as you are reaching the Hand Over guidepost.

Of course, you may be wondering if this all sounds a bit too tidy, and you would be correct. There are several scenarios that complicate the journey to connect, many of which can be predicted but some that may surprise you. Blood pressure measurement is one of the predictable circumstances. The first measurement, usually performed by your ensemble or team partner when they bring the patient into the exam room and prepare them for your clinical encounter, is often higher than usual, partly related to the "white coat" effect. When this is true, you will want at least two more measurements before deciding if any clinical action is needed. When is the right time to repeat the blood pressure measurements? One possible moment is when you reach the Connect guidepost. The patient is now comfortable, and you have not started exploring the present situation in depth and any anxiety that may provoke. Another time is prior to moving to the exam table, where you reach the Set Agenda guidepost. A third opportunity is prior to moving back to the chair after you've finished your exam. A fourth option is at the end of the visit, at which point a member of your ensemble or team could check the blood pressure. Choose based on the emergent circumstances of the encounter.

Another predictable scenario occurs when there has been some communication and preplanning prior to the clinical visit. There may have been a phone conversation or a web portal exchange that has provided enough information to already know there's something you want, such as a urine sample for analysis or a tick to examine. These can be collected by your ensemble colleague and examined by you before reaching the Connect guidepost. I recommend popping into the exam room to greet the patient, excusing yourself to do the sample exam, and then returning to complete the connecting. That quick pop-in appearance reassures the patient and enhances the sense of safety.

Then, we have the surprises. The patient who comes in feeling fine, but at check-in your colleague discovers a rapid irregularly irregular pulse and an unusually high blood pressure. Or the patient seeing you for what your office staff anticipated was a mild asthma exacerbation but, again at check-in, your ensemble partner discovers a disturbing pulse oximetry result. Do a quick check-in connection, clinical eye scan, order an electrocardiogram or nebulizer treatment, then return after they are done and complete the connecting. Always be ready to improvise.

You reach the Connect guidepost when you and your patient agree that you belong together for this clinical encounter and you are both ready to work. If, like me, you are challenged by remembering patients' names, consider using a "name game" to help you both personalize the encounter and remember the patient's name. Identify something unique and memorable about the patient such as a mole on their cheek, the kinds of socks or shoes they wear, or an idiosyncratic gesture, and associate that something with their name. This association paves the way to quicker name recall in future visits. That done, you have ritually closed this finger.

REFERENCES

1. Fine L, Rajput V. The smile is stronger than the handshake. *MedEdPublish*. 2020;9:68.
2. Brody H. *The Healer's Power*. Yale University Press; 1992.
3. Candib LM, Gelberg L. How will family physicians care for the patient in the context of family and community? *Fam Med*. 2001;33(4):298-310.
4. Candib LM. *Medicine and the Family: A Feminist Perspective*. Basic Books; 1995.
5. Frankel RM. Computers in the examination room. *JAMA Intern Med*. 2016;176(1):128-129.

Unit Two: The Journey to Set Agenda

Orientation

Surprise! I suspect you think the next step is to ask the patient why they are here today, the opening gambit for the history of present illness you learned during professional training. Not yet. Once you head down that trailhead, it is often difficult to pull back and elicit the rest of the agenda or frame the context for the encounter—to discern the patient's actual reason for connecting and the type of encounter by working through the second finger of the Clinical Hand, Set Agenda (see Figure 3.8). Once the patient and you have listed, prioritized, negotiated, and set the agenda, then you can embark on the pathways of clinical discovery and evaluation.

Doing the work of negotiating and setting the agenda ensures that both the patient and you address what matters most and helps to avoid the infamous "By the way. . ." comment just as you are about to end and leave the encounter.[1] Let's start with the wrist lines of guidance from the Clinical Hand (recalled in Figure 3.9) as understanding them in each particular encounter is a critical part of getting to the Set Agenda guidepost.

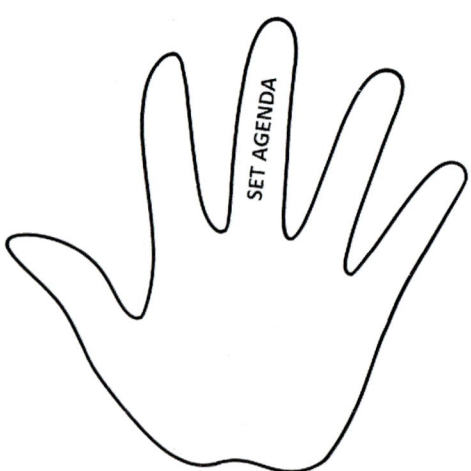

FIGURE 3.8. The Set Agenda Finger.

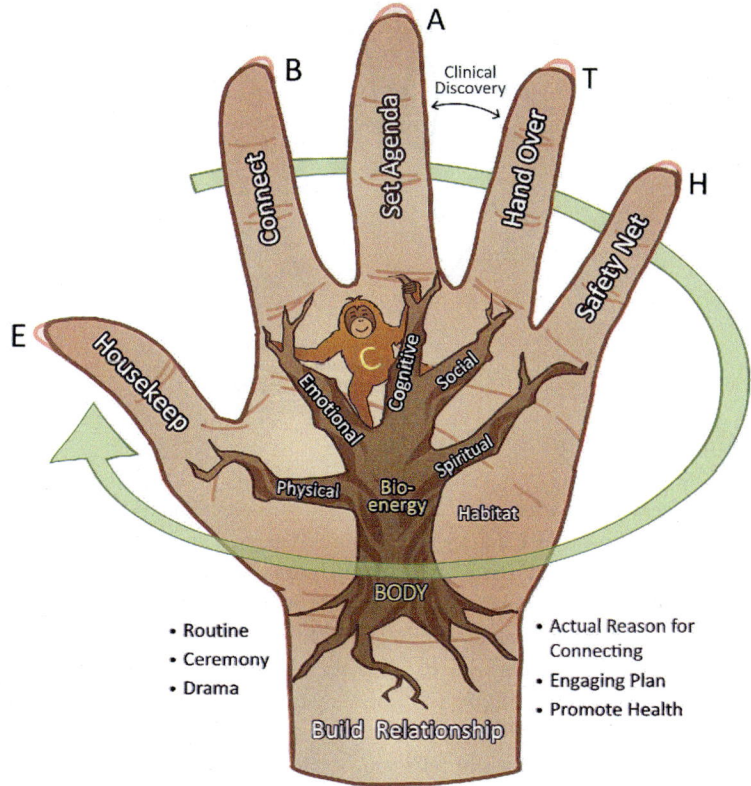

FIGURE 3.9. Clinical Hand Tool.

The Wrist Lines of Guidance: Three Goals and Encounter Types

Guiding Wrist—Goals of Encounter

On the ulnar side of the wrist within the Clinical Hand tool you will find the Guiding Wrist, the three goals for each encounter: address the actual reason for connecting; codevelop an engaging plan for the patient's concerns; and promote one health-related issue (see Figure 3.10). Remembering these goals will help us stay on time while meeting the functions of primary medical care.

Why do patients decide to visit with the generalist healer—what are their actual reason(s) for connecting? Knowing why the patient connects is vital to relationship-building, assures the patient that you are listening, and helps

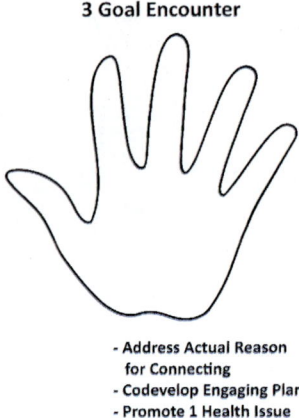

3 Goal Encounter

- Address Actual Reason for Connecting
- Codevelop Engaging Plan
- Promote 1 Health Issue

FIGURE 3.10. Guiding Wrist.

you connect your explanation(s) for the patient's concerns to their expectations on the Spiral of Healing. Addressing the actual reason for connecting is at the heart of goal-oriented care, relationship-centeredness, and shared decision-making. We must seek the actual reason for connecting because it rarely will be revealed directly by the patient.

Fortunately, the list of reasons is small.[2-5] All eight actual reasons for connecting are identified in Table 3.5. Knowing this list is fundamental and may be the most important diagnostic list to commit to memory.

For example, your patient tells you, "I think I sprained my ankle." What really motivated them to see you at this particular time for their ankle injury?

The first three reasons are directly related to the injury. It could be some underlying perceived threat such that they cannot stand the *worry* anymore. The patient checked the Ottawa Ankle Rules on the Internet, and they appear to be at risk of a fracture. If so, you need to address that worry and explicitly check for fracture. Or they cannot stand the *pain* anymore; it keeps them awake at night and has become intolerable. You need to address the pain and inability to sleep. Or the ankle discomfort is interfering with their dancing with friends at night; it has become a *problem of living*. For this to be serious enough to come to the doctor usually means there are some underlying interpersonal challenges related to the social life interference; they cannot do what they believe they must do. You need to address these functional concerns. Ask, "What else is going on in your life?"

Other possible reasons for connecting may be less directly connected to the injury; they may be externally or institutionally grounded or focused on general health concerns. For example, a patient may connect because someone

TABLE 3.5 — Actual Reason for Connecting

Intolerance of WORRY	Some Underlying Perceived Threat
Intolerance of PAIN	Nature and quality of symptoms become intolerable.
Problem of LIVING	Some interpersonal crisis; interference with social life
Social SANCTIONING	Someone else made me come in.
Sick Role LEGITIMATION	Someone doesn't believe I'm sick.
HEALTH Maintenance	Health check; need to get healthier
ADMINISTRATIVE Requirements	Need form or other health record completed
ACCESS Made Possible	Can finally afford to connect

else made them come in. This could be someone at their workplace, a parent, or a spouse. The patient brought up their ankle problem one too many times, and they were *socially sanctioned* to visit your clinic. Or they are connecting for *sick role legitimation*. Someone, often at school or their place of employment, does not believe their ankle is seriously injured, and the patient wishes—perhaps because the relevant institution requires—you to confirm the injury is present. In this case, you need to address some complication related to the sick role.

It is also possible that the patient's actual reason for connecting is to *improve their general health*. They wanted a wellness exam because they just celebrated their 75th birthday and hoped to start a new exercise program. Due to scheduling limitations at your practice, however, they could only get an appointment for an acute issue, so they chose their sore arthritic ankle as that gateway. You need to seize this moment for action toward better health.

The patient may only be there for *administrative* reasons—for example, to get an insurance form completed—or for a reason that combines both administrative and health-related concerns. For example, the patient needs a form filled out related to some travel they have planned, and because that travel involves hiking, they are also wondering about ankle strengthening exercises. You need to complete the form and provide guidance as needed. The patient may also have connected with you because they finally obtained insurance coverage and can afford *access*. The ankle has been troubling them for months, but they could not come earlier. You need to begin a healing relationship.

Put the list in Table 3.5 in your smart phone! The extra time to figure out the often hidden *actual reason for connecting* almost always saves time in the long run.

The second goal for every visit is the most obvious one: to codevelop an engaging plan that addresses the prioritized concerns identified as you both set the agenda. This is greatly aided by having working diagnoses or hypotheses for the prioritized concerns.

A third goal for each visit is to promote or address one health issue ideally related to one of the other two goals unless the focus of the visit is health maintenance/promotion to begin with. This is one way of speaking to the Elephant to facilitate behavior change, especially for those behaviors that are particularly resistant to change. For example, if your patient's concern is a possible ankle sprain and they are seeing you today because the pain is intolerable, it represents an optimal time to talk about their obesity and how beginning a strategy for weight loss will help in the rehabilitation of their ankle and prevention of future such injuries. Upper respiratory infections present an opportunity to discuss smoking cessation or to promote vaccines related to respiratory infections. If your encounter presents a window of opportunity for catching up on several health issues, choose one for your attention and have your clinical team/ensemble do one or two others. Be wary of trying to do too much and risking patient overload and forgetfulness, a cognitive threshold issue, or rising resistance.

Guiding Pulses—Encounter Types

The radial side of the wrist, the Guiding Pulses, of the Clinical Hand depicts the types of encounters: routines, dramas, and ceremonies (see Figure 3.11).[6] Ceremonies come in two forms: maintenance ceremonies and transition

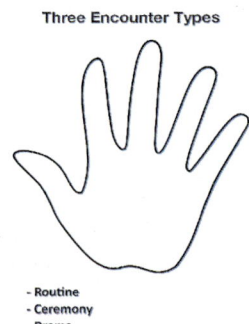

FIGURE 3.11. Guiding Pulses.

ceremonies. Knowing which type of encounter you are taking part in greatly facilitates staying on time and being realistic and your patient-centered management of the situation; it helps to keep your pulse on the situation.

In our generalist's craft of primary care healing, we do two fundamental tasks. We address life's afflictions, and we seek health. We address brokenness of some kind in the lives of our patients. We can mend it (i.e., fix, cure, repair) in many acute situations. We can redeem it (i.e., reframe, adapt, care) with most chronic conditions. We can use the brokenness for transformation (i.e., make a developmental leap toward better health) at moments when life seems to fall apart. We seek health for our patients and ourselves. We can nudge it along, promoting it in baby steps. We can accelerate or grow it in big jumps. We can protect it when it is at great risk. The encounter types represent these different task intentions, a part of aiming our power and redistributing it to patients. Table 3.6 presents an overview of the encounter types.

TABLE 3.6 Overview of Encounter Types

Encounter Type	Description	Intent
Routine	Simple, single issue, symptom lasting less than 2 wk Clinician and patient easily agree.	Mend brokenness. Promote/protect health.
Drama	Complex with uncertainty or new chronic diagnosis Potential turning point in patient's life	Transform brokenness. Grow health.
Ceremony	**Maintenance ceremony:** Stable chronic condition(s), health maintenance Clinician and patient easily agree. **Transition ceremony:** New unplanned drama	Redeem brokenness. Promote/protect health. Stabilize brokenness. Preserve health.

A *routine* is like cold, freshly squeezed orange juice or a simple, familiar melody. Routines refresh your day and keep generalist healers smiling because they are satisfying. We easily see how we help while staying on time. How do we know that a particular encounter is a routine (see Table 3.7)? A routine is simple: it involves a single issue where the symptoms have been occurring for less than 2 weeks and the actual reason for connecting is not sick role legitimation, sanctioning, or a problem of living, all of which complicate the dynamics of the encounter. Longer duration of the symptoms also adds complexity to the care evaluation and planning.

Direct communication is an early cue that the encounter is a routine. The talk and body language are "straight"; what you see and hear is what you get. Related to this is the notion of congruent or aligned triangulation, borrowed from navigators. This occurs when what you hear from the patient—what you see and touch in the patient's body language and during the physical exam—and what you feel in your gut—your inner awareness—are aligned.

TABLE 3.7 Features of Routines

ALL of the following are TRUE:
Presenting concern *is*:
- Simple, single, new
- Less than 2 wk old

Actual Reason for Connecting is not:
- Sick role legitimation
- Sanctioning
- Problem of living

Communication is direct.
Triangulation is congruent (i.e., what you see, hear, and feel are aligned).

Other Features
You and patient quickly agree on concern.
Narrative clues
- Acute or cyclic *vs* chronic
- Restitution instead of quest or chaos
- No overall change *vs* wanting to change life

Involves few plot complicators vs many plot complicators
Effectively addressed in 15-20 min or less

In short, you and the patient can easily agree on what the patient is experiencing. Table 3.7 summarizes the features of a routine.

From a narrative point of view, routines are nearly always about a single acute or cyclic episode, such as a sore throat, simple ankle sprain, an allergy or asthma exacerbation, or recurrent vaginal candidiasis. They are restitution narratives where the patient seeks a fix to the problem and not a quest or chaos narrative.[7] The patient wants no overall change to their life, just a return to the way things were. There are few plot complicators such as recent job loss, a marital affair, or alcohol dependence hindering a relatively easy solution.

It is helpful to recognize some nuances about routines. Delightfully, there are truly simple routines, like an uncomplicated "cold," an acute respiratory illness, or a small, clean laceration needing only glue or adhesive closure strips requiring no follow-up visit. There also are extended routines that will require one or two straightforward follow-up sessions, such as an ankle sprain or wound care for an uncomplicated dog bite. Finally, there are complicated routines: perhaps you are not the patient's regular clinician, or a patient currently involved in a drama (to be discussed later; see Table 3.8) such as newly diagnosed essential hypertension but now presenting with an upper respiratory infection. Otherwise routine encounters may also be complicated by a culture or language gap requiring interpretation by other people in the encounter session such as parents or caregivers. Though still routines, these minor complications are likely to increase the time needed for the encounter.

Routines are the bread and butter of relationship-building for clinicians and patients. When done well, both parties are satisfied and grateful. Power is shared, trust fertilized, boundaries respected. When patients come in for routines, they do not want other issues exposed or prodded. The mantra for clinicians is to keep a routine a routine. Save the stirring of the pot for dramas.

It is tempting for family physicians, or more often the administrators of their practices, to shift routines to other clinicians or to express care or urgent care centers to create more scheduled slots for chronic illness care. Overdone, that is a mistake and underestimates the value of routines as relationship builders. Routines are part of how first-contact access and continuity with a patient's personal generalist clinician add value to health care.

Dramas are entirely different. They sound like an opera filled with conflicts, emotion, confusion, excess, anguish, joy, and a wide range of music from stormy to lyrical. See Table 3.8 for a summary of identifying drama features.

The first clues to the encounter being a drama often appear as an internal sense of restlessness: you can sense trouble arising. Communication from the patient is often indirect; they have difficulty describing what is wrong.

TABLE 3.8	Features of Dramas

Any ONE of the following is TRUE:
The presenting concern is:
- Illness only or
- New chronic problem

The symptom(s):
- Has/have no observational or exam correspondences or
- Is/are a new diagnosis of chronic disease

Communication is indirect.
Triangulation is incongruent (i.e., what you see, hear, and feel do not align).
Actual Reason for Connecting is one of the following:
- Problem of living
- Sanctioning
- Sick role legitimation

Other Features
Complex, unresolved issues requiring multiple visits over time
The problem(s) exist in the patient's world and not only in the exam room or the computer screen.

Triangulation is incongruent—what you see, hear, and feel do not match. The patient says, "My head is splitting open with pressure!" while her affect remains flat and her hands relaxed by her side. Your intuitive sense feels puzzled. You wonder, "What is the patient trying to say? What is really going on here?" What is happening is drama. Your eye juggling tells you the problem(s) are not only here in the exam room but out there in the patient's life world as well. The symptoms frequently have no observational or physical exam correspondences. The actual reason for connecting is usually a problem of living, sanctioning, or sick role legitimation, and the narrative line suggests the patient is stuck in chaos. You cannot solve a drama in a single encounter. You need to join them, lean into the chaos, and shift the narrative toward a quest frame by using time across many visits and, often, a home visit.

Patients commonly bring new dramas to the clinical encounter as medically unexplained symptoms. Generalist clinicians initiate new dramas when they pronounce a new chronic condition diagnosis. Do not underestimate how dramatic the moment is when you tell a patient they now have a label, a problematic condition for the rest of their lives. Diabetes and hypertension, for example, can come to feel like medical routines to clinicians; we deal with them multiple times every day. They carry a frightening and devastating weight for patients. That new label changes how they understand their body, their identity, their future, their vulnerability, their insurability, and more. It is a drama; be there with them on this quest.

The specific clinical encounter wherein you share a new chronic condition diagnosis with a patient is a *transition ceremony*. The visits that follow constitute the drama. Transition ceremonies are new, unexpected dramas. They may involve a new, acute problem that is complicated and confusing. Thus, the encounter is no longer a routine or what was anticipated to be a maintenance ceremony. Instead, a new crisis or change in the chronic pattern is revealed. To the clinician, they feel like "a mess" or a "train wreck" and threaten to be "schedule busters" or "hidden time bombs." On your schedule, transition ceremonies look like either routines or maintenance ceremonies. You discover otherwise as you move with the patient from the guidepost of Connect to Set Agenda. Table 3.9 summarizes the identifying features of transition ceremonies.

Transition ceremonies are purposely designed to help you stabilize the patient, protect their health, prepare the patient for the extended upcoming drama with its longer time frame of care, and keep you on time. They are performed like a ceremony to ensure those goals are attained. Module 4 goes into detail on how to do routines, dramas, and transition and maintenance ceremonies.

There are two types of transition ceremonies (see Table 3.10).

TABLE 3.9 Features of Transition Ceremonies

Unexpected new drama
Sharing of new chronic condition diagnosis

Other Features:
- New, acute problem that is complicated and confusing and thus not a routine
- Anticipated maintenance ceremony that is actually a crisis or change in a chronic pattern
- A "mess!" A "train wreck."
- "Schedule busters" or "*Hidden time bombs*"

TABLE 3.10	Types of Transition Ceremonies
Type	**Description**
Heroic	Unplanned new drama or unclear final diagnosis
Labeling	New chronic disease label, e.g., Hypertension, Diabetes Mellitus, Lymphoma, Hypothyroid

Heroic transition ceremonies are unplanned, surprise new dramas. These situations often include unclear final diagnoses or working hypotheses by the end of the visit. That is okay since one of the goals of the ensuing drama will be to address that unfinished work. *Labeling transition ceremonies* are those in which patients learn they have a new chronic condition or disease. As noted earlier, labeling transition ceremonies are often neglected, even taking place over the phone or by email with increasing frequency. The latter is discouraged, but sharing bad news over the phone is possible[8] so long as it is done as a transition ceremony. Remember that power must be protected during transition ceremonies, and managing this successfully usually requires your presence.

Maintenance ceremonies are clinical encounters by exclusion, which means they aren't routines, dramas, or transition ceremonies. They do have inclusive criteria of high probability. This is by design so we, as busy clinicians, are less likely to miss a new drama. Table 3.11 summarizes the identifying features of maintenance ceremonies. Like routines, the communication is direct and the triangulation congruent (what you see, hear, and feel are aligned). More importantly, a maintenance ceremony is distinct from a transition ceremony in that it is not a new drama.

Maintenance ceremonies can lull you to sleep because, for any particular patient, the pattern and content of the clinical encounter appear repetitive, as if every visit is just like the one before it, and the one before that. They tend to involve either the ongoing management of stable chronic disease or uncomplicated health maintenance such as prenatal or well-child care. If not careful, both the patient and the clinician may be lulled by the pattern of the ceremony, slip into the well-worn script, and miss important changes and events between visits. Thus, do not think your clinical encounter is a maintenance ceremony until you have ruled out drama. For example, the patient's sister recently lost a foot to amputation because of diabetic complications, and the patient now wants to get more serious about tighter glucose control. That means a new drama. Do not miss the change.

> **TABLE 3.11** **Features of Maintenance Ceremonies**
>
> *ALL of the following are TRUE:*
> Communication is direct.
> Triangulation is congruent (i.e., what you see, hear, and feel are aligned).
> The encounter is NEITHER a:
> - Drama nor
> - Routine
>
> *ANY of the following are TRUE:*
> (Most, but not all, of these encounters will have the characteristics of maintenance ceremonies.)
> Stable chronic issues
> Uncomplicated health maintenance
>
> *Other Features*
> Typical characteristics:
> - Always the same ("Every visit is just like the one before it, and the one before that.")
> - Protocol driven (health maintenance or chronic condition guidelines)
> - Repetitive pattern
> - Shared symbols and beliefs
>
> Narrative clues:
> - Progressive, stable, or cyclic
> - No change

Many of the current EHRs risk tricking your brain into thinking *maintenance ceremony* because of how they template what you document. You enter the exam room for an anticipated well-child visit, so the EHR opens to a tidy template that creates your note with just a few clicks on the checklist. Beware! The well-child visit was scheduled 2 months ago. Since then, there were several bullying incidents at school that you uncover while discovering the actual reason for connecting. This is no longer a maintenance ceremony. EHR templates are helpful, but they can inadvertently close the mind to important new information. I rarely enter information into the EHR until after the agenda is set.

Maintenance ceremonies come in four types (see Table 3.12).

TABLE 3.12	Types of Maintenance Ceremonies
Type of Ceremony	**Description**
Growing	Slow improvement in function, quality of life, and patient empowerment "Friendly"
Decaying	Deterioration in disease status, function, quality of life "Scary"
Stuck	It all seems stuck. Clinician and patient exasperated "Hopeless"
Life Cycle	Related to life cycle changes • Well-child care and prenatal care • Well-adult care at life cycle transitions (i.e., marriage, menopause, older age)

Growing maintenance ceremonies are those with slow incremental progress in the care of chronic conditions. There is gradual improvement in functional status, quality of life, and patient empowerment. Think of these as "friendly" maintenance ceremonies. *Decaying maintenance ceremonies*, on the other hand, demonstrate gradual deterioration in functional status and quality of life. *Stuck maintenance ceremonies* are just that—they are characterized by neither improvement nor worsening of the patient's chronic conditions. *Life cycle maintenance ceremonies* are those related to health maintenance on the life cycle such as prenatal care, well-child care, and well-adult care. The intent for all maintenance ceremonies is change in the form of growth, but it is a very patient and subtle growth involving little nudges and the creation of openings and opportunities. The overall emphasis is *maintenance*.

Getting to the Set Agenda Guidepost

Now that you know the three goals for each visit and the type of encounter, you are ready to continue moving toward the Set Agenda guidepost. Going from the Connect checkpoint to Set Agenda generally takes about 5 minutes, or approximately 25% to 30% of the overall clinical encounter time. Take this time to elicit, negotiate, set, and summarize the full agenda. This prevents the "by the way" question at the end of the visit and expedites the visit overall. This kind of taking time *saves* time.[9,10]

Begin by identifying the patient's presenting concern, the one they used to schedule the appointment, and elicit any other concerns. This may include the list in their pocket or on their cell phone. If the patient is returning for a follow-up visit at your request, you also need to share your concerns and reasons for requesting their return. Do not forget to thank them for coming. With all the issues on the table, I often literally write them on the exam table paper. The patient and you begin negotiating and prioritizing what can be addressed given the time constraints of the scheduled clinical encounter. While doing the negotiations, you explore the actual reason for connecting and the patient's expectations for the encounter. A helpful question for identifying the actual reason for connecting and for prioritizing is, "What concerns you the most?" Additional useful questions are listed in Table 3.13, which overviews the content for negotiating and setting the agenda. Along the way, explicitly confirm the actual reason for connecting with the patient.

As the patient and you develop and negotiate the agenda, keep a trauma-informed approach in mind. When appropriate, frame questions as, "What happened to you?" as opposed to "What is wrong?" This whole process is a dance involving a search for new information about the actual reason for connecting, expectations and concerns, hypothesizing about the actual reason for connecting, and determining the type of encounter you've entered into. All this while negotiating, prioritizing, and preparing for the clinical discovery and evaluation part of the encounter. During this dance, I encourage you to review with your patient any information the EHR contains about their medications and prior visits: activities you may recognize as the Information Gathering, Share, and Educate steps of the POISED mnemonic discussed in Unit 1 of this module.

Soliciting patient requests can add more specificity to the actual reason for connecting and clarify some of the patient's expectations for the clinical encounter (see Table 3.14).[11] Is the patient present to seek medical information, experience therapeutic listening, obtain psychosocial assistance, get general health advice, receive biomedical treatment, and/or fulfill a bureaucratic need, such as obtain approval to participate in sports at the local high school? Knowing the patient's specific expectations for the visit beneficially informs the negotiating and prioritizing process while better ensuring the encounter will meet the patient's needs.

It should now be obvious why you need to take time negotiating and setting the agenda. If done well, you learn much that will inform later clinical

TABLE 3.13 Eliciting and Prioritizing the Agenda

Elicit Agenda	**Identify patient concerns.** • Presenting concern • Other concerns • Ask "What happened to you?" (not "What is wrong?") **Share clinician goals (esp. if return visit).** • Communicate clinician concerns. • Explain why you wanted the patient to come in for a return visit. **Identify patient's actual reason for connecting.** • "What worries you *the most about your* concern?" • "Why now?" • "What led you to get help now?" • "When did you decide to come in and get checked?" **Solicit patient requests (see Table 3.14).** • "How can I be most helpful to you?" • "What do you hope can happen at today's visit?" • "How can I help?" • "What kind of help were you hoping for today?"
Prioritize Agenda	Discern encounter type. Negotiate agenda. Keep a list of what didn't make the agenda.

discovery and evaluation. Helpful in that regard is to recognize and pay special attention to when patients signify "A LOT Moments" (see Figure 3.12) during which high-yield information is more readily available. These are moments when your patients are especially likely to reveal important information.

Notice these moments and use them to gently probe, to ask questions and discover the patient's inner chatter. They are teachable moments when the Elephant is more receptive and undecided.[12] Notice when the patient's breathing alters, the facial expression shifts, the body posture adjusts, or the

TABLE 3.14 Patient Requests

Medical Information	Wants to answer questions, "What ails me?" "What happened to me?" Needs label
Therapeutic Listening	Seeks magical comfort
Psychosocial Assistance	Desires a friend or hand holder
General Health Advice	Wonders, "What can I do?"
Biomedical Treatment	Seeking a prescription; something that will "fix it"
Bureaucratic Fulfillment	Needs to complete an administrative form

With permission from Like R, Zyzanski SJ. Patient requests in family practice: a focal point for clinical negotiations. *Fam Pract*. 1986;3(4):216-228.

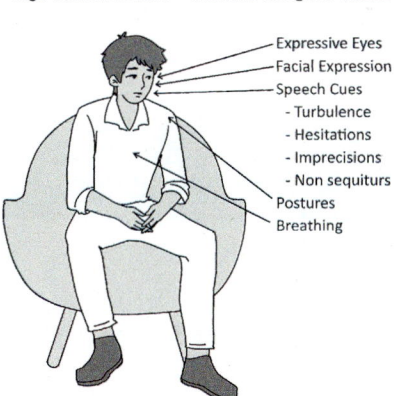

FIGURE 3.12. A LOT (High-Yield Information) Moments.

expressive eyes change direction. Attend when the patient's speech becomes more turbulent, which often means that sensitive or troubling material is seeking expression. Pay heed to speech hesitation or imprecisions such as, "You know what I mean?" No, we do not. So clarify for specificity. Also note non sequiturs like, "I've been constipated more lately. Macy, our dog, is more restless." These may signal worry, embarrassment, or sensitivity.

When you are finished prioritizing and negotiating the agenda for the day's clinical encounter, summarize the plan for the visit to open a negotiating process with the patient. There are often issues and concerns that did not make the agenda. Keep a list for later, and toward the end of the clinical encounter, decide if or when they can be addressed in the future.

The Set Agenda process is complete when the patient agrees with your summary, and you are clear about the actual reason for connecting and type of encounter (see Table 3.15). Of course, there is the rare occasion when the two of you cannot agree on an agenda, usually because the patient wants everything on the list covered. Focus on prioritizing the list and completing what you can within the scheduled time.

You have now accepted and validated the patient's experience. You have learned the expectations for the encounter, the first two parts of the Spiral of Healing. You are ready to shift the action to the examination table, into the clinically active space that will transport you to the third checkpoint in our ritual structure: Hand Over. Here, you will explore your patient's stories and engage in clinical discovery, evaluation, and sensemaking. Let's get moving!

TABLE 3.15 Indicators of Completing Set Agenda

Prior visits in EHR reviewed

Meds reviewed from EHR

Patient agrees with actual reason for connecting

Patient agrees with agenda summary
- Issues for today
- Issues for another day
- Type of encounter

EHR, electronic health record.

REFERENCES

1. Dugdale DC, Epstein R, Pantilat SZ. Time and the patient–physician relationship. *J Gen Intern Med*. 1999;14(suppl 1):S34-S40.
2. McWhinney IR. Beyond diagnosis: an approach to the integration of behavioral science and clinical medicine. *N Engl J Med*. 1972;287(8):384-387.
3. Zola IK. Pathways to the doctor—from person to patient. *Soc Sci Med*. 1973;7(9):677-689.
4. Like R, Zyzanski SJ. Patient satisfaction with the clinical encounter: social psychological determinants. *Soc Sci Med*. 1987;24(4):351-357.
5. Malterud K. Key questions—a strategy for modifying clinical communication. Transforming tacit skills into a clinical method. *Scand J Prim Health Care*. 1994;12(2):121-127.
6. Miller WL. Routine, ceremony, or drama: an exploratory field study of the primary care clinical encounter. *J Fam Pract*. 1992;34(3):289-296.
7. Frank AW. *The Wounded Storyteller: Body, Illness, and Ethics*. 2nd ed. The University of Chicago Press; 1997.
8. Mueller J, Beck K, Loretz N, et al. The disclosure of bad news over the phone vs. in person and its association with psychological distress: a systematic review and meta-analysis. *J Gen Intern Med*. 2023;38(16):3589-3603.
9. Stacey SK, Morcomb EF. Five steps to mastering agenda setting. *Fam Pract Manag*. 2021;28(2):27-31.
10. Mauksch LB, Dugdale DC, Dodson S, et al. Relationship, communication, and efficiency in the medical encounter: creating a clinical model from a literature review. *Arch Intern Med*. 2008;168(13):1387-1395.
11. Like R, Zyzanski SJ. Patient requests in family practice: a focal point for clinical negotiations. *Fam Pract*. 1986;3(4):216-228.
12. Flocke SA, Clark E, Antognoli E, et al. Teachable moments for health behavior change and intermediate patient outcomes. *Patient Educ Couns*. 2014;96(1):43-49.

Unit Three: The Journey to Hand Over: Exploring the Patient's Stories

Moving Toward the Hand Over Guidepost

Now we do the clinical work, the hands-on, intimate doctoring associated with the largest power differential in the visit and relationship. It is time to use the Relationship-Centered Clinical Method and Round Table of Evidence tools described in Module 2 (see Figure 3.13).

At this point, the encounter moves to the exam table, signifying a more sacred space. Ritually signaling and enacting space change enhances the patient's sense of safety. It is worth the extra effort. In a virtual clinical encounter, this is a moment to pause and have the patient make sure they are in a comfortable place and will not be disturbed. Check the doors; are all pets out of the room? Do they need to use the bathroom? When the upcoming clinical discovery and evaluation work is over, the patient will return to the chair if meeting in person. If virtual, they will take a deep breath, stand up and refresh, then resume their position in front of the computer screen. Next, you share what you have learned, and the two of you will reach common ground, make decisions, and formulate a plan together. This is the longest and most vulnerable part of the encounter, usually lasting 10 to 20 minutes. The human body recognizes the respectfulness, safety, and predictability of ritual structure and will often share more of itself in that space. Honor the ritual!

The Relationship-Centered Clinical Method is our main tool for helping us reach the Hand Over guidepost. This tool begins with weaving between the patient's stories, witnessing their experience, understanding the whole

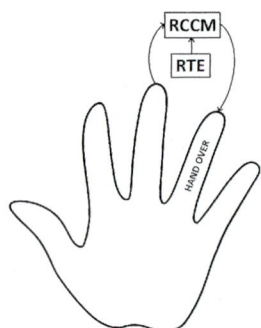

FIGURE 3.13. The Hand Over Finger. RCCM, Relationship-Centered Clinical Method; RTE, Round Table of Evidence.

person, and connecting their current concerns to their larger life story and context. (We actually began this process while approaching Set Agenda, the second guidepost.) This is where you utilize communication and listening skills, employ motivational interviewing techniques, and investigate within the patient's learning style and language. Cultural sensitivity and appropriateness are tantamount here.

Use of the Relationship-Centered Clinical Method moves you into clinical discovery, evaluation, and sensemaking as well as clinical problem-solving and framing—the diagnostic and management process. Using a "think aloud" strategy during this phase facilitates the patient's engagement and input as you expand shared understanding and sensemaking.[1] I find this especially helpful while doing the physical exam. Be careful to limit the thinking aloud to emotionally safe content.

Once you build feasible stories to make sense of the patient's concerns, it is time to find common ground, make shared decisions, and develop an engaging plan—the work of handing over. These are the moments of shared decision-making and setting goals. It is the time for sharing power. Here we convert the diagnosis-and-treatment strategy into patient goals and plans. Remember to match the treatment or care burden to the patient's capacity and resources. During all of this clinical activity, you are enhancing your relationship with the patient while being realistic. Throughout this process, you will be engaging with the EHR, so remember to be POISED (see Table 3.4)!

The description that follows for getting to the Hand Over guidepost will move through each part of the Relationship-Centered Clinical Method as if it is sequential. It is not! The overall work of this tool represents a living dynamic activity. The different parts of the process allow for the convenience of depicting the many recommendations, tips, and suggestions for each part. These parts are not as separate as they appear. In practice, you are weaving among them depending on what is revealed and how the clinical encounter unfolds. Improvise and adjust to what emerges. Be creative like health itself. Remember that the Five Fingers of Direction are the only required sequential actions; they are the ritual structure. All the other craft strategies are guides and suggestions to be used in service to your patient and their health. Note how the process of getting to the Hand Over guidepost flows from patient to doctor to collaborative, a rhythm like the ocean tides. Go with the emergent flow.

The journey to Hand Over is described over four units. Unit 3, the current one, covers exploring the patient's stories and understanding the whole person in context, the history-taking part of the Relationship-Centered Clinical Method. Unit 4 explains how to do clinical discovery and evaluation, including swinging on the Tree of Naming and Caring in the Palm of Hope.

Unit 5 explores using the Round Table of Evidence tool and the processes of sensemaking. Unit 6 completes our journey to the Hand Over guidepost and describes how to find common ground and make decisions. But before we grab our boards and surf the first part of the Relationship-Centered Clinical Method, let us briefly review a few observation and listening skills.

Observation and Listening Skills

The first part of the clinical action work requires engaging your best observational and active listening skills to enrich your ability to see and hear the bird in the bush, the stories in the patient's body. These skills are not explicitly part of the generalist's craft, but I have included two tables summarizing a few of the more important ones and exercises to practice them (see Tables 3.16 and 3.17).

TABLE 3.16 Enhancing Observation

Observational Skill	Exercises to Practice
Enhance Awareness	Do something different; keep shifting perspectives.
	Pay intermittent attention; keep senses moving.
	Beware of automatic vision, a special danger of continuity of care.
	Don't think a feeling; avoid naming until after the experience.
Build Explicit Awareness	Search for the rich and extraordinary in the ordinary.
	Overcome selective inattention.
Maintain Naivete	Always be a "tourist" and look for hidden gems.
Build Memory	Walk past the room and write down all you can see.
Introspection	Look at someone for 5 s and write down all your observations.
	Beware of stereotypes.
Develop a Wide-Angle Lens	Keep extending and moving the horizon of awareness.

TABLE 3.17 Enhancing Active Listening

Active Listening Skill	Description
Have Eye Contact	Occasionally shift away and return.
Don't Interrupt	Let the patient finish their thought.
Listen Without Judging	Do not jump to conclusions.
Stay Present	Do not start planning what to say next.
Nod Your Head	Make small comments such as "Yes," "Uh huh."
Don't Impose Your Opinion	Do not jump to conclusions.
Ask Questions to Clarify	Seek with specificity.
Paraphrase and Summarize	Use pause moments to confirm your understanding of what's being conveyed.

Data from Rogers CR, Farson RE. *Active Listening*. Industrial Relations Center of the University of Chicago; 1957; Gordon T. *P.E.T.: Parent Effectiveness Training*. New American Library; 1975.

A helpful proverb for both observation and listening comes from the world of birdwatchers and is attributed to John James Audubon (source unknown): "When the bird and the book disagree, always believe the bird."

Before leaving our discussion of observation and listening skills, let us recall the A LOT Moments described in Figure 3.12. In these high-yield information moments, expressive eyes and speech cues serve as signals that indicate the patient is internally accessing especially pertinent information. Figure 3.14 shares more details about what those expressive eyes might be signaling.[2]

The direction in which the eyes move often indicates a shift in how the brain is primarily processing information. When the eyes shift upward, suspect the patient is suddenly visualizing either constructed or remembered images. A shift to level suggests audio processing such as listening or constructing or remembering sounds. Looking down hints at processing feelings and an inner focus. Although more difficult to see, changes in the pupil can be valuable, assuming such changes are not pharmacologically induced. A dilating pupil indicates increased arousal and interest, whereas a constricting

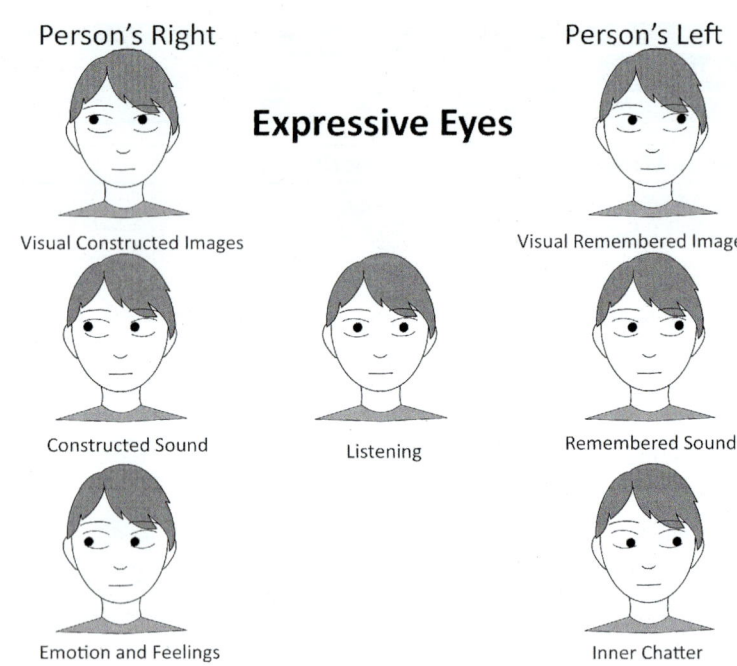

FIGURE 3.14. Expressive Eyes. (Adapted from O'Connor J. *NLP Workbook: A Practical Guide to Achieving the Results You Want.* Thorsons; 2001.)

pupil signifies something unpleasant or noxious. No wonder the common fear of the "evil eye" and the use of veils, dark glasses, hoodies, and shaded hats. On the other hand, a common misperception is that these eye movements can indicate deception. They do not.[3]

Speech also holds clues as to when patients are struggling with what and how much to share. When noticed, increase the sense of safety, then gently probe a little more. Table 3.18 shares some of those speech moments.

Think of these meta-models, a term from neuro-linguistic programming, as the activity of the linguistic unconscious.[2] When a patient is describing something, listen for what is missing, for the deletions and distortions. When a patient uses pronouns, do you know who/what they are referring to? Get specific. Patients also have linguistic cages that limit the possibilities. These come in the form of "I should" and "I can't" or statements of absolutes such as "I must. . . ." Expand those limits and refine the generalizations. Listen for when the patient is reading the minds of others and question it, or when they are avoiding their feelings or making a claim without a source. Question those

TABLE 3.18 Meta-Models as Speech Cues

Meta-Model	Description
Gathering Information	Know references
Specify deletions and distortions	Be specific What is missing?
Expanding Limits	No "should" or "can't"
Refine generalizations	Beware of absolutes
Changing Meanings	Mind reading Own feelings What is the source?

moments and change the meaning. Now, with our eyes and ears awake and tuned, we are ready to begin exploring the patient's stories.

Exploring the Patient's Stories

Much of what you need to know is embodied in the patient in front of you. You can learn to see, hear, and feel that knowledge. Our bodies are knowing bodies; trust them. The first part of the Relationship-Centered Clinical Method guides that work. Clinical discovery and evaluation begins with exploring the patient's stories of their health and maladies (see Figure 3.15).

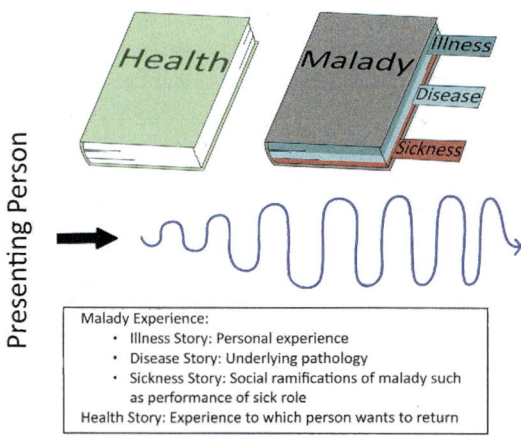

FIGURE 3.15. Weaving Among the Stories.

Use your observation and active listening skills to explore these health and malady stories and ascertain how to integrate person, context, health story, and the healing relationship.

Generally you will start with the malady story because that is why the patient is here with you and what is uppermost in their mind. But let us pause for a moment and ask ourselves, "Have I found my sacred silence? Am I mindfully attentive?" Our inner chatter sets the weather for our clinical work: stormy if cluttered and churning, mild if mindful. Our attitude sets the difficulty of the terrain: rocky and defensive or an open valley for learning. Settle your inner chatter of fears, worries, aggravations, and to-do lists, and clear the terrain of the boulders of staying in control and imposing your ideas. Let them flow by. Be still, be not afraid, allow ideas to emerge, stay with seeking. Remember the tools of the creative hero(ine) in Table 1.2. Answers are everywhere; have faith solutions will appear. The patient will help you. Be there with the patient, feeling free to improvise. Complete your deep breath.

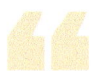

Now, Let Us Explore the Stories

The *malady experience* represents the story of body disorder, some type of body affliction or ailment with three dimensions or chapters in the book of malady: stories of illness, disease, and sickness.[4] The *illness story* is what the patient brings to the clinician. Illness refers to a person's subjective experience of their malady, the symptoms they perceive, how they feel. The *disease story* has at least two different understandings based on cultural context. Across cultures, disease refers to the dominant medical institutional theories and classifications of body disorders such as traditional Chinese medicine or Ayurveda in India. In Western countries, disease specifically refers to science-based biologically defined pathology and is standardized in the latest edition of the International Classification of Diseases (currently ICD-10 in the United States). The *sickness story* includes understandings of the sick role and what determines whether the body disorder is socially acceptable and/or suitable for medical treatment. Sickness represents the social and cultural conceptions and expectations related to the experienced malady. The sick role includes special rights and responsibilities that the social network and culture assign someone with a socially approved sickness.[5] In the United States, these have traditionally included the rights to be exempt from usual social roles and to be absolved of blame for any burden to yourself or others caused by your sickness. It also includes the responsibility to try to get well by seeking appropriate care. Always check for the many exceptions to this tradition depending on the sickness and cultural setting. For example, the absolution from blame does not always apply for substance use disorder in some settings where it is stigmatized.

You explore the disease story by using the seven parameters of the history of present illness learned in medical school, specifically location, quality, severity, timing, setting, alleviating and aggravating factors, and associated symptoms. Exploring the illness story includes both witnessing to the patient's experience and learning how they are currently making sense of that experience. FIFE (Feelings, Ideas, Function, Expectations) is a helpful mnemonic for remembering how to explore the illness experience (see Table 3.19).[6]

Ask about how their illness feels and what effect it is having on their function—their ability to do their everyday activities and what matters to them. Ask also about their expectations and concerns related to the illness and their ideas and explanations of what is wrong and what is going on. Culture and past experience greatly influence these ideas and attributions. What have they heard from family, friends, social media, and the Internet? The concepts of explanatory model and illness prototype and their associated questions[7] are very helpful in enriching your understanding of the patient's illness story and their related expectations. Cultural traditions offer patients many different explanatory models of illness experiences. LETS HEAR is a mnemonic for eliciting a person's explanatory model (see Table 3.20).[8-10]

Illness prototypes are cognitive characterizations of illnesses that individuals package and use to make sense of their illness experience. They come from past personal experiences, the experiences of others, and those met in multiple media formats like magazines, radio, and social media.[11] Table 3.21 highlights the three kinds of illness prototypes and the questions that elicit them.

Exploring the sickness story is aided by three questions (see Table 3.22). These questions will help you appreciate how the patient is navigating their social world.

Combining the illness, disease, and sickness stories gives you a rich understanding of the patient's overall malady story.

TABLE 3.19 Components of FIFE

F	Feelings
I	Ideas
F	Function (especially the effect on. . .)
E	Expectations

Data from Weston WW, Brown JB, Stewart MA. Patient-centred interviewing part I: understanding patients' experiences. *Can Fam Physician*. 1989;35:147-151.

TABLE 3.20 Eliciting an Explanatory Model

Letter	Item	Question
L	Label	"Do you have a name for your problem?"
E	Etiology	"What do you think caused your problem?"
T	Time	"Why do you think it started when it did?" "Do you think it will last a long time, or will it be better soon?"
S	Severity	"How severe is your illness?"
H	Natural History	"What do you think your illness does to you?" "How does it work?"
E	Effects	"What are the chief problems your illness has caused for you?"
A	Affects	"What do you fear most about your illness?"
R	Rx (treatments)	"What kind of treatment do you think you should receive?" "What are the most important results you hope to get from treatment?"

TABLE 3.21 Eliciting Illness Prototypes

Illness Prototype Type	Question
Personal	"Have you ever had anything like this before?"
Other	"Have you ever known anyone else to have something like this?" "Do you know anyone else with a problem like this?"
Media	"Have you ever heard or seen anything that refers to something like this on TV or radio, in magazines, on social media or the Internet?"

TABLE 3.22 Eliciting Sickness Story Features

Feature	Question
Social Support	"What help are you getting from others?"
Employment Issues	"Any problems at work accommodating your sickness?"
Social Expectations	"Any issues with what people are expecting from you?"

Do not forget the health story that existed before the malady took over the narrative. That health story of life in the River of Health is where the patient hopes to return. The goals and plan of care need to lead in that direction. Be realistic. You do not need extensive details. You want to know just enough to appreciate what the patient imagines health to look like and what changed when they shifted from health to ailment. Witness the malady experience while remembering what health represents for this person. You are weaving disease, illness, sickness, and health; you are crafting from biomedicine, embodied personal and social experience, and hopeful imagination. As you weave among these stories, begin exploring and deepening your understanding of the whole person in their context.

Understanding the Whole Person in Context

Right about now, you may feel a bit of panic. I get it. How can you possibly understand a whole person in context in less than 10 minutes? Relax, you cannot. Every encounter is an opportunity to learn more, to get closer to the patient and their stories. This is partly why relationship and continuity are so critical. Over time, with each encounter with a particular patient, you grow from the health and affliction stories to uncover a bit more of the underlying life story of this person. You build your understanding over time. Be like the crime solver in a good mystery novel. Who is this particular person? Each encounter is a new chapter in the story.

Why *story*? This is a good moment to pause and reflect on our repeated use of *story* as a narrative frame.[12] The simple answer is that stories connect and organize, and these processes are at the heart of generalism and primary health care. Stories are remarkably inclusive of what matters for the generalist's craft. They incorporate power; bridge biology and culture; address the four Cs of primary medical care—first contact access, continuity, comprehensiveness, and coordination; encompass the Ecological Clinical Map; differentiate encounter types; and hold the paradox of time (see Table 3.23).

From the cave walls of Lascaux to this year's Oscar winners, *Homo sapiens* are storytellers. Story is how the human brain makes sense, shapes identity, and organizes information into a meaningful form more easily heard by the Elephant, who is the true driver of human behavior change. Story is how we return to the River of Health. Storytelling needs the listener to be involved, to express empathy, and to become entangled as an active listener, all keys to being an effective generalist healer. We are ready to return to the clinical

TABLE 3.23 Story and the Generalist Craft

Feature	Description
Power	Sharing story facilitates locating, owning, aiming, and sharing power.
Biocultural	All care is biological; all care is cultural. Story connects the two.
The Four Cs of Primary Medical Care	Contact Access: Story is how we access each other.
	Continuity: Story connects when mobility and change disconnect.
	Comprehensive: Story has room for everything, even the incommensurable.
	Coordinated: Story is a means of sharing across sectors.
Ecological Clinical Map	Story holds all the circles of the ECM tool.
Encounter Types	Routine: People come to fix their story.
	Ceremony: People come because they are stuck in their story.
	Drama: People come because they have fallen out of their story.
Time	Story holds both Chronos and Kairos time.

ECM, Ecological Clinical Map.

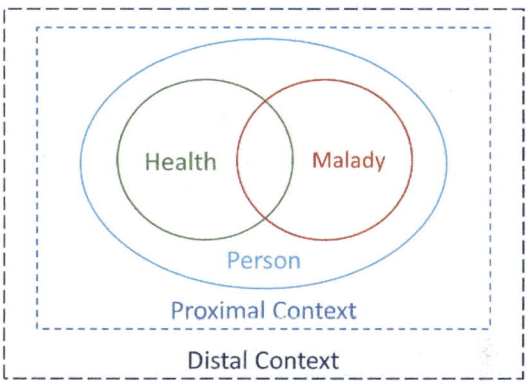

FIGURE 3.16. Understanding the Whole Person.

encounter and the healing relationship and to knit all this together in a life story (see Figure 3.16).

Understanding the whole person in context is a rich and never-ending quest. This is partly because none of us is really ever whole; we are always coming together, partly because we never stay where and what we just were. Understanding the whole person in context means connecting to the patient's life story and learning as you go. It means listening to what matters.[13] What are some of the pieces of the whole-person-in-context puzzle that make their life story? We can paint their picture from the outside by starting with the distal context: the institutions and places in which they are situated. Next, we add brush strokes of the proximal context of family and close friends, then finish by coloring the center, the person, with their multiple identities, recognizing all of them and how they change over time. Notice that the context boxes in Figure 3.16 are dotted lines. That is to highlight their permeability to each other and to the larger world.

Reflective Pause

Before exploring the details inside Figure 3.16, let us pause with a check-in on being realistic. There is always more that can be learned. But not all of it today. I am highlighting information that can be especially helpful in the primary medical care of a person over time using a generalist approach. Again, not all of it today. The detail is to prime your ability to recognize what may be important. But then prioritize and personalize based on the immediate circumstances and encounter. Apply the Windmill Sails of Generalism. Now, back to understanding the whole person and their contexts.

Let us start with the contexts (see Table 3.24). The *distal context* speaks to place, the many locations and ecologies where we and patients animate our lives. These include physical and structural institutions—for example, the economy, health care, government, media—and the pervading dominant culture. The distal context also includes the air, water, soil, animals, plants, and insects of our habitat. All these aspects of our distal context influence and shape our life story.

The *proximal context* consists of the people most involved in our lives and the more intimate spaces they inhabit. This includes everyday spaces—where we work, live, go to school—as well as our streets, our neighborhoods, and where we exchange goods and shop. Do we know where the safe spaces are? The proximal context also includes family and intimate friends. The mention of family can generate a range of emotions and bring a wide variety of configurations to mind. For our purposes as generalist healers, we will conceptualize family as a process (see Table 3.25).[14]

A family consists of those people who share affinity, intimacy, reciprocity, and continuity. This definition names the processes that matter in our life stories and in maintaining health while being inclusive of the many diverse forms that family exhibits on our planet. This diversity encompasses traditional nuclear families, extended families, LGBTQIA2S+ (lesbian, gay,

TABLE 3.24 **Understanding the Whole Person: Examples of Contexts**

Proximal Context:
- Family and intimate friends
- Finances and employment
- Education
- Leisure and play
- Religion and social supports

Distal Context:
- Community
- Dominant culture
- State of the economy
- Local health care system
- Media exposure
- Ecosystem and habitat

TABLE 3.25 Family as Process

Family Is Those People Who Share the Following:

Affinity	Some sort of bonding
Intimacy	Closeness and openness
	Special touching privileges
Reciprocity	Sense of trust and obligatory exchange
Continuity	Lasting over extended time
	Expectation of being there

Data from Carmichael LP, Carmichael JS. The relational model in family practice. *Marriage Fam Rev*. 1981;4(1-2):123-133.

bisexual, transgender, queer and questioning, intersex, asexual or agender, two-spirit, and + for other) families, families without children, foster families, adoptive families, communal families, orphanage families, blended families, single-person families, families with pets, and more. Families are relational systems and a major source of primary care. They can be places for stability and safety, places of change, places fraught with violence and abuse, and a mix of all three. Family structures include hierarchy, boundaries, multiple roles, and alliances and coalitions.[15]

A common pattern important for clinicians to recognize is scapegoating in the form of one family member being the symptom-bearer for unresolved family conflicts. Also common are patterns of triangulation such as when a child plays one parent against the other, and enmeshment where some family members are entwined with one another in unhealthy ways.[16] Notice these as you explore a patient's life story over time. The family circle[17] and the genogram[18] are fantastic tools for discovering family structures and patterns. It is important to remember that the first family genogram cocreated with the patient is always missing important information. As the healer–patient relationship strengthens over time and encompasses more trust, new information and family secrets emerge, so redoing the genogram at later opportune times can be elucidating. Genograms are especially valuable when you and the patient are involved in a drama.

The family life cycle[19] holds many insights for the discerning generalist healer (see Figure 3.17).[20] In every clinical encounter, I do a quick mental check on where the patient is on the life cycle. What developmental issues,

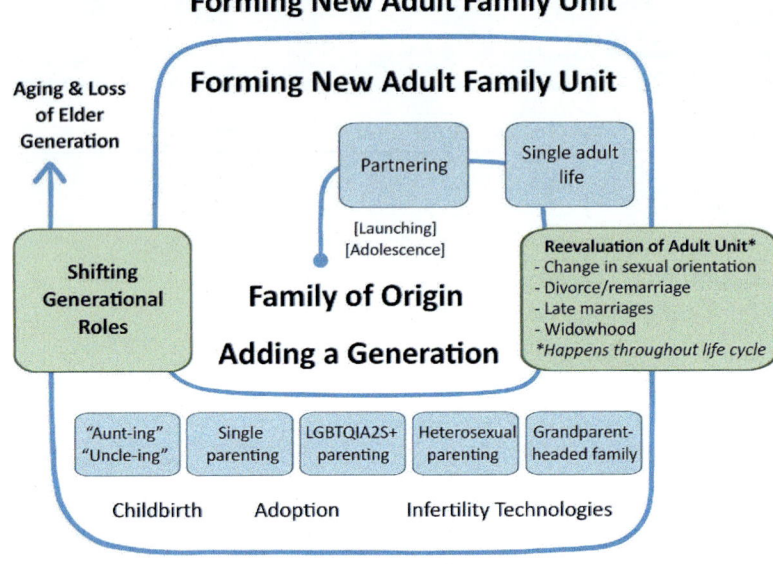

FIGURE 3.17. Family Life Cycle.

joys, or challenges commonly arise depending on where they are in that cycle, and how do those events intersect with current health and malady concerns? What are important tasks for the family at this time? What unresolved issues from past generations may be affecting the family in the present? Are we at an important anniversary date on the life cycle such as a miscarriage or death of a spouse? It is not unusual for people to become symptomatic on those occasions.

Since the family frequently serves as a primary unit of caregiving and support during malady episodes, it is helpful to assess their capacity for providing those services. The Family APGAR (see Table 3.26) is a simple measure for quickly assessing the capacity of the family when those services are most needed.[21] It measures five aspects of family capacity: adaptation, partnership, growth, affect, and resolve.

Learning the patient's life story now moves from contexts to the person in the center of Figure 3.16. One helpful approach consists of exploring a person's multiple identities of belonging beginning with the body. We all have a relationship with our body, both as a material home for our life and as a presentation of our self to those around us. How comfortable or not we feel

TABLE 3.26 — Features of the Family APGAR Measurement of Capacity

Feature	Description
Adaptation	Family's resources to adjust to change
Partnership	Family's communication and problem-solving skills
Growth	Space for emotional growth and access to role changes
Affect	Intimacy and reciprocity
Resolve	Determination, will, and effort to act on behalf of family

in our bodies profoundly shapes our health and how maladies manifest. Explore the patient's body identity, how they perceive themselves. Ask what they see when they look in a mirror. Inquire about body art (tattoos) and piercings and fashion. And remember that the "body keeps the score" related to past traumas.[22] Health and malady stories reside within the body identity.

Our personal identity includes family identity discussed earlier but is also composed of ecological, cultural, livelihood, and online identities. We are all hybrids. We live in many places: mansions, single-family homes, townhouses, apartments, makeshift shelters under a bridge, refugee camps, and so on. The ecologies and geography of those places shape our ecological identity. The geology, climate, flora, fauna, contaminants, air, water, and built structures all impact our health. Pay careful attention to where patients live, what is there, and how that matters to them. We come from many places, linked to us personally and ancestrally. Except for a few indigenous groups, we are all migrants. Those former "homes" and immigration stories make up part of our cultural identities. Ethnicity and the imposed structures of race do as well. Culture represents our human designs for living, our sense of "us," but be wary to avoid thinking of culture as a set of stereotypical traits. This is especially true in our globalized world in which nearly all of us share a mix of cultural backgrounds.[23] Hybrids indeed. Explore patients' cultural identities and your own.

Let us not forget livelihood identities, how each of us participates in the world to sustain our lives. That participation not only involves the work we do, our life as part of some workforce, but what else we do to sustain ourselves such as gardening, housekeeping, and childcare. It also includes what we offer to others and what we receive within the worlds in which we belong.

TABLE 3.27 Eliciting Livelihoods Identity

Relational Dimension	Definition	Question
Making	Making a living (what we make)	What do you do on a daily basis to sustain yourself? (both work and other)
Providing	Making others (what we give)	Who or what depends on you?
Receiving	Being-made by others (what we take)	Who or what are you dependent upon?

Our identity always exists within a web of belonging, of interdependence. Table 3.27 highlights some questions for eliciting the livelihoods identity of patients.[24]

Online self-presentations have emerged in recent years, especially among many younger patients, as an important aspect of personal identity and is well worth inquiry.

All of these identities—family, body, ecological, cultural, livelihood, and online—weave together, often with tensions in the fabric, to create a personal identity that embodies the health and malady stories.

Table 3.28 highlights how these stories come together to compose a whole person's evolving life story. This more encompassing narrative continually expands, changes, and deepens as your relationship with your patient builds over time, and you learn more with each opening window of opportunity.

An important reason for gathering all this information over time is to more clearly see your patient for who they truly are. Understanding the whole person helps you discover how to communicate with their Elephant and Rider to facilitate behavior change, especially when that change is dramatic. Thus, there are times you will want to assess a patient's readiness to change and how to help them along that journey. Table 3.29 describes six stages of change and some actions for moving on to the next.[25] Patients will be in very different stages for different behaviors. Assess accordingly.

Figure 3.18 illustrates the wheel of readiness to change. The wheel reminds us that relapse happens—sometimes often. It is important for you to appreciate relapse not as a failure but as part of the journey of change toward better health.

TABLE 3.28 — Highlights of the Whole Person's Life Story

Multiple Identities:
- Family identity
- Body (including trauma) identity
- Ecological identity
- Cultural identities
- Livelihood identity
- Online identity
- Others

Multiple Places:
- Livelihood, Personal, Other, Safe
- Migration story

Composing a Life Story:
- Incorporating health story (avoid medicalization)
- Learn a new story every encounter (windows of opportunity)
- Note hero stories, resilience stories, trauma stories

You now have an abundance of recommendations, questions, and strategies for understanding who the patient is and their health and malady stories, including their FIFE as well as their potential capacity to respond effectively with possible treatment burdens. Be realistic and apply these strategies with discretion. Do not use all the questions for every encounter. If it is a routine encounter, stay focused on the short agenda and learn only what you need to address the simple issue. When in a maintenance ceremony, learn a little something new each time that relates to what arises. Dramas will develop over many visits. The application of most of the strategies discussed here is encouraged over the course of those visits.

Recall the Windmill Sails of Generalism (recognize, prioritize, personalize). Recognize what is needed as the story emerges. Prioritize based on the agenda and what arises. And personalize based on the stories you are learning. Joanne Reeve, a general practitioner from Hull in England, suggests five elements to help focus your use of the simple rules as you weave among the stories.[26,27] Imagine helping your patient into a canoe and reentering the River of Health. Have you uncovered the *"creative self"* with the patient? Have you increased their *"power"* to the work of everyday life, that is, have you expanded their resources? Have you accounted for their *"flow of everyday life?"*

TABLE 3.29 The Six Stages of Change

Stages	Signal from Patient	Action
Pre-contemplation	Not yet acknowledging there is a problem needing a change	• Encourage self-exploration. • Personalize the risk.
Contemplation	There is a problem but not ready, unsure, or fearful of change	• Identify pros and cons. • Explore positive outcomes.
Preparation	Determined and getting ready to change	• Problem-solve obstacles. • Identify social support. • Take initial small steps.
Action	Taking steps and changing behavior	• Bolster self-efficacy. • Address feelings of loss.
Maintenance	Maintaining the behavior change	• Reinforce internal rewards. • Plan for f/u support.
Relapse	Return to old behavior; often feelings of disappointment, frustration	• Reaffirm commitment. • Identify triggers. • Recognize barriers to success.

Have you adjusted for any *"imbalance"* of resources and demands? Do you appreciate their identities and values? Is the patient positioned in the canoe for *"stability?"* Remember who owns the story—the patient. They are sharing with you to help them craft a plan that returns them to the River of Health. Hold it reverently.

Now that you know your patient's story, it is time to get physical.

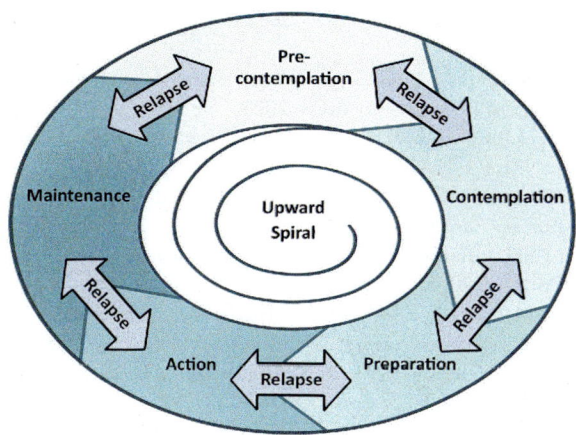

FIGURE 3.18. The Wheel of Readiness to Change.

REFERENCES

1. Noushad B, Van Gerven PWM, de Bruin ABH. Twelve tips for applying the think-aloud method to capture cognitive processes. *Med Teach*. 2024;46(7): 892-897.
2. Bandler R, Grinder J. *The Structure of Magic*. Vol 1. Science and Behavior Books, Inc; 1975.
3. Wiseman R, Watt C, ten Brinke L, et al. The eyes don't have it: lie detection and neuro-linguistic programming. *PLoS One*. 2012;7(7):e40259.
4. Hofmann B. On the triad disease, illness and sickness. *J Med Philos*. 2002; 27(6):651-673.
5. Parsons T. *The Social System*. Free Press; 1951.
6. Weston WW, Brown JB, Stewart MA. Patient-centred interviewing part I: understanding patients' experiences. *Can Fam Physician*. 1989;35:147-151.
7. Groleau D, Young A, Kirmayer LJ. The McGill Illness Narrative Interview (MINI): an interview schedule to elicit meanings and modes of reasoning related to illness experience. *Transcult Psychiatry*. 2006;43(4):671-691.
8. Kleinman A, Eisenberg L, Good B. Culture, illness, and care: clinical lessons from anthropologic and cross-cultural research. *Ann Intern Med*. 1978;88(2): 251-258.
9. Berlin EA, Fowkes WC. A teaching framework for cross-cultural health care—application in family practice. *West J Med*. 1983;139(6):934-938.
10. Miller WL. Models of health, illness, and health care. In: Taylor RB, ed. *Family Medicine: Principles and Practice*. 3rd ed. Springer-Verlag; 1988:35-42.
11. Young A. When rational men fall sick: an inquiry into some assumptions made by medical anthropologists. *Cult Med Psychiatry*. 1981;5(4):317-335.

12. Launer J. *Narrative-Based Primary Care: A Practical Guide*. Radcliffe Medical Press, Ltd; 2002.
13. Weiner SJ, Schwartz A. *Listening for What Matters: Avoiding Contextual Errors in Health Care*. Oxford University Press; 2023.
14. Carmichael LP, Carmichael JS. The relational model in family practice. *Marriage Fam Rev*. 1981;4(1-2):123-133.
15. Asen E, Tomson D, Young V, et al. *Ten Minutes for the Family: Systemic Interventions in Primary Care*. Routledge; 2004.
16. McDaniel SH, Campbell TL, Hepworth J, et al. *Family-Oriented Primary Care*. 2nd ed. Springer; 2005.
17. Thrower SM, Bruce WE, Walton RF. The family circle method for integrating family systems concepts in family medicine. *J Fam Pract*. 1982;15(3):451-457.
18. McGoldrick M, Gerson R, Petry S. *Genograms: Assessment and Intervention*. 3rd ed. W. W. Norton & Company; 2008.
19. McGoldrick M, Preto NG, Carter B. *The Expanding Family Life Cycle: Individual, Family, and Social Perspectives*. 5th ed. Pearson; 2021.
20. Foster E, Cohen-Katz J. Caring for the family: teaching systems and cycles in a family medicine residency program. In: Miller-Day M, ed. *Family Communication, Connections, and Health Transitions: Going Through This Together*. Peter Lang; 2011:323-348.
21. Smilkstein G. The family APGAR: a proposal for family function test and its use by physicians. *J Fam Pract*. 1978;6(6):1231-1239.
22. van der Kolk BA. *The Body Keeps the Score: Brain, Mind, and Body in the Healing of Trauma*. Viking; 2014.
23. Agar MH. *Culture: How to Make It Work in a World of Hybrids*. Rowman & Littlefield; 2019.
24. Miller E. *Reimagining Livelihoods: Life beyond Economy, Society, and Environment*. University of Minnesota Press; 2019.
25. Prochaska JO, DiClemente CC. Stages and processes of self-change of smoking: toward an integrative model of change. *J Consult Clin Psychol*. 1983;51(3):390-395.
26. Reeve J. Unlocking the creative capacity of the self. In: Dowrick C, ed. *Person-Centred Primary Care: Searching for the Self*. Routledge; 2019:141-165.
27. Reeve J. *Medical Generalism, Now! Reclaiming the Knowledge Work of Modern Practice*. CRC Press; 2024.

Unit Four: The Journey to Hand Over: Clinical Discovery and Evaluation

Clinical Discovery and Evaluation

Up until now, we have mostly been listening in dialogue with the patient: connecting, negotiating, and setting the agenda; exploring health and malady stories; and gaining a better understanding of the whole person in context. Now that we have fleshed out much of the background of the agenda issues, we are ready to begin actively figuring out what is going on and how we might help in restoring health. We are ready for clinical discovery and evaluation as we continue our movement toward the Hand Over guidepost. We are entering more sacred and intimate space for more probing questions and for touching, the physical examination (or its virtual equivalent), where we may feel the story in the body.

Touching Skills

Power resides in the human touch, especially in the context of affliction when patients come to us with hurting bodies and in a heightened state of expectation and fear. I am purposefully using the word *touch* instead of *examine* because the latter is unidirectional. The clinician examines the patient to learn something about the patient. Touching is bidirectional. The clinician touches the patient to both learn something and to transmit something—call it "healing intentions." We are locating, owning, aiming, and sharing power. The patient's "knowing" body also responds to the touch. This is why it is so helpful to touch the part that hurts—not only for examination reasons, but, more importantly, because it directly connects the patient and you at the vulnerable spot.

Touching and the exam, especially if explained as you go, become a means for organizing the body and its pain into a meaningful story that initiates the process of healing. Touching and examining with care, rhythm, and structure bring a little order and control in the form of clinical action. Perform accordingly. Table 3.30 reminds us to deliberately prepare the patient and ourselves for touching/examining. Keep your nails short and smooth at the edges and your hands warm and dry. Ensure physical support for the patient by offering a pillow, having them bend their leg, raising the back of the table, adjusting the lighting so it is not in their eyes. Personally support them with appropriate covering. If a friend or family member is in the room, give permission for them to hold the patient's hand. Eye contact and frequent check-ins

TABLE 3.30	Preparation for Touching (Examining) the Patient

Make your patient and yourself as comfortable as possible.
Cut fingernails short.
Keep hands warm, clean, and dry.
Support the patient physically, personally, and emotionally.

demonstrate emotional support and empathy as you touch the patient. What is the body trying to tell you? Table 3.31 highlights a few tips on how to touch and examine patients. Like kayaking in a river of rapids, enter when in the calm of an eddy and then move toward the rapids. If the pain is in the right lower quadrant of the abdomen, begin in the left upper quadrant and assuredly and rhythmically move to the right upper quadrant. Then, avoiding surprise, move on to the left lower quadrant and finally to the right lower quadrant. When appropriate, stroke in the direction of venous and lymph flow. Avoid hesitation and jerky motions. Stay in touch!

A surprisingly small number of physical exam maneuvers have a solid evidence base. So why still do them? Because they are evidence-informing, trust-inducing, and relationship-building.[1] Touching provides you with cues and clues while prompting patient memory, thus pointing to patterns of meaning that are critical for recognizing the Windmill Sails of Generalism. Touching is about knowing the patient, about embodying knowledge. The physical exam provides a view of the body from the outside in, whereas labs and imaging studies view the body from the inside.

TABLE 3.31	How to Touch (Exam) the Patient

Use contact and rhythm: Avoid surprise.
Begin where it doesn't hurt and move toward the pain.
Stroke with the flow: Follow dermatomes.
Use acupressure points.
Imagine topographic anatomy and be intentional.
Stay in touch: Maintain skin contact.

Notice when not to touch, or when to approach with heightened sensitivity. Be more careful when there is a prior abuse history, active paranoia, a history of posttraumatic stress disorder, or special cultural situations. For example, you might consider avoiding touching the head if your patient is from Southeast Asia. Use of a model, doll, or drawing can occasionally substitute in these circumstances.

Clinical Discovery

Let us begin the dance of clinical discovery, evaluation, and sensemaking (see Figure 3.19). To this adventure, we bring our body knowledge of anatomy, physiology, and pathology. We also bring our body stories of critical processes that help us anticipate, create, and intervene. We come with the amazing story of inflammation; the energetic tale of cyclic adenosine monophosphate; the mesmerizing saga of receptors, neurotransmitters, enzymes, and feedback loops swirling throughout and across our body systems sharing information; and the provocative genome and epigenetic story.

We also approach clinical discovery and sensemaking with our metaphoric understanding of the body as an ancient forest or garden and its remarkable adaptive and healing capacities, and we hold our own library of clinical experience and stories learned from colleagues. That said, the diagnostic and treatment planning processes for the generalist healer in primary care differ in some important ways from those traditionally taught in medical and nursing schools.

Here we part company with some of what you learned about diagnostic reasoning from medical specialists. Generalist healers in primary care are like wildlife trackers with a broad "investigative sensitivity"[2] and an enhanced style of attention. We begin by foraging for understanding, then use what we learn to generate a story—our form of a working hypothesis or theory.

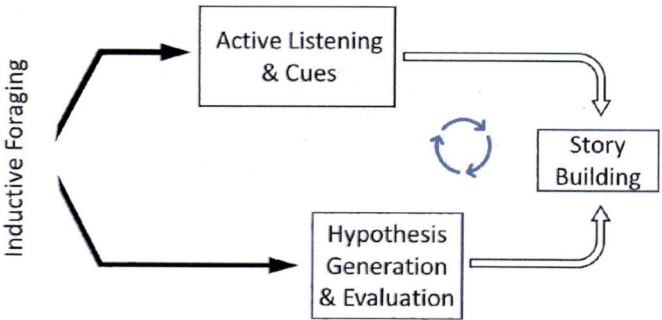

FIGURE 3.19. The Dance of Clinical Discovery and Sensemaking.

Thus, inductive reasoning looms large. Induction begins with an observation, continues by looking for supporting and disconfirming patterns, then arrives at a working hypothesis or theory; deduction, on the other hand, begins with a working hypothesis or theory, seeks support for it through observation, then confirms or rejects.

Practitioners of the generalist's craft actively invite patients to be partners in the work of inductive foraging. As artisans of the generalist's craft, we emphasize perceiving, knowing, and doing, but generalism is also a way of belonging that powerfully influences the other ways of perceiving, knowing, and doing. The generalist's craft is relationship-centered, which means that generalist healers cocreate a shared awareness and knowledge within a relational context. The purpose is to expand our field of shared understanding. Figure 3.20 illustrates this process using a modification of the Johari window.[3]

At the beginning of a clinical encounter, the clinician and patient have a limited awareness and knowledge that they share—public understandings that are known to both of them. But there is also important information the clinician has that is unknown to the patient: the clinician's experiential and medical knowledge that needs to be disclosed to the patient. Similarly, the patient has knowledge unknown or blind to the clinician that can be shared in the form of feedback to the clinician's questions. Finally, there is hidden knowledge, unknown to both, that require their collective exploration. Effective practice of the generalist's craft fosters learning conversations that facilitate disclosure, feedback, and collective exploration and expands the field of shared understanding.

You have been foraging from the beginning, uncovering information. You have encouraged your patient to freely share stories and explain the reason(s) for their visit and any concerns they have. This earlier foraging's intent was to

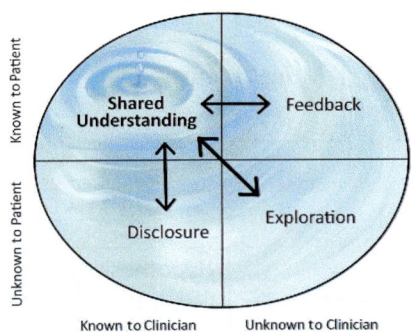

FIGURE 3.20. The Expanding Field of Shared Understanding from the Point of View of the Clinician.

develop the agenda and contextualize the identified concerns. Now you move your agenda items to the foreground. You shift the emphasis of your inductive foraging[4] toward searching for explanations and interventions. Think of it as free range reasoning versus fenced-in or caged reasoning.

A challenge from the first minute of inductive foraging is having the discipline not to leap to hypothesis generation. Hold the issues being addressed in mind. Stretch the horizon and scan widely across the view for the many cues that catch your senses. This is recognition work from the Windmill Sails of Generalism carried out in close communication with the patient. Listen and touch actively, being attentive and receptive. Listen and touch for feelings, and connect the feelings to the content being discovered. When conversing with the patient, use their language, their way of expression, and their words to reinforce their engagement. Foraging is greatly aided by attending to the high-yield A LOT moments described in Module 3, Unit 2 (see Figure 3.12). As cues accumulate, hunches are triggered, working hypotheses arise, and you start asking more directed questions and conducting more focused investigations. This direction of inquiry takes advantage of your memory, quick-thinking brain, and intuition. Figure 3.21 depicts these clinical discovery strategies and tactics.[4]

The diagnostic strategy moves from hypothesis-free inductive foraging and active listening, processes throughout which the patient was keenly engaged, to the recognition of cues and hunches that generate working hypotheses. With these come investigations that are more clinician-driven and aimed at deductively evaluating and challenging those hypotheses. This process ends with a final eco-scan that reviews what was seen on the initial

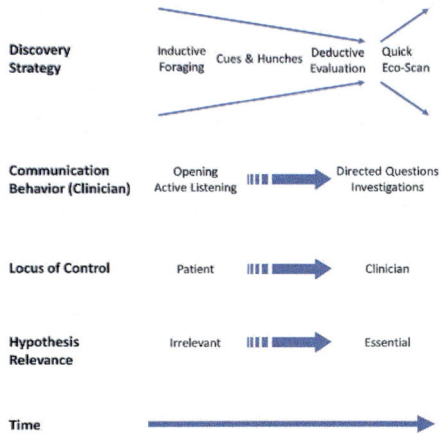

FIGURE 3.21. Clinical Discovery Strategies and Related Tactics.

foraging to make sure nothing important was overlooked, including any alternative hypotheses. As this is happening, you commence building the story that captures what's going on and the options for managing it.

Whew! Let's slow down and review the recognition processes inside the boxes about cues, hypothesis generation, and story-building from Figure 3.19 (see Table 3.32). Where others may settle for signs leading to diagnosis, our best healing thrives in the full story.

There are many sources for cues and hunches, beginning with self-labeling or when the patient names what is disturbing them. These labels often come from illness prototypes, especially past experience, suggestions from kith and kin, or the Internet. "I'm sure I've got strep throat; it's always like this." Descriptive questioning, which usually entails asking the patient to expand on one or more of the seven parameters of the history of present illness, often triggers important cues.

"Now that you ask again, I have noticed these stomach spasms seem to occur whenever we (my partner and I) talk about money issues." Stress and spasms are a cue for irritable bowel syndrome. Any other such associations you wonder? Certain visual, auditory, or other sensory cues can trigger a spot diagnosis[5] such as the target lesion erythema migrans rash of acute Lyme disease at the site of a tick bite, or the barking cough of pertussis, or a sitting 6-year-old child with drooling, high-pitched stridor and extended neck and chin cueing acute epiglottitis. A combination of thirst, feeling and looking unwell, and weight loss in an adolescent triggers the possibility of type 1 diabetes.[5] These presentations are also examples of pattern recognition where elements in the story and exam cue a pattern that triggers a working hypothesis.

Such pattern recall is often helped by illness scripts—a way to remember diagnoses often taught in medical schools.[6] Both a boon and a bane, heuristics, also referred to as rules of thumb, are our fast thinking brain's algorithms for making sense, and they are a major source of cues and hunches. Four common heuristics include anchoring, associational, availability, and representative rules of thumb. They offer useful cues and hypotheses, but can just as often be traps leading to premature closure. An *anchoring* heuristic is useful when you notice what comes up first and build upon it. It is helpful because what comes up first is often high-yield information, but your investigation should not stop there. The *associational* heuristic matches previous clinical situations to what you are observing. The *availability* rule of thumb refers you to what happened in the patient's last few visits, or to what happened in the hospital that morning. Again, these are good cues, but they should not mark the end of your exploration. The *representative* rule of thumb encourages you to match what you observe to similar things.[7] A patient presents with

TABLE 3.32 — Clinical Discovery Recognition Processes

Expand, Forage, Organize, Make Sense

Inductive Foraging	Patients encouraged to explore, explain, associate
	Clinician scanning
Cues and Hunches	Self-labeling
	Heuristics
	Pattern recognition
	Spot diagnosis
	Descriptive questions
	Illness scripts
Hypothesis Generation and Evaluation	Triggered routines
	Probabilistic reasoning
	Hypothetico-deductive testing
	Checklist routine (e.g., review of systems)
Sensemaking	Organizing what is learned in the story
	Creating clinical problem frame
Story-Building	What's the story of what's been happening?
	• Narrative types: Restitution, quest, chaos
	• Time patterns: Acute, cyclic, chronic
	• Plot themes, motivators, complicators, trajectories
	• Characters and setting

Prioritize

Time and Natural History	Urgency
	Probability and payoff
Patient Readiness	Liminal/teachable moment
Patient and Clinician Capacity	How much can be handled today?

dizziness and the smell of alcohol on their breath; the smell, representative of alcohol use disorder, leads you away from a more serious diagnosis of diabetic ketoacidosis.

It is important to remember that although heuristics can be useful, they are not reliable. They can provide helpful cues and hunches, but it is crucial to always seek more information before drawing any conclusions about the story you are building.

With several working hypotheses in hand, you begin to compare them while making sure nothing is missed. Hypotheses may trigger some learned routines—for example, sets of questions to ask that are specific to an organ system, symptom, or patho-mechanism that needs attention.[4] These are narrow arrays of questions that explore and rule out pathways and problems across an organ, symptom, or differential diagnosis. For example, a patient with a particular presentation of dizziness suggests problems in the inner ear and neurologic system that have no clear vascular cause, so you quickly do a cardiac exam and cardiovascular system review of questions. If uncertainty still nags, consider doing a full body review of symptoms. Both probabilistic reasoning and deductive reasoning work us through our hypotheses.

This is the moment when we move across our Windmill Sails of Generalism from the simple rule of recognizing to that of prioritizing. Prioritizing engages the concepts of probability and payoff. *Probability* concerns frequency and likelihood. How likely is a particular diagnosis? What is most likely? What is currently most common in the community? What are the particular hazards to which this person is exposed? *Payoff* raises the flag of urgency. What is the value of getting the correct diagnosis in this situation? Is there a diagnosis for which specific treatment is available and needed? What is essential not to miss at this moment in time? Will I lose the opportunity to prevent something more serious?

Remember the *red flags* impressed on us by our teachers. A thunderclap headache could be a hemorrhage in the head. Initial acute headache onset in someone over 50 years old suggests temporal arteritis or a mass lesion. Many red flag lists are now available in published guidelines. These are valuable in helping us work through any payoff concerns.[8]

A variant of red flags is *masquerades*.[9] These are common conditions that get forgotten because they can appear in many different disguises. Tuberculosis and syphilis were typical masquerades in the early to mid-20th century. Today, be on the lookout for masquerading depression, diabetes, alcohol use disorder, malignancy, self-abuse, anemia, and thyroid disorders.

Time to continue your story-building by moving to another Windmill Sail of Generalism—the simple rule of personalizing. Now we pull together what you have been learning. This includes what you know about the person, their life story, health story, what you uncovered regarding their malady story, as well as other items on the agenda. It also incorporates what you learned while foraging, accumulating cues, generating and evaluating hypotheses, and recollecting the words, metaphors, and explanations from the patient. All of these help to build a personal story for the patient about what is going on, the implications for treatment, and other care management strategies. One cannot underestimate the healing comfort of sensemaking.

The story is what you will share with the patient as you seek common ground and make decisions regarding the concerns, roles, goals, and care plans. The sensemaking explanatory story that you hand over to the patient, and they take home, has to feel personal for them. It addresses their actual reason for connecting and sufficiently satisfies their expectations. For example, it is not enough to suggest, "Gretel has strep throat, and I recommend a prescription for penicillin to be taken once a day for 10 days." Good counsel, but wrap the advice in a story. This was a routine visit with mother and daughter seeking restitution, a fix for an acute problem. Tell a short restitution narrative that ensures its complete and rapid resolution. Acknowledge other characters, setting, possible complications. Explain how you reached the diagnosis, where Gretel may have contracted it, what the implications for her siblings and parents may be, why the choice of antibiotic and the duration, what this all means for returning to school and everyday activities, and any other specific concerns that emerged during the encounter. This is Gretel's story. Make sure it is hers.

The Palm of Hope and Swinging on the Tree

Not every story includes a diagnosis. Many symptoms in primary medical care remain medically unexplained. Even without a clear diagnosis, you still need to frame the patient's problem so a management strategy can be developed. The Clinical Hand and supporting Round Table of Evidence tool come to our aid. Let's start with the Palm of Hope. It is a habitat holding a tree of health, the Naming and Caring Tree, with five limbs (see Figure 3.22).

Think of the limbs of the tree and the surrounding habitat as a web of multiple, reciprocal causation and multiple, reciprocally engaged caring supports: an ecology of cause and care. The limbs of the naming tree are a source for explanations, and the limbs of the caring tree give us management options. When you toss the knowledge gleaned from the clinical discovery and evaluation process onto the tree, where does it stick? Where are the bright spots to hang around when swinging from limb to limb? The tree represents the body

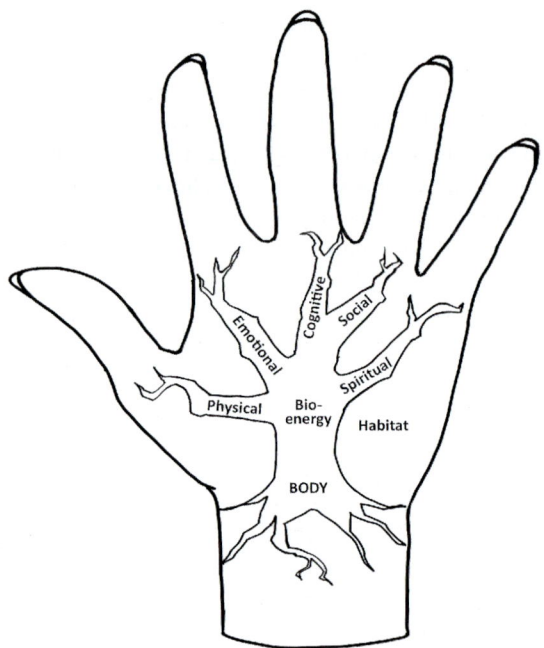

FIGURE 3.22. The Palm of Hope and the Naming and Caring Tree.

as a whole. Over the course of the human story, that body has been imagined as different cultural metaphors comprising body as animal cosmology from 60,000 to 11,000 years ago, body as garden from 11,000 to 300 years ago, body as machine throughout the 19th century up to about 1990, and currently, body as information system. Perhaps it is all of these, a combination of the many cultural metaphors that guide us. Each uses a different "science"—a different knowledge system and way of knowing—and all rest on the Round Table of Evidence.

The five limbs of the tree represent interdependent aspects of our body. I have given each a metaphoric representation that connects it to our evolutionary development and maps onto our body's pain systems. The *physical limb*, or snake limb, represents how our body exists and sustains itself and is shared by all animals. This is also the medical school limb, the limb of pathology, our organ systems and basic physiology, and it includes, like the snake, our brain, from the reticular formation down. This is the paleospinothalamic tract of the pain system that alerts us to trouble. The *emotional limb*, the bear limb, embodies how we pay attention with feeling via connections to the limbic brain and motor areas and is shared by all mammals. This is the neospinothalamic tract that helps us locate the source of pain with feeling. The *cognitive limb*, or human limb, pays attention to words, stories, and judgments with extensive connections into the neocortex. These cortical extensions help us make sense of our pain. The *social limb*, the tribal limb, registers how the troubles, ties, and traditions of our social lives impact our bodies—how they connect to our frontal cortex and greatly complicate our experience of pain. The *spiritual or* angel *limb* pays attention to the questions of ultimate concern that arise from our existence, straddling the consciousness of infinity and the experience of finite lives. It is represented by the descending pain pathways and their endorphins. The tree is rooted and placed within the context of a *habitat*, which refers to the places and ecologies where we live. All of these become sources for diagnosis and treatment, for naming and caring.

Diagnosis acts as a process infused with power and culture. Diagnoses designate the culturally defined boundaries of normal. This can help create a sense of order and may appropriately signify body trouble, but diagnoses can also fuel the medicalization of life.[10] When medical specialty organizations and the pharmaceutical industry keep expanding the criteria or lowering the diagnostic levels for markers of common conditions like diabetes, hypertension, obesity, and behavioral disorders, the number of "normal" people without a diagnosis shrinks. One of the roles for the generalist healer in primary care is to protect the population from such overmedicalization. We pay just as much attention to the harms as to the benefits. Diagnoses are labels. Yes, when patients have conditions disrupting their lives, we can name it, begin to bound it, organize it, make sense of it, and contain it so life and health are maintained or restored. But labeling also creates its own trauma that manifest in a myriad of ways, including increased absenteeism, marital distress, disturbing symptoms, and health care visits unrelated to the actual disease.[11] Diagnosis is a cultural construct, and it has the power to facilitate understanding prognosis, risk, and treatment. Remember that diagnosis is relational, a social event, a mythic moment. Locate, own, aim, and share the power of diagnosis as a fragile butterfly of knowledge. Use it well, remain open-minded, and keep the River of Health wide.

Treatment also acts as a process infused with power and culture. Allopathic treatments impart the combined powers of science and capitalism, a challenging tension for the generalist healer. It is essential for the generalist clinician to wisely and competently take advantage of the timely and powerful effectiveness of biomedical treatments. It is also important to not let that power overwhelm the value of working with the body's innate protective systems and the external natural systems with which they coevolved. The Round

Table of Evidence tool helps us in evaluating the different options. Treatment, like diagnosis, is relational. It is a social and cultural event that reinforces cultural values through aroused action. Watch any pharmaceutical ad for examples. Remember, as well, the meaning/placebo response, which bridges diagnosis and treatment by activating general medical effectiveness via expectancy, conditioning, and meaning. The craft you are learning does all of this by creating a socially sanctioned safe healing space with powerful emotional support where the patient gains a sense of mastery through explanations consistent with their worldview.

Let us see what naming and caring options are available on the limbs of the tree. Below, I share diagnostic mnemonics as a way to demonstrate and help you recall the many available possibilities for each limb. Table 3.33 presents a diagnostic mnemonic, ANCIENT DIVA, and some treatment selections on the physical limb of the Clinical Hand tree. This limb of the dancing snake, emphasized in medical schools and symbolized by the staff of Asclepius, resonates with the question, "When did you stop dancing?"[12] When swinging on this limb pondering diagnosis, I start with an anatomic scan and then begin my pathophysiology and illness scripts scans.

The emotion limb of the singing bear echoes with the question, "When did you stop singing?" Table 3.34 highlights a diagnostic mnemonic, TEL, and some treatment examples for the emotion limb. *Tell* is a word used in poker to

TABLE 3.33 Physical Naming and Caring

		Caring Examples
A	Anatomy	Pharmacology
N	Neoplasm	Surgery/Injections
C	Congenital/Genetic	Body therapies (e.g., physical therapy)
I	Infectious	Dancing/Tai Chi/Yoga
E	Endocrine/Metabolic	Exercise
N	Nutritional	Nutritional
T	Trauma	Herbs
D	Degenerative	Acupuncture
I	Inflammatory	
V	Vascular	
A	Allergic/Autoimmune	

TABLE 3.34 Emotional Naming and Caring

		Caring Examples
T	Threat: Anxiety disorders	Music/Art
E	Expression:	Solution-focused therapy
	• Substance use	Psychopharmacology
	• Somatoform and complex pain disorders	Rituals and ceremonies
		Humor
L	Loss: Affective disorders	Dream work
		Internal family systems therapy
		Other psychotherapies
		Spas and aromatherapy
		Light therapy
		Relaxation therapies

describe a behavioral shift—a nonverbal cue—that may signal the strength of a player's hand. *Tels* are also layered mounds of prehistory in the Middle East hiding stories from the past. It is often therapeutic to *tell* our emotions, to get them out rather than to store them inside as a burden. And work gently with denial/safeguarding, an important defense/protective mechanism. When you are faced with safeguarding in a patient, stop and shift your focus toward helping the patient build capacity for dealing with the wounds and associated emotions being protected. Be patient, and the singing will come.

Three axes of emotions all have motivational drive: the experience of threat and security, the experience of loss and attachment, and the expression of pain and pleasure. TEL names the "negative" end of these axes. Much of the psychopharmacology we currently use to treat these impacts the interconnected axis as a whole. When medication dampens threat, loss, or pain, it may also diminish the senses of security, attachment, and pleasure.[13] This is another reason why it is important to personalize treatment. And remember, for better or worse, that fear protects, anger defends against loss, and sadness releases tensions. Managing emotions is a lot like eye juggling.

The storytelling human swings onto the cognitive limb of the tree on the Clinical Hand wondering, "When did I stop being enchanted by my story?" People with developmental trauma often cannot tell their full story; they can only share a few frightening fragments. Table 3.35 presents a diagnostic mnemonic, I SEA, and a few examples of cognitive-related treatments. The intent

TABLE 3.35 Cognitive Naming and Caring

		Caring Examples
I	Illness prototypes: Self, other, media	Cognitive behavioral therapy
S	Self-image	Journaling
E	Explanatory models	Biofeedback
A	Attributions	Support groups

is to expand the horizons of patients' stories. The cognitive limb attends to what we say to ourselves, the words we use, the "thinking" that goes on inside the bubbles of our inner chatter, how we may or may not give meaning to our lives. As noted in the table, these cognitions include illness prototypes, our cultural explanatory models, self-images, and the many attributions and judgments we make about ourselves and others.

The social limb of the tree, the theatrical tribe, responds to the question, "When did you stop being honest in your relationships?" This is the limb of people, places, and things. Table 3.36 highlights a mnemonic for social diagnosis, TTTS, and some examples of social caring. The three Ts—troubles, ties, and traditions[14]—represent the most common social sources of malady.

TABLE 3.36 Social Naming and Caring

		Caring Examples
T	Troubles: Neighbors, livelihood, politics, religion	Drama therapy
T	Ties: Friends and family issues	Family therapy
T	Traditions: Gender, ethnicity, holidays	Pets
S	SCREEM resources (see Table 3.37): • Social • Cultural • Religious • Educational • Economic • Medical	Enhance SCREEM Social skills training Cultural healing traditions

Several institutional structures and their associated resources act as drivers for ensuring or diminishing the capacity for dealing with affliction. Their absence can both cause and worsen malady. The SCREEM mnemonic detailed in Table 3.37 names six of these drivers and their resources—social,

TABLE 3.37 The SCREEM Resources

Category	Resources
Social	Community agencies
	Government agencies
	Friends and neighbors
	Communication and transportation
	Impacts of structural racism
Cultural	Values and preferences
	Folk and lay care systems
	Explanatory models and illness prototypes
	Discourses of normalcy
Religious	Religious organizations
	Sacred spaces
	Ritual access
Educational	Schools: Access, curriculum, safety
	Adult education opportunities
	Music/art/sports/dance
	Public library
Economic	Income and benefits
	Banks, savings, insurance
	Housing and other assets
	Food security
	Commodities
Medical	Primary care
	Supportive care
	Emergency care
	Hospital care
	Disability care
	Home care
	Insurance

cultural, religious, educational, economic, and medical.[15] The treatment modalities on this limb address many of these issues, often focusing on creating new roles, new life scripts, and new settings. Cultural healing traditions include Ayurveda, traditional Chinese medicine, curanderismo, and indigenous traditional medicine. If your patient identifies with a particular ethnic tradition, inquire about any associated healing traditions.

The silent angel rests on the spiritual limb with the question, "When did you stop finding comfort in the sweet territory of silence?"[12] Table 3.38 features a mnemonic for spiritual diagnosis,[16] SAVE, and presents examples of spiritual healing options. Spirituality is deeply personal and often is connected with a particular religious faith. This calls for deep respect when inquiring about this aspect of a person's life. Do not underestimate the power of the spiritual limb during a patient's heightened vulnerability when suffering an affliction.

You might be surprised how many people undergo a spiritual crisis that impacts their health, from life cycle crises such as postpartum depression and midlife crises to life epiphanies including "born again" experiences and dramatic vocational changes. Visits with various kinds of spirits, including animal spirits, unseen beings, and angels, are also common human experiences, as is the feeling of deep emptiness as if you have lost your soul.

Fortunately, several tools for doing a spiritual assessment are available. I have found Open Invite to be one of the more helpful in the primary medical care setting.[17] It "opens" or introduces the topic of spirituality and "invites" the patient into a conversation about the topic. The *opening questions* include, "What helps you through hard times?" "May I ask about your faith or spirituality?" The *invite questions* focus on spiritual needs related to health, health

TABLE 3.38 Spiritual Naming and Caring

		Caring Examples
S	Soul *Story*: Life cycle issue, e.g., midlife crisis	Pastoral care
A	Soul *Awakened*: Epiphany/turning point	Shamanism
		Prayer
V	Soul *Visited*: Transpersonal, e.g., angel visit	Spiritual disciplines, e.g., confession and forgiveness
E	Soul *Escapes*: Soul loss	Gardening/Nature walks
		Healing ceremony

care decisions, and needed resources. The FICA tool[18] is also useful, with the mnemonic FICA (Faith, Importance, Community, Address) helping prompt you about areas of spirituality to assess.

The Clinical Hand's Naming and Caring Tree resides in a habitat. That geography also serves as a source of malady and health and holds the question, "When did you stop trusting the land?" Table 3.39 notes both diagnostic factors in the habitat and some examples of therapeutic interventions. The aide-mémoire PAW SCAB identifies many common features in our habitat that are both beneficial and an origin of malady.

Climate change significantly accelerates and promotes the role of these features in the production and maintenance of malady. Spending regular time in natural settings presumes the air is healthy and the place relatively safe. Check before prescribing. The Japanese have the concept, *shinrin yoku* (*forest bathing*),[19] and the oft-repeated refrain "go touch grass" in social media refers to leaving your screen and going outside. Good ideas!

Gardening in the earth is soothing and grounding. Trees and the land communicate through prolific root systems and mycorrhizal networks. Information spreads through the tree's cellular transport systems along with its sap.[20] This is depicted in Figure 3.22 as *bioenergy*. Though this construct is rarely noted in the biomedical literature, it is common in most cultural healing traditions, whether referred to as chi, qi, prana, or life force energy, and it is widely supported across populations worldwide. Traditional acupuncture is constructed on a belief in chi flow and correcting its blockage. Bioenergy is a useful concept in helping you and patients build healing stories for their maladies,[21] but recognize that it can also be a doorway into pseudoscience.

The Clinical Hand (see Figures 2.5, 3.1, and 3.9) portrays an ape with a prominent C on its chest hanging onto two of the tree limbs. Let me introduce

TABLE 3.39 Habitat Naming and Caring

		Caring Examples
P	Plants	Mitigate the problem
A	Animals	Move
W	Water	Advocacy
S	Soil	Spend regular time in natural settings: "Go touch grass"
C	Climate	
A	Air	
B	Buildings	

the Swinging Cultural Ape. The ape, as opposed to a human, reminds us of our evolutionary ancestry and the importance of evolution in understanding and appreciating why we, as human animals, are what we are and how we are connected to the story of life.[22,23] Our evolutionary heritage prompts us to respect the remarkable adaptive capacities, resilience, robustness, and antifragility properties of humans, as well as our diversity and interdependence with the rest of life. We are still evolving, as the steady emergence of new strains of different viruses attests.[24,25] Keep this in mind as you care for patients.

The C on the ape's chest stands for *culture*, the pervasive, often unconscious, human design template that guides much of our behavior. We are born sponges for culture, and by age 2 we have begun learning not only a language and its grammar but many of the unconscious expectations and ways of being within the world of people with whom we belong. The more accurate term is *bioculture* since culture weaves its way into our biology and vice versa, making the nature-or-nurture arguments irrelevant; the answer is always both.[26] Culture is why learning to be culturally sensitive and responsive matters.[27,28]

Culture is also what shapes the meaning of a symbol. Healing symbols, a type of ritual symbol, have special importance for the generalist's craft.[29,30] The stethoscope, exam table, and hypodermic syringe carry special significance. Ritual and healing symbols are bivalent, which means they have both an ideological or meaning-laden dimension and a physiology-action dimension. The stethoscope means clinician, listening, touching skin, detecting, power, secrets, heart, lungs, arteries, and intestines, and it provokes anxious physiologic reactions in muscle tone and heart rate and more. It is a powerful tool. When it connects you to the inner sanctum of the patient's body, remember this. Use it with care and reverence as you examine the patient. Share with them what it tells you. The exam table symbolizes a particular kind of place filled with a range of meanings including disease, hope, power, vulnerability, and violated taboos as well as being touched, probed, and viewed in a state of undress. Getting onto an exam table in a clinician's office triggers multiple physiologic responses and can trigger traumatic memories. The exam table is sacred space. Use it wisely and with deep respect. The hypodermic syringe also activates physiologic responses and symbolizes hope, fear, penetration, stabbing, power, and more. People's cultural backgrounds influence the many ways these healing symbols are perceived and received. Pay attention.

The biocultural ape poses in the tree clinging to two limbs as it prepares to swing to another. As generalist healers in search for a patient's malady and health story and possible care strategies, remember the mantra, "keep swinging." Swing across all the limbs and scan the habitat, remaining open and curious. Then hang out on the limbs that shine more brightly for the particular patient you are with. That brightness relates to the question associated with each limb. As you were doing your clinical discovery, evaluation, and sense-making work and then swinging through the diagnostic and treatment limbs, which question stirred your intuition? Has the patient stopped dancing and singing, become disenchanted with their own story, become less honest in relationships, lost comfort in silence, or stopped trusting the land? If the patient's response to one of those questions set your inner feelings aglow, spend more time on that limb. Check out those intuitive hunches with the patient.

Reflective Pause

Let us pause and check in on where you are in the clinical encounter. Remembering the ritual structure of the Clinical Hand, you reached the first guidepost and connected with the patient, then collaboratively set an agenda for the visit, getting to the second guidepost. Now on your way to the third guidepost, Hand Over, you've gathered pertinent information about the patient's malady stories, health and life story, and personal contexts. You've pursued specific diagnostic material to build a story that explains or at least offers additional next steps for explanation, and you are now searching for possible treatment and caring options. To help with this, you have swung through the tree limbs and habitat on the Palm of Hope. Being realistic, you improvised and did all this selectively. How did that selectivity happen?

Time to recall the agenda, type of encounter, and the Windmill Sails of Generalism for carefully selecting what tools and tips you apply in any given encounter. Focus on the agenda, and prioritize accordingly as you travel through the spiral of clinical discovery, where you inductively forage, recognize cues, generate hypotheses, and build the story. In a routine type of encounter, limit your search to the single simple issue, and you will quickly, within 5 to 10 minutes, make sense, confirm the diagnosis, and prepare several treatment options. In a maintenance ceremony, again let the goals for today's agenda set the pace and shape the field of view where you will search. Prioritize and personalize to the moment. Depending on the number of issues on the agenda, this can usually be done in 10 to 15 minutes. Dramas are different. The time spent will depend on how much time you scheduled. Limit what you pursue to that time frame, and be clear when negotiating and setting the agenda. The content of each drama encounter depends on where you are in the overall drama. Module 4 will go into this in more detail. All of this seems like so much, but it becomes manageable and fun when you remember to recognize, prioritize, and then personalize. You can breathe again. Now, back to treatment and care planning.

REFERENCES

1. Seki SM, DeGeorge KC, Plews-Ogan ML, et al. Physical exam: where's the evidence? A medical student's experience. *Fam Med Community Health.* 2020;8(1):e000284.
2. Morizot B. *Ways of Being Alive.* Polity Press; 2022.
3. Luft J, Ingham H. The Johari window, a graphic model of interpersonal awareness. Proceedings of the Western Training Laboratory in Group Development. University of California Press; 1955.
4. Donner-Banzhoff N. Solving the diagnostic challenge: a patient-centered approach. *Ann Fam Med.* 2018;16(4):353-358.
5. Heneghan C, Glasziou P, Thompson M, et al. Diagnostic strategies used in primary care. *BMJ.* 2009;338:b946.
6. Custers EJFM. Thirty years of illness scripts: theoretical origins and practical applications. *Med Teach.* 2015;37(5):457-462.
7. Klein JG. Five pitfalls in decisions about diagnosis and prescribing. *BMJ.* 2005;330(7494):781-783.
8. Ramanayake RPJC, Basnayake BMTK. Evaluation of red flags minimizes missing serious diseases in primary care. *J Fam Med Prim Care.* 2018;7(2):315-318.
9. Murtagh J, Bird S, eds. *Murtagh's Cautionary Tales.* 3rd ed. McGraw-Hill Education Pty Ltd; 2019.
10. Illich I. *Limits to Medicine: Medical Nemesis: The Expropriation of Health.* Penguin Books, Ltd; 1976.
11. Sims R, Kazda L, Michaleff ZA, et al. Consequences of health condition labelling: protocol for a systematic scoping review. *BMJ Open.* 2020;10(10):e037392.
12. Arrien A. *The Four-Fold Way: Walking the Paths of the Warrior, Teacher, Healer, and Visionary.* HarperOne; 1993.
13. Langley C, Armand S, Luo Q, et al. Chronic escitalopram in healthy volunteers has specific effects on reinforcement sensitivity: a double-blind, placebo-controlled semi-randomised study. *Neuropsychopharmacology.* 2023;48(4):664-670.
14. Gubrium JF. *The Mosaic of Care: Frail Elderly and Their Families in the Real World.* Springer Publishing Company; 1991.
15. Smilkstein G. The family in trouble—how to tell. *J Fam Pract.* 1975;2(1):19-24.
16. Koenig HG. *Spirituality in Patient Care: Why, How, When, and What.* Templeton Foundation Press; 2002.
17. Kuckel DP, Jones AL, Smith DK. The spiritual assessment. *Am Fam Physician.* 2022;106(4):415-419.
18. Puchalski CM. The FICA spiritual history tool #274. *J Palliat Med.* 2014;17(1):105-106.
19. William F. *The Nature Fix: Why Nature Makes Us Happier, Healthier, and More Creative.* W. W. Norton & Company; 2017.
20. Simard S. *Finding the Mother Tree: Discovering the Wisdom of the Forest.* Alfred A. Knopf; 2021.

21. Hintz KJ, Yount GL, Kadar I, et al. Bioenergy definitions and research guidelines. *Altern Ther Health Med.* 2003;9(3 suppl):A13-A30.
22. Condemi S, Savatier F. *A Pocket History of Human Evolution: How We Became Sapiens.* The Experiment LLC; 2019.
23. Tattersall I. *Understanding Human Evolution.* Cambridge University Press; 2022.
24. Fabrega H Jr. *Evolution of Sickness and Healing.* University of California Press; 1997.
25. Lieberman DE. *The Story of the Human Body: Evolution, Health, and Disease.* Pantheon Books; 2013.
26. Carroll J, Clasen M, Jonsson E, et al. Biocultural theory: the current state of knowledge. *Evol Behav Sci.* 2017;11(1):1-15.
27. Culhane-Pera KA, Reif C, Egli E, et al. A curriculum for multicultural education in family medicine. *Fam Med.* 1997;29(10):719-723.
28. Dobbie AE, Medrano M, Tysinger J, et al. The BELIEF Instrument: a preclinical teaching tool to elicit patients' health beliefs. *Fam Med.* 2003;35(5):316-319.
29. Helman CG. *Culture, Health and Illness.* 5th ed. Hodder Arnold; 2007.
30. Stein F. *American Medicine as Culture.* Westview Press; 1990.

Unit Five: The Journey to Hand Over: Sensemaking

The Round Table of Evidence and Information Mastery

The Round Table of Evidence

We've just finished swinging through the tree of the Clinical Hand and imagined what is troubling the patient, and we've started preparing some treatment options. Now, what is the evidence for treatment? What other options might there be? What does the patient think? How do we make sense of what we have learned? Time for us to leave the sacred space around the exam table and move to the Round Table of Evidence where we find an ecology of knowledge from multiple sources (see Figure 3.23).

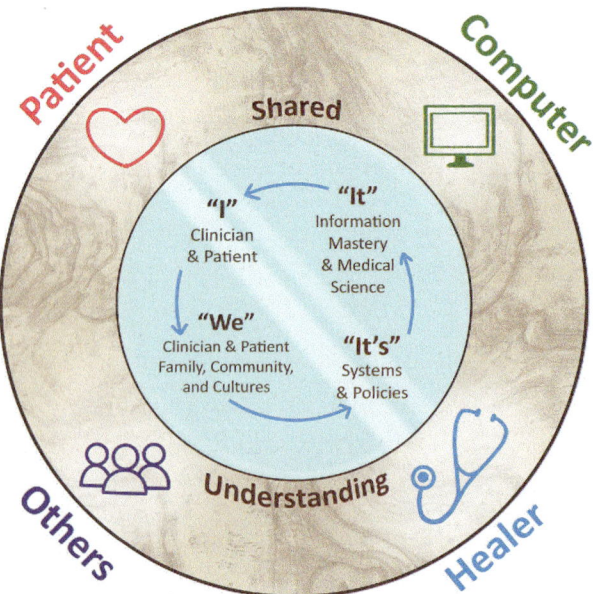

FIGURE 3.23. The Round Table of Evidence.

Everyone gathers around the table, even the computer "spirit." Depending on the situation, family members or a friend, a member of your clinical ensemble, and even a specialist you contacted virtually may be there. And more than likely, a computer screen and keyboard are available and visible to all. At the Round Table of Evidence, everyone explores and evaluates the evidence for the multiple diagnostic and treatment options that have emerged. Collaboratively, you reach a shared understanding from which to begin the work of Finding Common Ground and making decisions. This is relationship-centered, evidence-informed primary medical care. The Round Table of Evidence tool expands on the models of evidence-based medicine taught in most medical schools that focus on the application of research evidence by taking into account the clinical state and circumstances, patient preference, and clinical expertise.[1,2] It does this and more, incorporating multiple evidences and knowledges, the tools of information mastery and sensemaking, and contextualizes them.

The ways of knowing and evidence inhabiting the ecology of knowledge at the center of the table are represented by the Generalist Wheel of Inquiry (see Figure 3.24).[3,4]

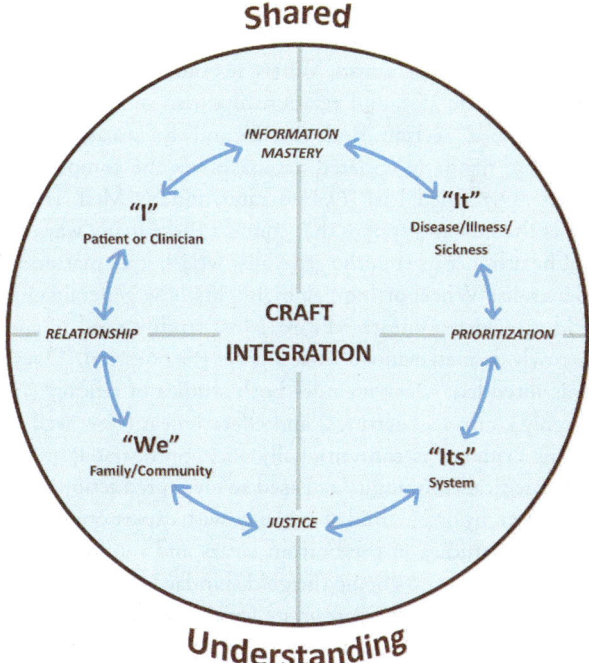

FIGURE 3.24. The Generalist Wheel of Inquiry.

The upper half of the wheel refers to knowledge about individuals, and the lower half highlights knowledge about the collective. The left side of the wheel focuses on inner, conscious perspectives, and the right side of the wheel focuses on the outer or external observed world. The resulting four sections of the wheel answer different questions and require different ways of knowing, resulting in different types of knowledge. The upper left inner/individual section of the wheel, the "I" perspective, offers insights into the question, "What are the words?," that derive from qualitative and self-reflective methods for understanding. Most current health care research focuses on the upper right outer/individual, or "It," section of the wheel and answers the question, "What are the numbers?" This is the territory of biomedicine, epidemiology, and most clinical research using quantitative methods. Where these two top sections of the wheel intersect is the domain of information mastery. The question, "Who benefits?," is addressed in the lower right outer/collective section, the "Its" perspective, and uses mixed methods and multiple voices to generate knowledge about systems, organizations, and policy. The intersection of the two outer sections is the realm of prioritization. Finally, the lower left inner/collective section of the wheel, the "We" perspective, answers the question, "What else?" This section requires qualitative, mixed methods, and many voices as it witnesses the knowledge of family, community, and clinical team experiences. Where it bounds the "Its" section is the world of policy and justice, and relationships rise to importance where it intersects with the "I" section. Both the "It" and "Its" areas of the wheel are easily accessed in regularly updated databases via the computer, for example, UpToDate, DynaMed, PEPID, Epocrates, and NatMed. The generalist's craft serves as the hub and spokes that connect these many ways of knowing in service of health. Let us spin the generalist wheel; it all matters!

The Generalist Wheel of Inquiry highlights how generalism adds value to the world of evidence-informed care. Most studies used to generate our current narrowly defined evidence base answer the question, "Does it reliably do what was intended?" This includes both studies of efficacy (how well it works in highly controlled settings) and effectiveness (how well it works in practice). This evidence is conventionally and appropriately understood in the specialist medical community as based solely on reductionist science and adheres to a hierarchy or pyramid of evidence with expert opinion, case series, and observational studies in the bottom layers and randomized controlled trials and systematic reviews being the gold standard at the top.[5] The Round Table of Evidence tool, more appropriate for the generalist primary medical care setting, embraces an ancient forest standard where all the evidence is welcome and evaluated within the contexts of those gathered at the table as an ecology of knowledge. Generalism asks for much more and addresses the questions, "Who benefits?" and "What else?" Generalists also consider when to use general therapeutic approaches and when to use targeted methods (see Table 3.40).

The Round Table of Evidence is individualized and tailored for the patient, emphasizes judgment over rules, builds on the healing relationship, and incorporates public health concerns.[6] It considers multiple cultural points of view. Western medicine assumes a single universe, and the cause of an ailment is something physically wrong within the person. The goal is to unmask what is wrong and correct or mitigate using scientific approaches. But some other cultures presume multiple universes, such as the three-tiered universe of the shaman. The cause of affliction might be an intentional attack by a spirit being. The diagnosis might involve identifying the invisible being who signifies the need for a major life change, in which case treatment involves creating a new sense of belonging and forging new social group affiliations.[7] There are research and resource literatures for integrative, complementary, and alternative medicine that can be helpful.[8-10] Generalist healers and their patients bring all of this to the table. It is all evidence. The three Windmill Sails of Generalism offer a framework for describing how this works in each clinical encounter: recognize the evidence that matters for the visit, evaluate and prioritize that evidence, and contextualize and personalize it for use by the patient to find common ground and codevelop an engaging plan.

TABLE 3.40 Additional Evidence Questions for Generalists

Who benefits?
What harms?
What costs?
What burdens?
What are the patient's capacities and resources?
How well does this treatment approach fit with the patient's past experiences?
How well does this treatment approach fit with different patients and their different beliefs and values and goals?
What about interactions?
What about ecological effects?
What about evolutionary perspectives?
What are other options?
How does this treatment approach compare to other options?
What about my own past clinical experiences?

Let us start by finding and recognizing the evidence that matters for the encounter. Searching for evidence at the round table with your patient affords an opportunity to educate patients on how to search the Internet and differentiate the useful from the problematic. Seize the moment. Table 3.41 summarizes the types of evidence explored at the round table and some of the sources for that knowledge.

TABLE 3.41 Types and Sources of Evidence

Types of Evidence	Sources of Evidence

Values and Preferences	Patient, family, and friends
	    Cultural traditions
	    Spiritual beliefs
	    Attitudes toward health care
	Clinician
	    (As above)

Patient Capacities	Patient
	    Health literacy
	    Access-to-care needs
	    Competing responsibilities
	    SCREEM (Social, Cultural, Religious, Educational, Economic, Medical) resources
	    Health behavior

Community Capacities	Health system Legal system Political context
Clinical Circumstances	Patient Severity, complications, location

Expertise	Patient
	    Body wisdom
	Clinician
	    Clinical experience
	Others

Habitat Features	Patient
	    Knowledge of neighborhood, etc.
	Computer
	    Maps, contamination sites, parks, transportation schedules, etc.

TABLE 3.41	Continued
Research Evidence	Medical and social science literature Complementary and alternative medicine literature Integrative medicine literature

With the evidence gathered, it is time to evaluate and prioritize. I usually begin with the four questions shown in Table 3.42.[11] These apply to information regarding diagnostics, studies, treatments, and more.

What are the numbers? Critically examine what numbers and statistics were used and whether the assumptions underlying the statistics or measures fit the reality of the questions and your situation. Ponder what is missing. A common mistake in the medical literature is oversimplifying and obscuring the biomedical story by inappropriately using a measure of central tendency (mean, median, or mode) when the distribution of the variable, like blood pressure in some populations, is not normal or Gaussian but has a long tail of outliers. Number needed to harm is frequently neglected. Table 3.43 proposes a few quick questions to ask of quantitative studies in the medical literature.[12]

What are the words? Pay special attention to how results are described. Note what is missing or where something is being exaggerated. Table 3.44 suggests some questions to better evaluate qualitative studies in both the medical and social science literature.[13]

Science is, for better and worse, a human endeavor. Power, money, and associated conflicts of interest seep into medical research to warp what questions get studied, what gets published, the content of clinical guidelines, and more. Thus, *Who benefits?* This question especially applies to drug trials and marketing efforts. Follow the money. The fourth question looks beyond the immediate focus of the question being studied. *What else?* Think about the ecological and longer-term possible consequences. Pay special attention to the interdependences.

TABLE 3.42	The Four Questions for Information Evaluation
What are the numbers?	Numeracy
What are the words?	Literacy
Who benefits?	Policy
What else? (follow the ripples)	Ecolacy

TABLE 3.43	Questions for Evaluating Quantitative Studies

Is the sample randomized?

Is the study design appropriate for the hypothesis?
  Experimental: RCT—intervene, observe effect
  Observational: Case–control—match groups, observe
  Longitudinal: Cohort—follow participants over time
  Cross-sectional: Each participant only examined once

Who's in, who's out, how big, and who said, "No"?

Are the measures reliable and valid?

What are potential confounders, e.g., historical effects?

What are the Type 1 (statistical significance) and Type 2 errors (power)?
  Minimum standards: $P < .05$; $\beta < 0.20$

Are the statistics appropriate? Is the distribution of key variable normal?

RCT, randomized controlled trial.

TABLE 3.44	Questions for Evaluating Qualitative Studies

Is the method appropriate for the question?
  Observation for behavior
  Interviews for perceptions
  Documents for historical information

Is the sampling strategy information rich? Is data saturation achieved?

Is iteration evident, and does it include seeking disconfirming evidence?

Are the findings/story convincing beyond superficial description?

Is reflexivity evident?
  Do you know the author(s) presuppositions?
  How was the author(s) changed by the study?

Information Mastery

Information mastery is a practical package of tools for helping generalist clinicians in primary care find and evaluate the medical literature and resonates well with the Round Table of Evidence. Based on the guiding principle that some information or evidence is more useful than others to clinicians and patients, information mastery helps us find, evaluate, and use that evidence through the application of four concepts. The first concept advises us to search for and read only POEMs, or Patient-Oriented Evidence that Matters.[14] POEMs provide information or evidence that helps a patient live longer or better. This is in contrast to DOE, or Disease-Oriented Evidence—information about disease and treatments that does not include evidence of meaningful patient outcomes. Table 3.45 contrasts POEMs and DOEs.[15]

The second concept in information mastery is the usefulness equation, which states that the usefulness of evidence equals the relevance of the results to the clinical situation, multiplied by the validity of the information, divided by how much work it takes to obtain the evidence.[16] Four critical questions help you achieve that usefulness (see Table 3.46). The team behind

TABLE 3.45 POEMs Versus DOEs

Patient-Oriented Evidence That Matters
(Outcomes directly related to patient's experience)
- Quality of life
- Mortality
- Pain (including Pain scale)
- Mobility
- Recovery time
- Length of hospital stay
- Cost

Disease-Oriented Evidence
(Surrogates for patient's condition)
- Cardiac biomarkers
- Blood pressure reading
- Low-density lipoprotein, high-density lipoprotein
- Blood sugar
- Bone density
- Body mass index
- Other laboratory tests

TABLE 3.46 — Questions to Identify Useful Information

Will this information have a direct bearing on outcomes my patients care about?
Is the problem common in my practice?
If valid, will this study require changing my practice?
Is the study valid?

information mastery, led by Allen Shaughnessy and David Slawson, developed multiple teaching tools and worksheets for optimizing its usefulness that can be found at the Center for Information Mastery website at Tufts School of Medicine, Department of Family Medicine. One of those tools, STEPS (Safety, Tolerability, Effectiveness, Price, Simplicity), aids in evaluating and comparing pharmacotherapeutics. Table 3.47 shows the STEPS to take when assessing a drug.[17]

Concept three highlights the need for resources to hunt for information at the point of care,[18] such as the computer databases noted earlier and some kind of keeping-up resource that finds information that is both relevant and valid.[19] The fourth concept is clinical jazz, the music of the generalist's craft where we harmonize and riff on the mix of best available information at the Round Table of Evidence. Highly recommend becoming an information master!

TABLE 3.47 — STEPS for Evaluating Pharmacotherapeutics

Item	Description
Safety	Long-term or serious side effects
Tolerability	Bothersome side effects Pooled drop-out rates
Effectiveness	How well it works in real-life settings Comparative effectiveness trials
Price	Include cost of monitoring side effects
Simplicity	Ease of administration and storage

Data from Shaughnessy AF. STEPS drug updates. *Am Fam Physician*. 2003;68(12): 2342-2348.

Sensemaking

The patient and you have successfully recognized and gathered the evidence related to the clinical encounter and prioritized that which is most useful. Now is the time for personalizing and tailoring, for the contextualization of care and sensemaking. Contextualizing care refers to making sure the care strategy considers the patient's circumstances, attitudes, and behaviors.[20] Here is where you account for the particulars of the patient's situation: the recent death of a pet, needing to care for a spouse who suffered a stroke, loss of the family's only car, difficulty swallowing pills, or fear of injections and vaccines. This is how you move from caring to healing.[21] Sensemaking is the process we use to incorporate the prioritized evidence with the personal and contextual to finish building our explanatory story and care options. According to Karl Weick, "The basic idea of sensemaking is that reality is an ongoing accomplishment that emerges from efforts to create order and make retrospective sense of what occurs."[22] Note how this differs from decision-making, which is a rational process of choosing between defined options. Sensemaking is the process of reducing ambiguity so that situations can be understood, problems defined, and plausible options delimited. Sensemaking engages the Elephant and the Rider of Changing Behavior, whereas decision-making speaks only to the Rider (see Figure 2.4). Reframing the earlier quote from Weick, the basic idea of generalist primary medical care is that health is an ongoing accomplishment that emerges from efforts to create order and make retrospective sense of the embodied experiences of patients. Sounds great, but how do we do it?

Hang in there because before I delve into doing sensemaking, I have one more concept to introduce pertaining to scale. As a generalist clinician in the 21st century, I am increasingly being recommended treatments that alter human genes and being told to assess and intervene on the social and ecological drivers of health. Really? There is no easy answer to that question, but I recommend that generalist healers in primary care focus their energy on more sensible scales. All living beings evolved sensory means for interacting and learning within their environments. This suggests that life together works out better when each organism acts within the purview of what it can sense. In other words, when they act within "sensible scales" (see Figure 3.25).

I use the term *sensible* here because this is the scale range for which our brains and bodies, our senses, coevolved, and because they are within the range where we are most capable of making sense. For humans, these include the system scales between local community and cell (visible using simple microscope) and serve as a caution for generalist healers in primary care. Likewise, communities, corporations, and nation-states have their own appropriate senses for their own sensible scales. Direct human action above the

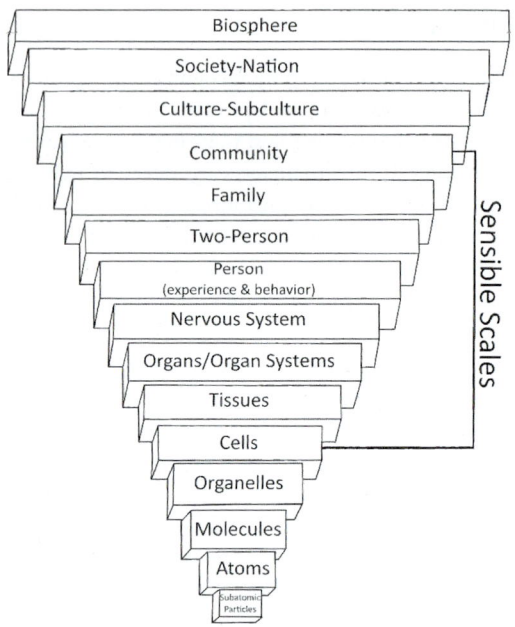

FIGURE 3.25. Sensible Scales for Generalists.

system level of local community or below the level of cells greatly increases the risk of unanticipated consequences. When intervening at the organelle and molecular levels, referral to specialists should be considered because this is often where specialists work. Collaboration becomes critical. When intervening at or above the community level, the limitations of the clinical office setting require connections with community organizations and public health. With that caveat established, we are ready to do sensemaking.

Sensemaking begins with determining the time frame being considered—the next few days, week, months? Then you practice another form of eye juggling: With one eye, you look to identify who else is here, referred to as social anchoring, and you look for cues as to what is out there and where to direct your attention. With another eye, you look at yourself, your identity, who you are, and what you know. With the third eye, you look back, employ retrospection, and reflect on what you've done before in similar situations, activating your well of clinical experience. Then, you invite the patient to participate in this process, producing collaborative sensemaking. Using these three viewpoints, you organize a "good-enough" explanation, a plausible one, and explicitly identify the actions that can be taken and the reality those actions create, referred to as *enactment*. This good-enough sensemaking story and these treatment options move into the work of Finding Common Ground and Making Decisions to Hand Over as the patient's healing story and engaging plan. Table 3.48 summarizes this sensemaking process and highlights important elements gleaned while exploring the health and malady stories, understanding the whole person in context, working through Clinical Discovery and Evaluation, swinging on the Naming and Caring Tree, and collaborating at the Round Table of Evidence.

TABLE 3.48 The Sensemaking Process in the Clinical Encounter

Sensemaking Element	Exploring Stories Understanding the Whole Person	Clinical Discovery Tree Swinging
Looking Out Social Anchoring and Cues	Patient Colleagues Health and malady stories FIFE and illness prototype (IPs) Life cycle stage Genogram *Proximal and distal context* Livelihoods identity	Computer Evidences Cues and hunches Hypotheses Tree limb possibilities
Looking In Identity	Family Healer's journey Clinical expertise	
Looking Back Retrospection	Past shared experiences Patient's past illness experiences	Clinical experience Critical incidents Illness scripts
Making Sense Plausibility and Enactment	Good-enough explanatory story Care/treatment options Shared understanding	
Finding Common Ground and Making Decisions Hand Over Healing Story and Engaging Plan		

FIFE, feelings, ideas, function, expectations.

This is a critical moment of integration in the clinical encounter, and the process, as presented, can feel a bit abstract and overwhelming. It is challenging work and needs practice, but it is also one of the most gratifying stages of practicing the generalist's craft. Let's illustrate with an example.

You are seeing 48-year-old Pedro Rodriguez for the third time in the past 15 months. He has been followed at the clinic for 7 years, but when his prior personal primary care physician, a family medicine resident, graduated over a year ago, she transferred their relationship to you. You've seen him only once since your introduction at the time of transfer; since then, he has missed three scheduled appointments. You have been worried about him and have mixed feelings when you see his name on your schedule alongside the words, "abdominal pain." You like Pedro, a proud and remarkably resilient man, but he is tight-lipped, has serious problems and health risks, and you have struggled to develop a relationship. Preparing for the visit, you review the chart, recalling his problem list of hepatitis C with compensated early cirrhosis, essential hypertension, osteoarthritis, and history of right subdural hematoma. His only prescribed medication is amlodipine 5 mg once a day. The most recent clinical data from his last visit 9 months ago include a hemoglobin A1c of 5.9, fasting glucose of 110, blood pressure of 156/94, and waist circumference of 41 in. As you approach the exam room, your ensemble colleague, Mika, who brought Pedro back to the room, recorded his initial vital signs and checked in on why he was here today. She reports that he looks more worried than usual and says he is here because of several recent falls. She lives in the same neighborhood as Pedro and shares some gossip from a friend that Pedro's having problems at home with his wife, Olivia, and children, Isabella and Mia. You ask about the vital signs, and she says they're fine except the blood pressure is up at 165/102. You sigh. The elevated blood pressure, the gossip, and the disconnect between his appointment reason for the encounter and the one shared with your colleague points to a possible new drama. You prepare for a possible transition ceremony. You take a deep breath, open your hand, recenter your intentions, knock on the door, and turn the knob. The encounter begins, and you initiate the ritual structure and the move toward the guidepost of Connect. Let us zoom forward in time.

You connect and, collaboratively with Pedro, set an agenda. You both agree this is a new drama and, thus, a transition ceremony. His actual reason for connecting is not the abdominal pain or the falling, although they worry him. It is a problem with living, and he was sanctioned to come by his wife, Olivia, to address "drinking too much." He desperately fears losing his family and, uncharacteristically, cried when he brought this up. You BATHEd him before proceeding to finish negotiating and setting the agenda. You note that he mentioned being pleased to see Mika, your clinical associate, again. The final Set Agenda was to address the alcohol drinking and begin planning for dealing with family issues, along with your desire to rule out potential serious problems causing the falls and abdominal pain. This took 10 minutes. During the weaving of what was learned while setting the agenda; exploring stories and understanding the whole person in context; and clinical discovery and evaluation craft work, you learn that he struggled with alcohol in the past but kept it a secret from the doctors at the clinic. He went to a local Alcoholics Anonymous (AA) group recommended by a friend 8 years ago and has been abstinent since—well, until 8 months ago when his 28-year-old son, Carlos, from a prior partner was arrested for selling fentanyl as a member of a local gang. Since then, Pedro had fallen twice at home when drunk, the last time being 2 weeks ago, after which he scheduled this appointment. He denied head injury and headaches. The abdominal pain began about 6 months ago when his wife found out about his 28-year-old son. Pedro had kept this a secret from Olivia, his wife of 25 years, until Olivia's friend reported seeing Pedro at the jail. Pedro's life was shattered, and he had felt too ashamed to see you, which is why he had missed his prior appointments. His family, which also includes 20- and 25-year-old daughters Isabella and Mia, is his biggest concern. The abdominal pain was spasmodic and associated with intermittent constipation but not with meals. He denied melena, bright red blood, vomiting, lightheadedness, or syncope. He is not eating well. He has been out of work for a year since his layoff from a local warehouse firm. He does have Medicaid insurance. His parents are still alive and just scraping by in Puerto Rico; he has not seen them in 3 years and worries about them. There is no alcohol on his breath. He has been erratic in taking his amlodipine. Your brief neurologic exam along with heart and lung auscultation and palpation of the abdomen reveals no remarkable findings. A stool guaiac was negative. The lowest of two additional blood pressure measurements was 160/98. When swinging on the tree from the Clinical Hand tool, the cognitive and spiritual limbs were brighter. Pedro has become disenchanted with his story and frightened in the territory of silence. Only a few types of evidence have been briefly explored. A quick computer check on red flags for gastrointestinal bleeding or subdural hematoma is reassuring. You still remember a patient where you initially missed a subdural hematoma, and she ended up in the emergency room 2 days later requiring emergency surgery. You have been in the room for 16 minutes of a 20-minute scheduled visit. What do you do, practitioner of the generalist's craft?

Table 3.49 summarizes some of the key parts of the sensemaking process, including working hypotheses and pertinent evidence, for this clinical

TABLE 3.49 The Sensemaking Process for Pedro's Clinical Encounter

Sensemaking Element	Exploring Stories Understanding the Whole Person	Clinical Discovery Tree Swinging
Looking Out Social Anchoring and Cues	Pleased to see your associate, Mika Past medical history: htn.; hepatitis C with early cirrhosis; osteoarthritis; h/o subdural hematoma Meds: amlodipine 5 mg once daily Stories: Prior alcoholism with h/o AA success; son, Carlos, arrested for drug sales; poor medication adherence FIFE: ashamed; wants to stop drinking and save family; not functioning well Proximal and distal context: Medicaid: Life cycle: children leaving home; Family: "secret" son revealed; wife Olivia feels betrayed; parents struggling in Puerto Rico; Livelihoods identity: laid off work	Computer: red-flag check OK Cues and hunches: no signs or symptoms of GI bleed or mass effect from subdural; falls when drunk; no weight change; blood pressure high Hypotheses: Alcohol binge; losses with depression; possible spiritual crisis; susto; irritable bowel Tree limb possibilities: Physical: alcohol complicating cirrhosis; htn.; arthritis Emotional: threat of loss Cognitive: self-judging; loss of self-esteem Social: more isolation; income loss Spiritual: soul loss
Looking In Identity	Family: father died at 50 from alcohol complications Healer's journey: 3 y out of family medicine (FM) residency; doing craft at clinic with FM residents Clinical expertise: still doing hospital and birthing care	

Looking Back Retrospection	Past shared experiences: few; secrets Patient's past illness experiences: alcohol bingeing; subdural; chronic liver disease	Clinical experience: full-time: full scope with vulnerable, diverse population Critical incidents: missed subdural dx. Illness scripts: head injury; GI bleed; alcoholism; depression; irritable bowel; hepatitis C: hypertension

Making Sense
Plausibility and
Enactment

Good-enough explanatory story:
Pedro's children are now adults and leaving home; his parents are struggling in Puerto Rico, and he can't help them since unemployed, and then his "secret" son, Carlos, is arrested for drug dealing. He starts binge-drinking alcohol. His wife, Olivia, discovers the "secret" son. Pedro develops abdominal pain but keeps drinking, falls twice when drunk. Poor eating. A proud man now mired in shame, a shell of himself. Alcohol and stress worsening liver disease and increasing bleeding risk, both GI and intracranial, and also further elevating blood pressure. Despite high risk, you don't suspect active GI or intracranial bleed. Pedro knows he must stop drinking and restore family trust. Suspect depression, spiritual crisis, possible cultural syndrome of susto (soul loss), and irritable bowel.

Care/treatment options/questions:
Obtain blood work including metabolic profile, complete blood count, prothrombin time. Continue amlodipine; monitor BP. Consider CT scan of head. Consider prediabetes diagnosis. Call friend from local AA for connection and return for daily meetings for next week starting today. Possible referral to hepatitis clinic. Consider introducing to behavioral health therapist. Reschedule for 30-min first "drama" visit in next 3-5 d. Consider family conference and/or home visit within month.

Finding Common Ground and Making Decisions
Hand Over Healing Story and Engaging Plan

AA, Alcoholics Anonymous; BP, blood pressure; CT, computed tomography; FIFE, feelings, ideas, function, expectations; GI, gastrointestinal.

encounter with Pedro Rodriguez. The time frame for your sensemaking is the next week given the high risks of the situation. You have crafted a plausible explanatory story and have several care plans and questions to share with Pedro.

This is a good time to remind yourself about flow and improvisation. So far, all the activity from the Set Agenda guidepost toward the Hand Over checkpoint may seem sequential, like the figure depicting the Relationship-Centered Clinical Method (Figure 2.7). It is not. Up to Finding Common Ground, we weave back and forth both within and between the boxes on exploring, understanding, and discovering before sitting at the Round Table of Evidence. But even there, we may jump back to those other activities all depending on the flow of the interactions. You are improvising, recognizing windows of opportunity as they arise. Just like the Windmill Sails of Generalism, where recognize, prioritize, and personalize are not necessarily sequential but more like the paddles of a windmill (see Figure 2.3) always spinning depending on the movement and direction of the wind. This whirling motion within the Relationship-Centered Clinical Method slows down when we wrap up the sensemaking with an explanatory story and treatment options. Sensemaking completed, it is time for Finding Common Ground and collaborative decision-making.

REFERENCES

1. Haynes RB, Devereaux PJ, Guyatt GH. Clinical expertise in the era of evidence-based medicine and patient choice. *ACP J Club*. 2002;136(2):A11-A14.
2. Sackett DL, Rosenberg WM, Gray JA, et al. Evidence based medicine: what it is and what it isn't. *BMJ*. 1996;312(7023):71-72.
3. Stange KC, Miller WL, McWhinney I. Developing the knowledge base of family practice. *Fam Med*. 2001;33(4):286-297.
4. Stange KC. Ways of knowing, learning, and developing. *Ann Fam Med*. 2010;8(1):4-10.
5. Wallace SS, Barak G, Truong G, et al. Hierarchy of evidence within the medical literature. *Hosp Pediatr*. 2022;12(8):745-750.
6. Greenhalgh T, Howick J, Maskrey N; Evidence Based Medicine Renaissance Group. Evidence based medicine: a movement in crisis? *BMJ*. 2014;348:g3725.
7. Nathan T, Stengers I. *Doctors and Healers*. English ed. Polity Press; 2018.
8. Mortada EM. Evidence-based complementary and alternative medicine in current medical practice. *Cureus*. 2024;16(1):e52041.
9. Vincent C, Furnham A. Complementary medicine: state of the evidence. *J R Soc Med*. 1999;92(4):170-177.
10. Jonas WB. The evidence house: how to build an inclusive base for complementary medicine. *West J Med*. 2001;175(2):79-80.

11. Hardin G. *Filters Against Folly: How to Survive Despite Economists, Ecologists, and the Merely Eloquent*. Penguin Books; 1985.
12. Straus SE, Glasziou P, Richardson WS, et al. *Evidence-Based Medicine: How to Practice and Teach EBM*. 5th ed. Elsevier; 2019.
13. Crabtree BF, Miller WL. *Doing Qualitative Research*. 3rd ed. Sage Publications, Inc; 2023.
14. Slawson DC, Shaughnessy AF, Bennett JH. Becoming a medical information master: feeling good about not knowing everything. *J Fam Pract*. 1994;38:505-513.
15. Slawson DC, Shaughnessy AF, Ebell MH, et al. Mastering medical information and the role of POEMs—patient-oriented evidence that matters. *J Fam Pract*. 1997;45(3):195-196.
16. Shaughnessy AF, Slawson DC, Bennett JH. Becoming an information master: a guidebook to the medical information jungle. *J Fam Pract*. 1994;39(5):489-499.
17. Shaughnessy AF. STEPS drug updates. *Am Fam Physician*. 2003;68(12):2342-2348.
18. Ebell MH. How to find answers to clinical questions. *Am Fam Physician*. 2009;79(4):293-296.
19. Shaughnessy AF. Keeping up with the medical literature: how to set up a system. *Am Fam Physician*. 2009;79(1):26.
20. Weiner SJ. Contextualizing care: an essential and measurable clinical competency. *Patient Educ Couns*. 2022;105(3):594-598.
21. Weiner SJ. *On Becoming a Healer: The Journey from Patient Care to Caring about Your Patients*. Johns Hopkins University Press; 2020.
22. Weick KE. The collapse of sensemaking in organizations: the Mann Gulch disaster. *Adm Sci Q*. 1993;38(4):628-652.

Unit Six: The Journey to Hand Over: Finding Common Ground

Finding Common Ground and Making Shared Decisions

Conceptual Strategies for Finding Common Ground

We have almost reached the guidepost of Hand Over, but first, the patient and you must both agree on what is happening and what is next. We begin the work of Finding Common Ground and Making Decisions. This entails collaborative or shared decision-making and, sometimes, explicit negotiation. The patient and you need to reach agreement on three areas of common ground: the concerns, goals of care, and roles (see Figure 3.26).[1] What are *the agreed-upon concerns*, problems, and their priority? What are the goals of care, and are they linked to the patient's life story? What are each of the participants' roles, and what will they each do before the next connection?

This is where diagnosis and treatment strategy is converted to goals and a plan for the patient to take home. You convert your clinical action, what you learned, and your suggestions for care into an engaging plan, aiming power. Now intentionally share power and personalize. This is also where you again information gather, share, and educate from POISED when using the EHR with the patient.

Before elaborating on how to find common ground on concerns, goals, and roles, I highlight six conceptual approaches and associated skills that facilitate this part of the generalist's craft. Clarifying an understanding of harm is the first. Story embraces the complexities of life, and those complexities include the inevitability of harm. As healers, most of us were told, somewhere in our training, to follow the precept *"Primum non nocere,"* or "first, do no harm." What does that really mean? It is impossible. There is no harmless action, no

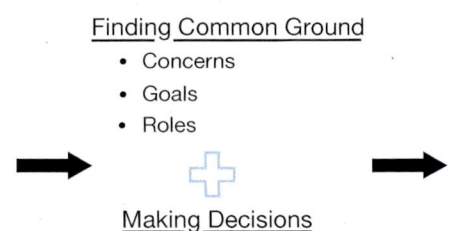

FIGURE 3.26. Finding Common Ground.

harmless intervention. Harm is a value-based concept since all actions are interactions and cause multiple changes, some of which will be harmful to something somewhere in the ecology of life. Call them inevitable side effects. All actions are relational and power-full. This is why the appropriate and wise use of power is a moral imperative for healers. Story enables this empowered wisdom. Better advice is to "minimize harm and optimize benefit" and "pay attention to the ripples." Remember the four questions: What are the numbers? What are the words? Who benefits? What else?

The second conceptual strategy to help us find common ground is to reconsider the second finger of the Clinical Hand tool, the guidepost of Set Agenda. That checkpoint finger signals us to address the actual reason for connecting and the issues set forth in the agenda as we develop the plan.

Finding Common Ground is a collaborative effort between the patient and you, and if the agenda was set collaboratively, and if you used a "think-aloud" strategy while implementing the Relationship-Centered Clinical Method, then the collaboration is conversational, goes well, and is easily achieved. The conversation advances even more fluidly with the use of effective communication skills, motivational interviewing, cultural sensitivity, awareness, and accommodation of the patient's health literacy,[2,3] and by connecting to the patient's learning style and language. Kolb's experiential learning cycle (see Figure S2.1) serves as a third helpful conceptual strategy[4] as it offers clues for identifying a patient's learning style during clinical discovery. The cycle delineates four modes of experience. *Concrete experience* and *abstract conceptualization* are how we emotionally engage a task, the perception continuum from feeling to thinking. *Reflective observation* and *active experimentation* are how we approach a task: the processing continuum from watching or observing to doing. How patients answer the questions, "What brings you here today?" and "What have you tried to help the concern?," provides clues. The first prompts perceptual responses (i.e., "My throat is scratchy, and I'm coughing so hard I can't get any work done")—specific descriptions suggesting the concrete experience mode. "I think I have a strep throat" is conceptual and consistent with the abstract conceptualization mode. The second question, about what was tried, requires a processing response. "I asked some friends and checked online" reveals the reflective observation mode. "I tried some over-the-counter pills and steam" reflects taking personal action: the active experimentation mode of doing. The best learning happens when all four modes are activated, but starting with the patient's dominant style helps motivate the Elephant of Changing Behavior and eases translating the plan into action.[5]

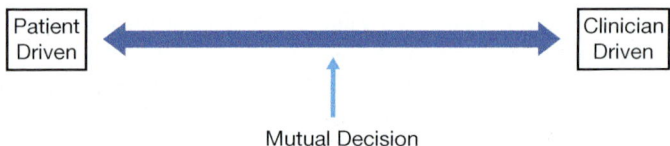

FIGURE 3.27. Continuum of Decision-Making.

The fourth conceptual framework is the Continuum of Decision-Making (see Figure 3.27). This figure reminds us that shared decision-making is a continuum. Severity of an ailment tends to move the arrow of mutual decision closer to being clinician-driven, as does older age of the patient. There is much cultural variation around how much patients want to be involved in decision-making. When people are well or younger and view the encounter as more transactional, they often prefer that decisions be patient-driven. As you share power, the arrow of mutual decision is likely to move toward the center, but start where the patient prefers.

Sometimes Finding Common Ground becomes contentious, especially when you feel strongly about what needs to happen next and the patient does not agree or vice versa. This is even more likely when there is a deep cultural divide.[6] At these times of conflict, the fifth conceptual strategy, the use of principled negotiation[7] and positive criticism,[8] can be helpful. Table 3.50

TABLE 3.50	Tips for Principled Negotiation and Positive Criticism

Principled Negotiation
Separate people from the problem: The patient is not the problem.
Focus on interests and interdependences, not position: Do not get stuck defending a particular means or solution.
Generate a variety of options and possibilities: Keep swinging on the Naming and Caring Tree.
Use agreed-upon criteria to judge the solution.

Positive Criticism
Protect self-esteem: Avoid destructive labels.
Choose the right words: Provide a positive intent statement.
Involve the patient: Listen, check it out, never assume.
Use their words.
Bring motivation into negotiation: Encourage readiness to change; identify incentives; How am I motivating? What's in it for the patient?
Stay cool, calm, collected: Manage arousal, humor; condition relaxation.

summarizes some of the more valuable tips for Finding Common Ground in the primary care clinical encounter using this strategy. Keep the problem that is generating the conflict "out there" where both of you can work on making sense and changing it. Remember the patient's goals and values; keep learning, and beware of defending. Invent options for mutual gain. How would you both know the situation is improving? When you believe the patient needs to hear some critique, such as when you observe a parent slapping their child when misbehaving, pay special heed to the positive-criticism tips.

The sixth concept to facilitate finding common ground is the capacity-to-burden ratio from minimally disruptive medicine.[9,10] Many of the questions suggested in our discussion of exploring the health and malady stories and understanding the whole person in context help assess the patient's capacity to successfully implement a given care plan. The SCREEM resources on the social limb of the Naming and Caring Tree also evaluate capacity. Equally important is appreciating and assessing the burden required for enacting a given treatment strategy. The tolerability, price, and simplicity prompts from the STEPS evaluation framework for pharmacotherapeutics does that for different drug therapies. Remember to match the burden of care to the capacity of the patient through shared decision-making.

Applying the six conceptual strategies as needed, we are ready to find common ground regarding concerns, goals, and roles.

Concerns: Problems and Priorities

Concerns in the Relationship-Centered Clinical Method refer to the explanatory story for the problems and priorities emerging from the clinical encounter. Ideally, the problems and concerns were identified when the agenda was set. But new concerns might have surfaced during the remainder of the visit and as priorities were established. You have built a story to explain the identified issues. That story should address the actual reason for connecting and respond to the patient's expectations. Now, you share it with the patient and listen for their feedback and questions. At the same time, you introduce care options that reflect your understanding and prioritization of the story. Again, seek feedback and questions from the patient. Before proceeding to make decisions about treatment, make sure you both agree on the explanatory story(s), and shift attention to defining the goals that will help shape the final treatment plan.

Goals: Goal-Oriented Care and Personalizing

What are the goals of care? There are at least two different time scales for answering this question. One looks toward the horizon of life and your life story and imagines what matters most, your core values, and how this influences

TABLE 3.51	Goal Types

Prevention of premature death and disability
Optimization of current health-related quality of life
Optimization of personal growth and development, including specific life goals
Improving chances of good death
Living as long as possible

Data from Mold JW. *Goal-Oriented Medical Care: Helping Patients Achieve Their Personal Health Goals*. Full Court Press; 2020.

your thinking about health and malady. Table 3.51 offers a list of five types of goals that help us be more explicit about these life span–level goals.[11]

Life cycle ceremonies of maintenance such as Medicare annual wellness exams or other health maintenance visits are an excellent time for having these discussions. I build these in as part of the agenda for these visits. A values history facilitates this conversation (see Table 3.52).[12]

These long-term goals are very helpful in guiding the determination of the short-term goals of care for specific malady episodes. Short-term goals are shaped by the patient's initial expectations for the clinical encounter and what has been uncovered during the visit. The goals need to address the identified concerns, be explicit, and make achievement of them easily recognizable by the patient and you. Once the short-term goals for the clinical encounter are clear, the patient and you advance to codesign your plan of care for reaching the goals.

TABLE 3.52	Values History

Which best fits you?
- "I want to live as long as possible, regardless of the quality of life that I experience."
- "I want to preserve a good quality of life, even if this means that I may not live as long."

What is a good quality of life for you?
- What activities do you enjoy?
- What makes you laugh or cry?
- What goals do you have for the future?
- What makes life worth living?

Wait! This is probably not what you learned in medical school. You can probably recite the drill: "Get the right diagnosis, then prescribe the evidence-based treatment." That drill is not part of the generalist's craft in high-quality primary medical care. Its common usage partly explains why 50% of prescribed medications are either not taken or taken incorrectly.[13] The patient never owned the plan. Recall the Elephant and the Rider of Changing Behavior (see Figure 2.4). The plan must speak to and be heard by the patient's fast-thinking brain; it needs to be emotionally charged. Cocreating the explanatory or diagnostic story, spending time together at the Round Table of Evidence recognizing care options, Finding Common Ground collaboratively, prioritizing, mutually setting goals, and then personalizing and tailoring the treatment plan does just that. It motivates the Elephant, directs the Rider, and shapes the path. Making health using the generalist's craft, especially swinging on the limbs of the Naming and Caring Tree, helps us avoid overmedicalization and inadvertently creating unnecessary dependency. Even when you have a definitive medical diagnosis and there is a specific medication's use supported by multiple randomized controlled trials, that drug may not be the best choice for the patient you are seeing given the circumstances and contexts of their life at this particular point in time. Recall the many treatment options on the limbs of the Naming and Caring Tree. Include them in your considerations. Tailor the plan to minimize burden and match capacity, to resonate with the patient's world—their life, malady, and health stories—to optimize developing self-care skills, minimize medicalizing, and meet the goals of care (see Table 3.53).

Sometimes the severity and risk of the disease warrants prescribing a specific drug despite initial patient resistance. More often, there is time to explore other potentially helpful options to gain the patient's trust, encourage further learning, and create opportunities to shift directions in the future. Recognize the situation; prioritize and personalize. Do the craft and perform the improvisational clinical jazz of the generalist's craft. Almost magical!

TABLE 3.53 **Questions to Guide Tailoring the Care Plan**

Does the plan minimize burden and match patient capacity?
Does the plan resonate with the patient's world?
  Their life story?
  Their malady and health stories?
Does the plan develop the patient's self-care skills?
Does the plan meet the mutually generated goals of care?

Roles

Once the patient and you agree on a management plan, the next lift in doing the craft carries you into defining everyone's role in enacting the plan. What is each person's specific "homework," and when is it due? This work includes you and any involved members of the practice ensemble, the patient, any family or friends, and any others implicated in the plan. Table 3.54 highlights this work of establishing roles.

We are almost ready to Hand Over care to the patient and send them back into their life, but not quite. Did you keep that list of possible items that did not make the agenda? New issues for the future may have surfaced during the clinical encounter that have not been directly addressed because they were not prioritized. Briefly review that list with the patient and decide on what the follow-up for those items might be. Document that list!

Table 3.55 depicts the explanatory story and plan for Pedro Rodriguez that resulted after Finding Common Ground and Making Shared Decisions. You will note some additions to the explanatory story in the table—highlighted in yellow—where Pedro wanted emphasis and in light blue where you, the clinician, had your own specific concerns. The patient rejected the diagnosis of susto (soul loss) and was defiantly resistant to a diagnostic label of depression. The plan pays attention to your clinical worries about head trauma, gastrointestinal bleeding, blood pressure, glucose, and depression, but it also emphasizes the patient's concerns about his alcohol use, his family, and his dignity. Also note how his personal connection to your clinical ensemble partner, Mika, is incorporated. Pedro's actual reason for connecting has been addressed, and his expectations have been met. The first pass on the Spiral of Healing is fulfilled.

TABLE 3.54 Roles

What is everyone's specific "homework," and when is it due?

Who?
- Patient and family
- Clinician and practice ensemble/team
- Others in larger health care team
- Medical record
- Community

Don't forget to document the roles!

TABLE 3.55 Pedro's Explanatory Story and Engaging Plan

Explanatory Story
(Patient additions highlighted in yellow and clinician's in light blue; issues still controversial highlighted in gray; issues dropped marked with strikethrough.)

Pedro's children are now adults and leaving home; his parents are struggling in Puerto Rico, and he can't help them as much as he'd like since unemployed, and then his "secret" son, Carlos, is arrested for drug dealing. He starts binge drinking alcohol. His wife, Olivia, discovers the "secret" son. "All hell breaks loose." Pedro develops abdominal pain but keeps drinking, falls twice when drunk. Poor eating. A proud man now mired in shame and humiliation, a shell of himself. Alcohol and stress worsening liver disease and increasing bleeding risk, both GI and intracranial, and also further elevating blood pressure and blood sugar. Despite high risk, don't suspect active GI or intracranial bleed. Pedro knows he must stop drinking and restore family trust. Suspect depression, spiritual crisis, ~~possible susto, a cultural syndrome,~~ and irritable bowel.

Problem List Additions:
- Alcohol bingeing
- Family conflict
- Abdominal pain
- H/O falls

Engaging Plan (Concerns and Goals)
Goals:
- Stop all consumption of alcohol.
- Restore sense of dignity: Find employment; help parents.
- Restore family's trust in him: Gain wife and children's forgiveness; family will meet Carlos.
- Better blood pressure control
- Stabilize liver disease.

Treatment Plan:
- Call friend from local AA for connection and return daily for next week; recommend family attend Al-Anon (given contact information).

(continued)

> **TABLE 3.55** *Continued*
>
> - Labs: Metabolic profile, complete blood count, prothrombin time—fasting tomorrow AM
> - Meds: Continue amlodipine at same dose; start multivitamin once a day.
>
> Follow-up:
> - Reschedule for 30-min first "drama" visit in next 3-5 d.
>
> Note: Decided to hold on prediabetes diagnosis, CT scan of head, referral to hepatitis clinic, introduction to behavioral health therapist
>
> Roles
> Clinician: Will follow up with phone call or portal note on lab results and check in within 2 d; give behavioral health therapist heads-up about patient.
> Clinical Associate (Mika): Will do "teach-back;" will make phone call with patient to AA friend before leaving today; will assure f/u appointment within next 5 d; will check in via phone call or portal in next 2 d.
> Patient: Will begin daily AA meetings starting today; will resume daily amlodipine and add multivitamin; will get fasting blood work tomorrow AM; recommend family attend Al-Anon.
> Patient's Family: Will consider becoming part of Al-Anon group.
>
> Future
> Introduce patient to behavioral health therapist at next visit.
> Consider family conference and/or home visit within month.
> Reconsider hepatitis C clinic in future.

AA, Alcoholics Anonymous; CT, computed tomography; GI, gastrointestinal.

Sometimes, the explanatory story remains uncertain, and no evidence-informed management option is identifiable. What then? Keep swinging on the Naming and Caring Tree. Remember those five limbs and the habitat. Look for supportive, nonspecific care options that strengthen the patient's capacities, restore some order, provide an active plan until time and diagnostic efforts bring more certainty to the situation. Examples include music such as chanting or art, nutritional changes, journaling, nature walks with friends. There are so many options on the Naming and Caring Tree. There is never a situation where you cannot help. Keep swinging!

TABLE 3.56	Indicators of Completing Hand Over

Match care burden with patient capacity.
Utilize teach-back.
Share power and motivate patient with engaging plan.
Debrief re: Electronic health record content.
Say goodbye with reassurance.

Getting to the Hand Over Guidepost

Hand Over is almost complete. One last step to help reinforce the plan and ensure the patient's understanding is to utilize the "teach-back" technique[14,15]: share the plan with the patient, then encourage them to use their own words to describe the plan back to you. If a procedure is part of the plan, ask them to demonstrate it. Throughout this activity, pay special attention to health literacy. I encourage training clinic staff in this technique so they can do this with the patient after you have left the clinical encounter.

Debrief with the EHR, the last step in POISED. Let the patient know what you are putting in the medical record, then print the after-visit summary and any patient education materials for the patient to take with them. Table 3.56 notes a few quick checks to indicate reaching the guidepost of Hand Over.

This phase ends when you print the patient visit summary and Hand Over care to the patient, demonstrating the sharing of power. Your ritual work is almost done. Time to head for the Safety Net guidepost.

REFERENCES

1. Brown JB, Weston WW, Stewart MA. Patient-centred interviewing part II: finding common ground. *Can Fam Physician*. 1989;35:153-157.
2. Hersh L, Salzman B, Snyderman D. Health literacy in primary care practice. *Am Fam Physician*. 2015;92(2):118-124.
3. Taggart J, Williams A, Dennis S, et al. A systematic review of interventions in primary care to improve health literacy for chronic disease behavioral risk factors. *BMC Fam Pract*. 2012;13:49
4. Kolb DA. *Experiential Learning: Experience as the Source of Learning and Development*. 2nd ed. Pearson Education; 2015.
5. Green LA, Seifert CM. Translation of research into practice: why we can't "just do it." *J Am Board Fam Pract*. 2005;18(6):541-545.

6. Fadiman A. *The Spirit Catches You and You Fall Down: A Hmong Child, Her American Doctors, and the Collisions of Two Cultures*. Farrar, Straus, and Giroux; 2012.
7. Fisher R, Ury W, Patton B. *Getting to Yes: Negotiating Agreement Without Giving In*. 3rd ed. Penguin Books; 2011.
8. Weisinger H. *The Power of Positive Criticism*. AMACOM-AMA Publications; 2000.
9. May C, Montori VM, Mair FS. We need minimally disruptive medicine. *BMJ*. 2009;339:b2803.
10. Leppin AL, Montori VM, Gionfriddo MR. Minimally disruptive medicine: a pragmatically comprehensive model for delivering care to patients with multiple chronic conditions. *Healthcare (Basel)*. 2015;3(1):50-63.
11. Mold JW. *Goal-Oriented Medical Care: Helping Patients Achieve Their Personal Health Goals*. Full Court Press; 2020.
12. Doukas DJ, McCullough LB. The values history. the evaluation of the patient's values and advance directives. *J Fam Pract*. 1991;32(2):145-153.
13. Brown MT, Bussell J, Dutta S, et al. Medication adherence: truth and consequences. *Am J Med Sci*. 2016;351(4):387-399.
14. Bodenheimer T. Teach-back: a simple technique to enhance patients' understanding. *Fam Pract Manag*. 2018;25(4):20-22.
15. Yen PH, Leasure AR. Use and effectiveness of the Teach-back Method in patient education and health outcomes. *Fed Pract*. 2019;36(6):284-289.

Unit Seven: The Journeys to Safety Net and Housekeep

The Safety Net Guidepost

Getting to the Safety Net guidepost represents a cognitive clinical discipline (see Figure 3.28).

Safety netting is a conscious self-check-in where you perform a prognosis review and an appraisal of the patient's safety as you leave the clinical encounter, especially if there is still some diagnostic uncertainty or the situation has an especially high risk for a troublesome outcome.[1] I usually do this after teach-back as I push the key for printing the after-visit summary.

In many ways, you have been safety netting throughout the clinical encounter. Being transparent during clinical discovery and evaluation, repeatedly tailoring and addressing patient expectations and concerns, paying attention to the capacity-to-burden ratio, and ensuring Hand Over of an engaging plan, you were safety netting. It is built into the generalist's craft. Reaching the Safety Net guidepost, however, means adding one more cord to the weave of the Safety Net. This last prognostic pass helps prevent premature closure, reminds you of your continuity commitment, reinforces patient safety, and helps you keep learning. It's also the last two, "checking" and "trial and learn," of five elements of Joanne Reeve's "Wise Framework" for doing the knowledge work of medical generalism.[2] Checking refers to not missing or overlooking something and not making inappropriate assumptions, while trial and learn suggests need to plan for follow-up and potential revision in understanding. The first three elements, "data collection," "exploration," and "explanation," all happened if you've done the generalist's craft.

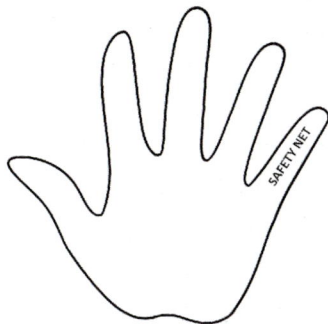

FIGURE 3.28. The Safety Net Finger.

The critical question is to ask yourself, "What do I think is going to happen?," and then to ponder what you would do if it does not. The intent is to ensure you do not miss those early moments in the natural history of a disease where intervention can prevent serious disability or mortality, such as early-onset herpes zoster or pulmonary embolus. It helps you sort out when to watchfully wait or delay and when to get aggressive; when to refer; and when to do diagnostic testing. Do not miss dramas disguised as routines or maintenance ceremonies, especially when you are running late on your schedule and are tempted to save time. Table 3.57 summarizes the indicators for reaching the Safety Net guidepost. Your time with the patient ends. The ritual closes for the patient. You acknowledge that with a reassuring goodbye, a nod making eye contact, or, if appropriate, a handshake.

If you are a clinician in training, precepting your case to your instructor is a form of safety netting. When precepting, especially early in your training, you usually present your story to the preceptor just before you begin Finding Common Ground. Be careful not to transfer your role as the personal clinician for the patient to the faculty. Take the risk: put an explanatory story together and propose a plan. Where you are uncertain, ask key or directed questions. Listen openly, and adjust your story and plans accordingly. Remain the clinician for this encounter.

Let us return to our clinical encounter with Pedro Rodriguez one last time. You left Pedro in the exam room with Mika, the clinical associate he

TABLE 3.57 Indicators of Completing Safety Net

Prognosis Review
- What do I think is actually going to happen?
- What if it doesn't happen that way? How will I know if I'm wrong?
- What is my backup plan?
- Did I miss something important?
- Do a quick "red flag" check.
- Does the patient know when, for what, and how to reconnect?
- Does the patient have an adequate Safety Net in place?

Precepting (if applicable)
- Present an organized story.
- Ask "key questions."
- Listen openly.
- Remain the clinician.

trusts, and are checking your documentation in Pedro's record. You do a prognostic review in your head and suddenly pause. Darn, you forgot to check on whether Pedro was taking any medications for his arthritis that might aggravate gastrointestinal bleeding. You briefly rejoin Pedro and Mika and learn that Pedro is not taking anything for his arthritis. Whew! You add that to your note, and as you look to see who is next on your schedule, you bump into your thumb on your Clinical Hand, where you see the word, *Housekeep*. Your ritual is not yet done.

The Housekeep Guidepost

Just as we invested considerable energy at the beginning of the healing encounter by preparing and setting intention, we invest recharging energy at the end as we Housekeep (see Figure 3.29).

The "houses" that may need cleaning include the *administrative house* of documentation, the *clinic house* and its ensemble of healers, and your *personal house*, the one that just completed a clinical encounter and will soon be in another. If it is the end of the day, you are preparing your personal house to go home to family, or to walk your dog, or to meet friends, or just to have some alone time. All those houses benefit from clearing, best after each visit. Never skip this part of the ritual!

Begin by completing any necessary EHR documentation or forms related to the session. And recognize that, depending on your EHR system, your schedule, and your current time frame, full completion may not be possible at the moment. Leave notes of critical information you do not want to forget if documentation will be completed later, whether by yourself or by others. After the documentation, housekeeping is quite simple to do, and so cleansing! Wash your hands with mindfulness. Wash your hands not only

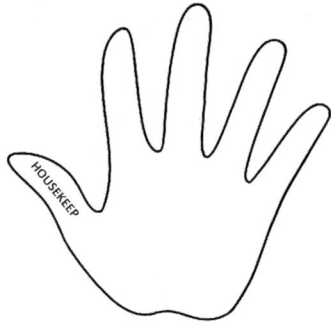

FIGURE 3.29. The Housekeep Finger.

TABLE 3.58 Tools for Housekeeping

Mindful handwashing
Cup of tea
Squeeze ball
Tiny "flushing sound" toilet
Handkerchief
Styrofoam airplane
Looking at funny GIFs/memes
Scrolling through pictures
Short walk
Conversation with colleague
Many others

to prevent the spread of infection, but to prevent any ghosts from the prior visit to appear in the next. How do you feel after the visit? My own reactions range from experiencing great joy to feeling like a failure. Patients can trigger unhappy memories from your family-of-origin story through counter-transference.[3] The intense work of the encounter can exhaust us, or the excitement of the craft invigorate us. Regardless, these feelings need to be experienced and then cleared so as not to influence the next encounter. Many visits only require mindful handwashing, but those that are especially taxing or carry considerable emotional weight may need an even deeper cleansing.

Table 3.58 lists some of my tools for housekeeping. This extra minute spent on bringing the ritual structure to a close saves many more as the day marches on. What are your props and/or practices? Do they help you smile? Have fun? Good housekeeping helps prevent errors and burnout and enhances your life outside of clinical practice. No one wants you arriving home dragging a bag of the day's emotional laundry.

The last Housekeep check is with your clinic ensemble. How are they doing? What happened while you were in the exam room? Housekeep with each other. You all are now ready for the next visit. Table 3.59 identifies the checkpoints and actions for reaching the Housekeep guidepost.

Here, we are at the beginning of our next great adventure. Another patient awaits. These tools of the generalist's craft will help you thrive as a healer. They will support you in the Practice of Hospitality as you enact the disciplines of fidelity, thought, and community. Go forth, celebrating abundance, mystery, and grace ….

TABLE 3.59 Indicators of Completing Housekeeping

Documentation check	Critical computer work, paperwork
Visit check	How was that encounter for me?
Personal check	How am I doing?
Office/Ensemble check	What's happening around me and with my partners?
Mindful handwashing	Cleaning and opening for the next encounter

REFERENCES

1. Friedemann Smith C, Lunn H, Wong G, et al. Optimising GPs' communication of advice to facilitate patients' self-care and prompt follow-up when the diagnosis is uncertain: a realist review of "safety-netting" in primary care. *BMJ Qual Saf.* 2022;31(7):541-554.
2. Reeve J. *Medical Generalism, Now! Reclaiming the Knowledge Work of Modern Practice.* CRC Press; 2024.
3. Stein HF. *The Psychodynamics of Medical Practice: Unconscious Factors in Patient Care.* University of California Press; 1985.

MODULE 4

Doing the Encounter Types

Introduction

A major feature of primary medical care is the guaranteed uncertainty of the situation awaiting the generalist healer behind the next opened portal. There are no boundaries to what problems may present, no barrier between you and the surprise and thrill of the unexpected. One of the early tasks of the generalist healer in a clinical encounter is to quickly assess the situational context and match it with an appropriate response when enacting the generalist's craft. Are you in a routine, maintenance ceremony, transition ceremony, or drama? Module 3, Unit 2 introduced these types of encounters and how to identify them. This module expands on that and describes how to perform each using the strategies of the generalist's craft.

The moment a clinical encounter begins, check the wrist lines on the radial side of your Clinical Hand and start assessing the patient and the story(s) they bring to the encounter. Begin Sensemaking. The Cynefin (pronounced kuh-NEV-in) framework developed by Dave Snowden in 1999 offers a helpful means for doing this Sensemaking (see Figure 4.1).[1] *Cynefin* is a Welsh word meaning both "habitat" and "familiar," and the framework is a conceptual tool designed to help you find your sense of place by making sense of where you are and the situation you are in (see also the Ecological Clinical Map, Figure 2.5). You begin at the center of the Cynefin framework in uncertainty and confusion. Always start there! Do not presume to know before you have spent a bit of time there. Figure 4.1 shows four different situational contexts surrounding the uncertainty.[1-3] The challenge is to discover which of those four you are in. In the Cynefin framework, the *obvious* (also called "simple" or "clear" in the literature) corresponds with a routine clinical encounter. *Complicated* aligns with a maintenance ceremony, *complex* links to a drama encounter, and *chaos* matches with a transition ceremony. Let us briefly explore each of these worlds.

Each of the domains in the Cynefin framework represents a different situational context, each with distinctive characteristics and preferred ways of managing the problems found there, just like the types of encounters. Table 4.1 summarizes these differences and includes examples from the

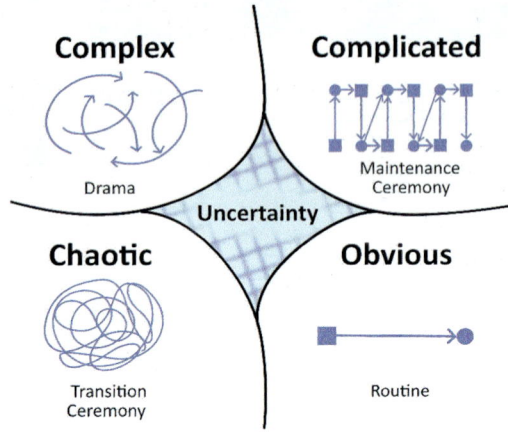

FIGURE 4.1. Cynefin Framework: Making Sense of Situations.

TABLE 4.1	Domains of the Cynefin Framework Within Primary Medical Care	
Domain	**Characteristics**	**Examples**
Obvious	Simple, shared understanding Known knowns Clear cause and effect Sufficient parts adequate Fact-based management, best practice Coordinate if assistance is needed Sense, categorize, respond **Routine** encounter	Upper respiratory infection Strep pharyngitis Simple ankle sprain Mild concussion Otitis media Tick bite <24 h ago Acute back pain after gardening
Complicated	Expertise required Known unknowns Knowable cause and effect Whole is the sum of its parts	Controlled hypertension, diabetes, asthma, depression, and/or acne History of cancer follow-up Stable chronic kidney disease

TABLE 4.1 Continued

Domain	Characteristics	Examples
	Range of right answers	Well-child care; prenatal care
	Cooperate if assistance is needed	Medicare wellness exam
	Sense, analyze, respond	Sports physical; driver's license exam
	Maintenance ceremony encounter	
Complex	Unknown unknowns	Recurrent abdominal pain
	Whole is greater than sum of parts	Early visits for new chronic disease
	Cause and effect are never clear	Chronic Lyme; long COVID
		Unexplained headaches
	Effective strategies emerge	Multiple symptoms unexplained
	Collaborate if assistance is needed	Relapsing multiple sclerosis
		Progressive dementia
	Probe, sense, respond	Substance use disorders
	Drama encounter	Early depression or anxiety care
Chaos	Unknowables abound	Initial visit for complex situations
	Protect life and health	
	Rapid response	Possible child or older adult abuse
	Direct intervention to establish order	Worst headache ever
	Act, sense, respond	Acute abdominal pain
	Transition ceremony encounter	Difficulty breathing

primary medical care setting. An obvious situation is just that: the patient and you quickly have a shared understanding of the concerns. You both know what is important to know. Cause and effect are clear and obvious, the solutions are fact-based, and best practices apply. This is the domain of a routine clinical encounter. The patient's concern is simple, single, and present for less than 2 weeks, and you both easily agree on what is happening.

Communication is direct, and triangulation is congruent (what you see, hear, and feel all align). Together, you and the patient can easily aim and share power as you mend and fix the brokenness and protect and promote health.

A *complicated* situation is similar in that cause and effect are discernible, but there are many moving parts; extra work and some special expertise are required; and there are often a range of possible right answers. Again, the patient and you easily agree on the issues and goals. In the primary medical care setting, complicated situations appear in the form of stable chronic conditions and health maintenance episodes. Managing chronic diseases is a complicated process of slowing down or even reversing the pathophysiologic processes seeking to disrupt healthy physiology while maintaining quality of life, minimizing care burden and side effects of treatments, and advancing self-management skills. The presence of several chronic conditions in the same patient only further complicates, and the encounter may begin to approach the boundary with complexity. Health maintenance such as prenatal care and well-child visits also necessitates paying attention to the unique circumstances of each patient's health and life world as you both seek to enhance health. The intent for aiming and sharing power is to redeem the brokenness and promote and protect health.

Complex situations deny easy predictability. There are unknown unknowns, making connections between cause and effect problematic. Triangulation in the clinical encounter is not congruent (what you see, hear, and feel do not align). Working toward meaningful understanding and effective care strategies requires recognizing the many strands of explanatory forces and identifying emergent patterns. When present with patients experiencing this kind of complexity, you are in a drama. New chronic illness, an exacerbation of a chronic condition, or the presence of critical aspects of the malady that remain unexplained are all dramas and potential turning points toward greater health or worsening affliction. Here, the intent for aiming and sharing power is to transform brokenness and grow health.

Dramas usually begin in *chaos*. When the patient first learns they have a chronic disease, or when their diabetes spins out of control, or when they develop multiple symptoms at the same time that family and work crises erupt are all situations of chaos, new dramas, in need of a rapid intervention—a transition ceremony. Transition ceremonies are warranted when, as a generalist healer, you find yourself in a situation of chaos. Little appears knowable. The patient is lost in their malady and seeks a rapid response, the establishment of some order, a direct intervention. If the clinical action is successful, this situation moves into complexity and a series of future drama visits. Here the power is aimed and shared toward preserving health and preparing for transformation.

Before describing how to do each of the encounter types, let us return one more time to the familiar uncertainty that resides at the center of the Cynefin framework in Figure 4.1. It was your point of departure, yes, but I advise you to return there several times during the clinical encounter, especially if you think you are in a routine or maintenance ceremony. Step back into uncertainty just before you set the agenda. Is this indeed a routine or maintenance ceremony? Or is there some lingering uncertainty? Check in with uncertainty again as you begin clinical discovery with inductive foraging. Am I discovering anything novel that suggests a new drama is surfacing? Step back into uncertainty at least one more time at the Hand Over checkpoint and as you weave a Safety Net. If at any point you realize this "refreshing" routine or maintenance ceremony may actually be a new drama, stop and switch to a transition ceremony. The high volume and demands of primary medical care can surreptitiously guide us toward routines and maintenance ceremonies. Once locked in, the routine and repetitive scripts reinforce entrainment, and we miss the cues of important changes with the patient and their condition(s). Multiple check-ins with the territory of uncertainty will help you resist these impulses. In simpler language, always beware the chaos and the drama. Expect them. Have a high degree of discernment of whether you are indeed in a boobie-trap-chaos-drama situation. And then keep asking, "What else?" as you Set Agenda to catch any chaos-drama whiffs. (As an aside for apprentices of the generalist's craft, the reverse is often true. When your diagnostic skills are thin, many routines and maintenance ceremonies can look like dramas. Your faculty and mentors will help.)

Routines

Patients experience joy when routine encounters are done well by their generalist healers. The guidelines are easy enough—make sure it is a routine, keep it a routine, and be precise with the treatment. Great performance of a routine encounter, however, takes practice in enacting the disciplines of the generalist's craft in primary care. Remember the Clinical Hand's five guideposts, ritual structure, and the three visit goals; they fully apply. Do not take shortcuts; move through each guidepost. Take a little extra time getting to the Set Agenda checkpoint, and make sure the encounter in which you are engaged is a routine and not a new drama. As you explore the patient's health, malady, and life stories, consider a quick scan of family and friends. Table 4.2 offers suggestions for asking about family and friends in a routine.

As you begin clinical discovery, start with inductive foraging, even when the diagnosis seems clear. Do a quick but wide scan of the horizon as a check that it might just be more than a routine visit, and only then prioritize on

> **TABLE 4.2 Remembering the Family in Routines**
>
> "Who's at home?" (or "Who's hanging out with you?" if the patient is unhoused)
>
> "Anything new at home (or '. . .with your family or close friends?')"
>
> "Does anyone in your family (or close friends) have concerns about your situation/problem?"

the single issue of the agenda. A good example is a presentation of flu-like symptoms such as fever, runny nose, scratchy throat, headache, cough, and body aches. It is January, flu is prevalent in the community, and you have already seen several positive test cases of influenza today. Your patient presents with classic symptoms. Routine, right? Probably, but hidden among your hundred-or-more seasonal flu cases will be one that is not: the zebra. Those rare mimics include the acute retroviral syndrome of HIV infection, viral meningitis, acute Lyme disease, epicarditis, and thrombotic thrombocytopenic purpura. Finding the rare others is why you do the wide horizon scan. While foraging, do a quick check on travel, high-risk behaviors, bruising, recent contacts and their age and health, and activities. Always be ready to jump from a routine to a transition ceremony if new information so indicates.

Reassured the encounter is still a routine, proceed to confirm the diagnosis or concern, and reach common ground with the patient on the treatment plan. Here are a few tips along the way: Be sure to touch the concern during your exam. Be generous in your use of ritual objects and healing symbols like the stethoscope and otoscope. Express confidence. Remain culturally sensitive and tailor or personalize your approach and care options to fit the patient and their capacity. It is okay to use the language of biomedicine; it has some symbolic power. But always translate that language and match the patient's health literacy. The goal is to Hand Over what you know to the patient, to share the power of knowledge. Keep the script acute and avoid creating dependency. You want the patient to have and enact their own cure.

A special caveat concerning treatment plans in routine encounters is to emphasize precision in the prescription. The purpose of that precision is to prevent an acute simple concern from becoming a complicated or complex chronic one. This is especially true when pain is a prominent symptom.

TABLE 4.3	Precise Treatment
Take	Take this medicine every ___ hours × ___ days.
Do	Do ___ exercise/action ___ times every ___ hours × ___ days.
Do	Do ___ amount of the following activities each day and increase them as follows ___.

Fordyce's randomized controlled trial of acute pain treatment demonstrates this effect.[4] In the study, all the patients were given the same medications and recommended the same activities and exercises. Group A was told to let pain be the guide for using the medication and doing the activities and exercises. Group B was given strict, precise instructions. There were no differences between the two groups after 6 weeks. But 1 year later, Group B participants had significantly fewer work absences, less health care utilization, and less impairment. The precise instructions appeared to prevent the development of complex pain. Table 4.3 shows instructions on how to prescribe precise treatments. Consider this table before sending your next prescription to the pharmacy with the directive to take as needed.

As you Hand Over the explanation and care plan to the patient, remember to address the actual reason for connecting and promote a health habit related to why they came. Do not forget the Safety Net, especially the prognostic check. Table 4.4 summarizes a few key points to ensure that you master routine clinical encounters and nudge patients back into the River of Health.

TABLE 4.4	Mastering Routines
	Beware of missing a new drama.
	Keep it a routine.
	Touch the concern(s).
	Use precise treatment.
	Remember the family.

Maintenance Ceremonies

Maintenance ceremonies are now the most common of the encounter types in most primary care offices. Why? More of us live longer, and more of us are older. These two factors combine to generate lots of chronic conditions needing primary medical care support. Let us investigate how to become masters at performing maintenance ceremonies. Most maintenance ceremonies are scheduled as such based on your suggestion. As you meet with the parent(s) of a newborn who you recently delivered, you recommend well-child visits at 3 to 4 days, optimally as a home visit, and at 1, 2, 4, 6, 9, and 12 months over the next year. You encourage patients with chronic problems to reschedule in 2 to 3 or even 6 to 12 months for follow-up depending on the severity and/or complications related to the patient's current status and circumstances. When you see these patients' names on your schedule, you presume: *maintenance ceremony*. Be wary, and do not presume. Life happens between visits. Rule out a new drama before drawing a conclusion. During a program of mixed methods research on diabetes management, Patrick O'Connor discovered a cohort of patients who had been getting their care from primary care physicians and suddenly switched over to an endocrinologist without the primary care physician's knowledge. Why? Something had changed in the patient's life, some epiphany such that they now wanted more aggressive care of their diabetes, and their primary care doc did not notice the change.[5] Patient and doctor got stuck in the scripts of their maintenance ceremonies and missed the new drama.

As you prepare for your possible maintenance ceremony, clarify intentions. Recall why you invited the patient into the clinic and review your short- and long-term goals for them. Where is the patient on their walk toward better health? Remember and enact the ritual structure of the five guideposts. Welcome the patient back during your greeting, thank them for returning, and connect with remembrances from past experience. As generalist healers, we engage in what Kathryn Montgomery calls, "a medicine of neighbors."[6] We do not practice our craft with professional detachment nor as friends, although we might be friends outside the clinical encounter. Neighborliness preserves both the clinician's and the patient's boundaries while at the same time creating space for learning, chance, difference, surprise, and intimate contact.[6]

Once connected, begin your negotiation and Set Agenda time by asking about what has happened since the last visit. As the clinician, your memory of the patient is episodic—constructed visit by visit. Your patient's memory builds primarily between visits. Probe that memory. Find out about their recent experiences, including any major changes in their health, and how they think about them. Ask if they have anything new they would like to address.

TABLE 4.5	Remembering the Family in Maintenance Ceremonies

"How's (your friend/family member, e.g., your mother, partner)?"
"What's new at home or with your family/close friends?"
"Does anyone in your family/circle of friends have concerns about your health (or symptoms, child, or pregnancy, etc.)?"
"You're doing a great job with ____."
"Say hello to ____."

Even in maintenance ceremonies, patients have an actual reason for connecting and expectations about the visit. Identify them. Inquire about family and friends. See Table 4.5 for examples of questions that will help you gather this information. Be sure to include affirmations when warranted, such as, "You are doing remarkably well caring for your child, especially given your tight finances."

The patient and you may also have collaborative relationships with one or more specialists providing occasional consultations. Review any related information or questions. Incorporate the patient's agenda along with reviewing your goals for the visit. The agenda is a negotiated agreement.

Create sacred space as you shift toward exploring the stories and clinical discovery. Shift mood and voice tone and use ritual objects. Perform a maintenance ceremony like the ceremonial walk of a labyrinth. Enter the space, intensify, diminish, summarize, and then return to everyday space, a space of neighborliness. Develop a routinized approach, including the role and expectations of your clinical ensemble partner(s)—this is especially important for health maintenance and life cycle ceremonies, which can be heavy with protocol-driven expectations including immunizations, prevention counseling, screening. Tailor the ceremony to the patient and their circumstances. Do good clinical jazz. Maintenance ceremonies are an opportune time to enhance your understanding of the whole person, to learn a bit more of their life story and their proximal and distal contexts. Emphasize the enhanced relationship and context learning parts of the Relationship-Centered Clinical Method during maintenance ceremonies.

While implementing the Relationship-Centered Clinical Method, evaluate whether any chronic conditions are progressing, stable, or improving. Explore where the patient is having success with the care plan and where there are stumbling blocks. Look for early symptoms and signs of complications.

If you are conducting a life cycle maintenance ceremony, check on potential issues for the patient's stage in the life cycle, such as identity during adolescence, menopause at midlife for women, empty-nest feelings as the last child leaves home, or retirement plans and adjustments at a first Medicare annual wellness visit. Finding Common Ground is a good moment to review both malady goals and longer-term life plan goals. Incorporate any health promotion here. Hand Over is also where you optimize enabling patient self-management capacity and skills. Work on converting all maintenance ceremonies into growth ones, recognizing this is usually subtle growth, little nudges toward better health. Table 4.6 highlights important tips for mastering maintenance ceremonies.

The Safety Net process for maintenance ceremonies benefits from a quick checklist review for the age-, gender-, and sex-appropriate health maintenance protocol and/or for the appropriate chronic disease guideline suggestions. Ideally, you would check them during preparation for the clinical encounter and again as you reach the Safety Net guidepost. Do not forget to Housekeep, especially if you just experienced a "hopeless" maintenance ceremony where both you and the patient felt exasperated, as if you were "treading water" in their care. Consider bringing this case to your next Balint group.

In summary, maintenance ceremonies take place in complicated space. Unlike the obvious, clear space of routines entailing you to sense, categorize, and respond with "best practice" care, maintenance ceremonies call on you to sense and then analyze the situation before choosing among options for your recommended response. Maintenance ceremonies represent the unheralded, everyday garden work of weeding, pruning, watering, soil enrichment, and, yes, even pest management that are part of the process of growing better health. A satisfying process indeed!

TABLE 4.6 Mastering Maintenance Ceremonies

Make sure the encounter is not a new drama.
Review your goals and incorporate the patient's agenda.
Invoke ceremony.
Emphasize patient self-management.
Focus on growth; nudge toward health; build capacity.
Remember the family.

Dramas

Dramas are the grand opera of primary medical care and unfold over several, often many, clinical encounters. They involve the habitat and all five limbs of the Naming and Caring Tree, including song, dance, theater, story, silence, and land; great staging; exaggeration of emotions and melodrama; and the big themes of life splashed onto the everyday with touches of history and mythology and theology. All with a prelude and multiple acts and scenes. Welcome to the big stage of Clinical Opera! But there is no fixed libretto to follow here. The opening prelude is a transition ceremony during which you are introduced to the opera's main characters and the confusing swirl of drama and themes that surround them. I will describe how to manage transition ceremonies in the next section, but here we focus on all the ensuing scenes, when you learn what the important issues and challenges of the drama are and how they entangle, then how the stories turn and clarify and stabilize—or not. Doing dramas requires your best mindfulness and attending, patience, respect, empathy, and creativity. These are the masterworks of improvisational clinical performance. Let us explore how to stage dramas.

Dramas represent potential turning points in patient's lives. For some, the drama follows a trajectory of decline and is marked by the inability to return to an earlier functional status or quality of life. For some, a new life story may need to be shaped (e.g., following a major cerebrovascular event resulting in permanent paralysis). For others, the drama can trigger significant behavioral change resulting in improved quality of life (e.g., following a myocardial infarction prompting weight loss, greater physical activity, and reduction in alcohol intake).

Dramas also come with great variation in duration. Some, like a new diagnosis of hypertension, may only need three to four visits before becoming stable maintenance ceremonies, whereas others involve significant diagnostic uncertainty and difficulty mobilizing needed resources, for example, many substance use disorders can last more than a year, necessitating many visits and multiple collaborators. Three factors that greatly facilitate effective dramas are continuity of care, shifting patient expectations regarding time frame, and developing shared understanding of complexity through use of the Naming and Caring Tree (see Table 4.7).

A drama constitutes a complex and highly relational series of visits over time. Continuity of care becomes crucial. Stepping into the middle of a drama as a "stranger" clinician is disconcerting to all parties and usually disruptive. Of course, always being available as the personal clinician is not practical—thus the recommendation to partner with *a colleague for dramas, especially* those with a likely longer time frame. This is an excellent opportunity for

TABLE 4.7 Facilitators of Effective Dramas

Facilitator	Description
Continuity of Care	Same personal clinician at most visits Consider partnering with a practice colleague Frequent discussions among clinical ensemble
Shift Patient Expectations of Time Frame	From immediate or short to longer—Match expectations to reality Need for multiple visits Drama illness trajectory useful visual aid (see Figure 4.2)
Develop Shared Understanding of Complexity	Multicausal, no simple fix Address all five limbs on the Naming and Caring Tree and its habitat Clinical Hand is a useful visual aid.

a physician to partner with an advanced practice clinician such as a nurse practitioner or physician's assistant. Depending on the presence of behavioral factors, a drama often benefits from close collaboration with a behavioral therapist. If scheduling issues prevent continuity for a particular visit, preparing the new "understudy" clinician for the upcoming clinical encounter is crucial. Everyone gains when there are frequent discussions about the drama in the form of huddles and/or case conferences among the clinic ensemble.

Once patients have decided to bring their concerns to a primary care clinician, they are usually hoping for a short-term solution. Dramas, by definition, don't contain that option. They take time. An important part of the early work in a drama is to help the patient shift their expectations to a longer time frame. Ideally, this process begins at the transition ceremony during which the drama was first identified. Figure 4.2 depicts a prototype drama illness trajectory that serves as a useful visual aid in helping patients appreciate the time frame for their drama and the necessity for multiple visits.

I have found it particularly helpful to introduce this figure at the first drama visit following the transition ceremony. The trajectory of a drama mirrors the mythologic hero's journey from innocence, or a relative state of health, to crossing the threshold into the world of affliction, where you undergo trials and gain allies along the pathway that will return you to everyday life with

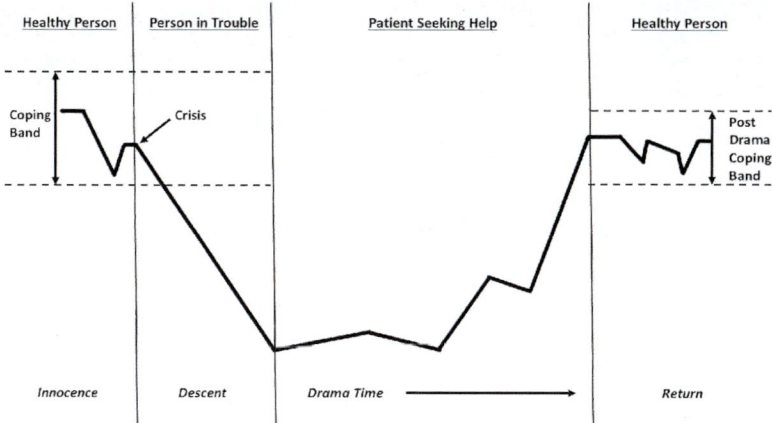

FIGURE 4.2. Drama Illness Trajectory. Adapted from Smilkstein G. A model for applying behavioral science to family practice. In: Rosen GM, Geyman JP, Layton RH, eds. *Behavioral Science in Family Practice*. Appleton-Century-Crofts; 1980:18.

lessons learned and a changed self.[7,8] You are both on a quest narrative. In the figure, you will notice the transition from person to patient, reminding us that patients are people flattened by malady in their life. The coping bands in Figure 4.2 denote the patient's adaptive capacity, their robustness, resilience, and antifragility. They represent the width of the patient's River of Health. Within our coping bands, we vacillate around some perception of "normal." During dramas, that perception often needs to be altered, and a new "normal" created. The post-drama coping band can be narrower or broader, and the same, worse, or better relative to health. We accompany the patient on this journey, which is also a journey of locating, owning, aiming, and sharing power. Along the way, pay attention to where you are; consider mapping it. The trajectory depicted in Figure 4.2 resides within a landscape. How supportive of healing is that landscape? How are you influencing that landscape on behalf of the patient? What resources are you helping to mobilize, and what help are you getting to do so?[9]

There are four valuable components in performing healing dramas: the three stories of symptoms, family, and life; the five limbs of the Naming and Caring Tree and its habitat; the two healing teams, consisting of the clinic ensemble and the patient's support team; and time. Table 4.8 highlights these and other important tips for mastering dramas. Dramas are complex situations with lots of important hidden information. Sometimes the patient

TABLE 4.8 Mastering Dramas

Listen to the *Symptom(s)* Story.
Listen to the *Family(s)* Story.
  Draw and use Genogram.
Listen to the *Life* Story(s).
  Draw and use Life Space Diagram.
Swing on all the Tree Limbs.
- Treat the *Physical.*
- Treat the *Emotional.*
- Treat the *Cognitive.*
- Treat the *Social.*
- Invoke the *Spiritual.*

Rewrite the Stories.
Use Multiple Visits Over Time.
Expand the Clinical Ensemble.

hides this material because they think it is not related, other times because it triggers traumatic memories, and still others because there is not enough trust to risk divulging secrets. Thus, dramas begin with probing for information of multiple kinds, then making sense and responding. Let us walk through a generic overview of how dramas evolve.

The craft of performing dramas is similar to creating and caring for a new garden on thin soil. You study and learn about the soil, then start, and never stop, with weeding. You care for the symptom story. Next, you build and nourish the soil; you work with the family story. And then you plant the seeds of new life. You work with the life story. What does this look like back in the clinic? Spend extra time understanding the person and their proximal and distal contexts, then dig deeply into the symptom story since that's usually what brought the patient to you. Go well beyond the standard history of present illness parameters. Elicit all the symptoms and their histories. Remember the principles of trauma-informed care. Ask "What happened?" and not "What is wrong?" Determine what settings produce the different symptoms. Listen to the language the patient uses to describe their symptoms, their images of illness, and pay heed to any symptom–emotion–body location associations. Explore for connections to past trauma. Elicit any cultural models and personal scripts. Swing through all the naming or diagnostic limbs of the Naming and Caring Tree. Observe and listen for patterns. What is the larger story being shared? How do the different threads weave together? As you build the symptom stories, begin addressing them with carefully aimed care strategies that won't mask possible clues. Prioritize improving function and quality and any specific causal factors that are discovered.

Before moving from the symptom story to the family and life stories, I want us to pause and note the relationship between encounter types and narrative types. Earlier, in Module 3, Unit 2, and coming up in Module 5, I associate routines with a restitution narrative, transition ceremonies with a chaos narrative, and dramas and maintenance ceremonies with a quest narrative. Viewed from a distance, these generally align, but, within dramas, the association can become more complicated, especially as it relates to the symptom story. Hip fracture in older adults offers a good example. Older adults who experience a hip fracture have a 5- to 8-fold increase in mortality within 3 months of the fracture.[10] Many factors contribute to this disturbing outcome, but a surprising one is the patient's narrative concerning the fracture and its care. Those who perceive their broken hip as a mechanical, fixable problem (restitution narrative) do better than those who perceive otherwise (quest narrative).[11] An older adult with an acute hip fracture is certainly a new drama encounter, but this study reminds us that, sometimes, managing the symptom story as a restitution narrative may be beneficial. As the patient's rehabilitation progresses and more attention shifts to the family and life stories, using quest narratives for them becomes appropriate. Keep this in mind as we now address how to codevelop family and life stories with your patients.

Along the way, begin exploring the patient's family story. Table 4.9 offers some questions for the family inquiry. Dramas are also an excellent time to

TABLE 4.9 Family Questions in Dramas

Who's in your family?
What's new or changed in your family?
Who are your major support systems in your home or your family?
What other support systems do you have?
Who is there conflict with?
Was your family of origin a safe place?
Are you safe at home now?

draw a genogram and review it with the patient while also discussing the symptom stories and exploring possible connections. Current symptoms often find their source and trigger in past childhood and family trauma. Do not forget personal and family pets.

Once a more coherent drama story starts to emerge, return to and expand on the patient's life story. Learn more about the proximal and distal contexts, especially their SCREEM resources. Doing a life space drawing with the patient is often helpful with life story development.[12,13] Meanwhile, keep swinging on the Naming and Caring Tree (see Figures 2.5, 3.1, and 3.9) and try to involve all five limbs. Doing so helps attune the many aspects of the person as body and story in their habitat and healing landscape. Together with the patient, rewrite more coherent stories, and begin shifting from the symptom to the emerging life story as you find common ground.

And sometimes the drama gets stuck. Despite trying all the above, you still feel lost, as if something important *is missing*. Table 4.10 suggests some breakthrough tactics for these circumstances.

If the drama continues to persist, ask the secondary-gain question, "How might the drama be helping the patient?" Dramas can activate important supports and help the patient find more agency and belonging, but for some people, especially those who started with thin adaptive capacity, leaving the drama and risking the loss of those supports can be frightening. Also remember that too much health care nurtures learned helplessness. Dramas are the penultimate test of the clinician's mastery of the generalist's craft and a source of great joy. We witness a broken life find its dance steps and singing voice, rediscover their story, feel safe with their tribe, become comfortable with silence and their land. We witness healing.

TABLE 4.10 Breakthrough Tactics for Dramas

Tactic	Description
Home visit	Engage the context; bring stories together.
Family meeting	Convene family and significant friends.
Patient homework	Give the patient (and others) some work to do and bring to next session.
Expand the team	Engage community agencies, resources.

Transition Ceremonies

New dramas almost always lay hidden in your daily schedule, usually as an acute visit. They are unexpected schedule busters and call for a transition ceremony. What patients want most when life falls apart and they lose their wings is support. They need the *clinikos*, the place of support and the clinic ensemble awaiting them there with that support in the form of safety, comfort, and hope, the three goals of a transition ceremony. On the surface, transition ceremonies rarely appear ceremonial. They look hectic, intense, often a bit scattered, just on the edge of chaos. Actually, they are situations of chaos for the patient, and that chaos can easily capture you unless you act within the structure of ritual. Craft a series of linked rituals into a ceremony that builds a nest within the storm.[14]

Think of each phase between the first three guideposts of the Clinical Hand as a separate ritual enacted with empathic calm and surefootedness. Connect with confidence and a reassuring style. Listen intently, with compassion but unruffled, as you negotiate and Set Agenda, a short one focused on the chaotic concern(s). Create clear ritual markers between the phases. Use the different ritual spaces within the exam room. Set apart the Clinical Discovery and Evaluation time on the way to Hand Over, and touch the concern(s) with confidence, even though you are probably not feeling it. Have the patient get fully dressed and return to the comfort of a chair before completing the Hand Over. Use ceremony to create order and safety. The patient's body will notice. By bounding the liminal space, you help contain the chaos of the story. When in a chaotic situation, act first to establish order, then sense and respond (see the case of Pedro Rodriguez in Module 3, Unit 5). Transition ceremonies are ceremonies for crossing over from chaos into complexity and the start of the multiple visits of a drama.

Table 4.11 identifies the aims of transition ceremonies. The first two aims prioritize protection. Stabilize the patient's clinical status. If they need oxygen or a nebulizer treatment, set it up. If they require an electrocardiogram, do it before proceeding with further questioning.

First and foremost, transition ceremonies are a time for protecting the patient and containing the chaos. Thus, stabilize the current status, then protect the patient from further harm before the next visit, the initiating of the drama. That further protection often involves initiating a new pharmaceutical, conducting an intervention (see the call to initiate AA meeting attendance in Pedro Rodriguez's case in Module 3, Unit 5), assigning homework for the patient such as keeping a journal of their symptoms, or setting up a diagnostic test or consultation. Usually, these actions, including the follow-up

> **TABLE 4.11 Aims for Transition Ceremonies**
>
> Stabilize the situation: Protect patient before initiating the new drama.
> Protect from further harm (check for "red flags").
> Decrease anxiety.
> Identify initial themes of the drama.
> Offer a transitional explanation (safety, comfort, hope).
> Begin reconnecting the patient to family/community.
> Enable agency (instill faith).

visit, happen within the next week or less. Paradoxically, these actions decrease the patient's immediate anxiety; their body recognizes the order being built. During the transition ceremony, you are also listening and observing the underlying themes potentially driving the drama and chaos.

The last three aims delineated in Table 4.11 serve to reinforce the first four. Offer a transitional explanation with underlying messages of safety, comfort, and hope, and begin the work of reestablishing belonging by specifying some connection with family or friends. Begin the work of restoring the patient's sense of agency by assigning them tasks that address their concern(s) between now and the next visit. And do not forget that transition ceremonies are often when dire diseases first present. Do not miss them!

Over half the time spent in transition ceremonies happens between the Connect and Set Agenda guideposts. Most of that time is spent listening. Transition ceremonies are the one time when exploring the patient's malady stories from the Relationship-Centered Clinical Method slips over into the phase before setting the agenda and gets incorporated into expanding on eliciting the patient's concerns for the visit. Spend extra time listening to the background of the patient's malady story and listening for the feelings that accompany it. Be sure to elicit what frightens and troubles them the most and what is happening. Do not forget to accept and validate what you hear; the patient must know you acknowledge their story, their experience. Remember, you do not need to accept their explanation. When you finally get to the exam and history-taking, prioritize touching the fright and troubles and on ruling in or out possible "red flag" conditions. Breathe into the patient's fear when listening to their lungs by slowing their breaths. Use ritual objects like the

> **TABLE 4.12** **LATE—Mastering Transition Ceremonies**
>
> L   Listen to the background of the story and for feelings.
> A   Address fear: What frightens and troubles the patient the most?
> T   Touch the fright or trouble.
> E   Express hope and enact an initial plan that builds on what you've heard and the patient's strengths—Don't promise!

stethoscope and share what you discover. Highlight what is good with their body as you also uncover what is amiss. Express hope, and give them something to do that is a creative extension or enhancement of what they shared when asked how they have handled it so far. Build on their strengths with a simple new touch. Reassure without promising. Too much is unsettled to warrant promises; offering them risks breaking trust. Table 4.12 summarizes the keys for mastering transition ceremonies in the form of the mnemonic LATE: Listen, Address the fear, Touch the trouble, and Express hope and enact an engaging plan. Arrange for an extended-visit follow-up for the first drama session. When the actions of LATE are applied, it will not be too late for the patient—and you are less likely to be late for your next appointment.

In many ways, transition ceremonies are a big BATHE[15] (see nails on Clinical Hand). Since many transition ceremonies are scheduled as acute visit appointments, the patient may be seen by a clinician other than their personal practitioner due to schedule availability. What to do? Perform a transition ceremony as described but with a few special caveats. Mention the patient's personal clinician by name during connecting time. Refer to them again whenever appropriate throughout the clinical encounter. Transfer the care back to the patient's regular personal clinician at the Hand Over when you schedule the follow-up visit unless the patient states otherwise. During housekeeping, send a note to that clinician with a summary of the visit to help them prepare for the initial drama visit. If you cannot send the note, then create a reminder to do so before the end of the day.

Transition ceremonies cross over on the bridge of safety, comfort, and hope. You are preparing and making it safe for future transformation. A transition ceremony is where power is protected. You use your clinical hands to hold a sacred space for your patient, who has left the River of Health and fallen into deep mud. Be the generalist healer who is there to rise up under, with compassion (suffering with), to offer safety, comfort, and hope!

REFERENCES

1. Kurtz CF, Snowden DJ. The new dynamics of strategy: sense-making in a complex and complicated world. *IBM Syst J*. 2003;42(3):462-483.
2. Sturmberg JP, Martin CM. Knowing—in medicine. *J Eval Clin Pract*. 2008;14(5):767-770.
3. McLeod J, Childs S. The Cynefin framework: a tool for analyzing qualitative data in information science? *Libr Inf Sci Res*. 2013;35(4):299-309.
4. Fordyce WE, Brockway JA, Bergman JA, et al. Acute back pain: a control-group comparison of behavioral vs traditional management methods. *J Behav Med*. 1986;9(2):127-140.
5. O'Connor PJ, Crabtree BF, Yanoshik MK. Differences between diabetic patients who do and do not respond to a diabetes care intervention: a qualitative analysis. *Fam Med*. 1997;29(6):424-428.
6. Montgomery K. *How Doctors Think: Clinical Judgment and the Practice of Medicine*. Oxford University Press; 2006.
7. Campbell J. *The Hero with a Thousand Faces*. 2nd ed. Princeton University Press; 1968.
8. Hawkins AH. *Reconstructing Illness: Studies in Pathography*. Purdue University Press; 1993.
9. Miller WL, Crabtree BF. Healing landscapes: patients, relationships, and creating optimal healing places. *J Altern Complement Med*. 2005;11(suppl 1):S41-S49.
10. Haentjens P, Magaziner J, Colón-Emeric CS, et al. Meta-analysis: excess mortality after hip fracture among older women and men. *Ann Intern Med*. 2010;152(6):380.
11. Borkan JM, Quirk M, Sullivan M. Finding meaning after the fall: injury narratives from elderly hip fracture patients. *Soc Sci Med*. 1991;33(8):947-957.
12. Blake RL, Bertuso DD. The life space drawing as a measure of social relationships. *Fam Med*. 1988;20(4):295-297.
13. Cushman RA, Crabtree BF, Miller WL. Life-space diagrams and genograms as measures of social support in the elderly. In: Norton PG, Stewart M, Tudiver F, et al, eds. *Primary Care Research: Traditional and Innovative Approaches*. Vol 1. Research Methods for Primary Care. Sage Publications, Inc; 1991:162-168.
14. Mead M. *Blackberry Winter: My Earlier Years*. Reprint ed. Kodansha USA, Inc; 1995.
15. Stuart MR, Lieberman JA III. *The Fifteen Minute Hour: Efficient and Effective Patient-Centered Consultation Skills*. 6th ed. CRC Press; 2019.

MODULE 5

Deepening Practical Wisdom

Overview

Practice, practice, practice! Historically, primary medical care has been called general practice. It still is in many parts of the world. I love the simple honesty of it. We are generalists, caring for whatever the health-related concerns may be, and always practicing our craft, making it better. Modules 3 and 4 presented the essential practical wisdom of the generalist's craft in primary care. Keep practicing what you learned there. As you practice, your practical wisdom will deepen. Module 5 shares some additional perspectives and tips, some add-ons to the Clinical Hand and its supporting tools to further deepen and enrich your practice.

Module 5 is premised on the idea that you learn through practice, embracing the major principle underlying Donald Schön's theory of reflective practice.[1,2] Learning develops from recognizing the importance of context and reflective conversation, both with yourself and with colleagues and patients. Schön's model of reflective practice recognizes the importance of what he terms *knowledge in action* (see Table 5.1).

Baseline tacit knowledge underlies most professional activity. For us, it represents the once tacit knowledge of the generalist's craft now made explicit in this *Field Guide*. Reflective practice builds on this knowledge in action using two modes of reflection. The first is *reflection in action*, where you evaluate, learn, and adapt your behavior within ongoing clinical encounters as you do the generalist's craft. Think of this as the reflective clinical jazz improvisation mentioned several times in Modules 2 to 4. Patients are often energetic participants in these reflective conversations. *Reflection on action* is the second mode of reflective practice and refers to explicit retrospective reflection after a clinical encounter. You step back and critically evaluate actions taken and any subsequent outcomes. You dive deeply into the what, how, and why of the encounter, gleaning new insights and understandings and nuances about the generalist's craft. Consider journaling. Gather with some colleagues for reflective conversations. Join a Balint group. The tips and perspectives shared here in Module 5 represent examples of new ideas generated out of reflection

TABLE 5.1	**Model of Reflective Practice**	
Reflective Practice	**Definition**	**Reflective Questions**
Knowledge in Action	Tacit knowledge of the profession (made explicit by *Field Guide*)	What do I already know about the situation? How can I use it to be helpful?
Reflection in Action	Reflective learning while doing (clinical jazz improvisation)	What is happening? What am I feeling? What other factors are involved?
Reflection on Action	Reflective learning in retrospect	What happened? Why did it happen that way? How will I change what I'll do in the future?

on action by experienced masters of the generalist's craft in primary care. Try them. Keep practicing. Develop and share your own.

Ecological Clinical Map Add-Ons

Patient

I assisted in the birth of Felicity's daughter Julia in 1983 as her family physician, and I diagnosed Julia's Hodgkin lymphoma in 2016 (from which she is currently disease-free). During the 40 years of partnering with Julia as her personal physician, I came to recognize several different ways that Julia presented herself. And they were more than expected developmental changes. There were many aspects to Julia, as is true of all the patients I've developed relationships with over time. Indeed, I've discovered the same is true when reading patients' stories about their illness and healing journeys.[3] Their self-told tales and my own experiences revealed four different aspects, or "faces," of individuals who visit us as generalist healers. Nearly everyone has all four faces. They include the individual as patient, or *patiens*; as techno-consumer; as person; and as human animal[4] (see Figure 5.1). You will greet all of these

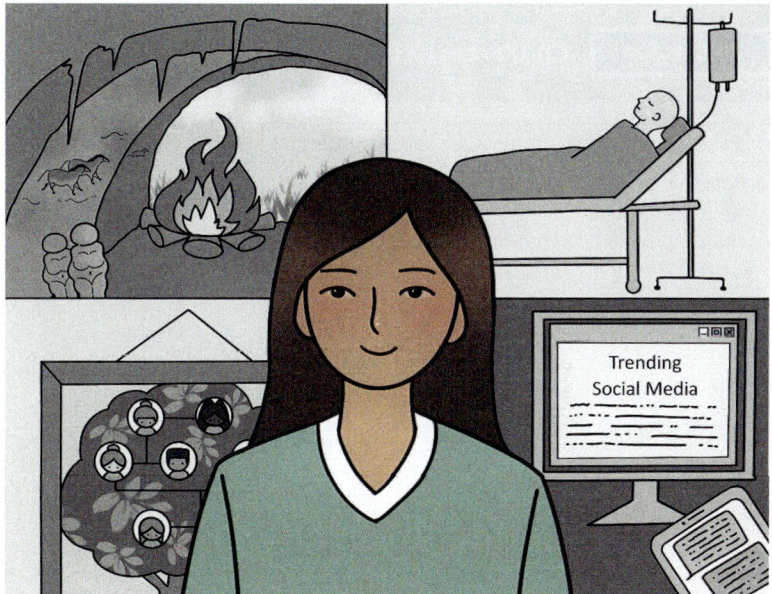

FIGURE 5.1. Four Faces of Patient. (Clockwise from upper right: patient, techno-consumer, person, human animal.)

faces in your clinical encounters. Recognizing which face presents itself at any given moment helps you know how best to respond.

I refer to the four presentations of self as "faces" for three reasons. The face is what our eyes first behold when we greet someone. Face is also a critical aspect of our presentation of self in public settings; it is the image we project, the mask we wear. Finally, I mean "face" as alterity or otherness, as an ethical obligation, as the complex other we encounter face-to-face, becoming aware of the other's mortality and vulnerability and feeling called upon to respond.[5] The four faces awaken a moral imperative to care. It is also a wonder to see the many different ways people represent these four aspects or faces of self. Table 5.2 highlights some of the characteristics of the four faces of patients.

Most individuals appearing before us in the clinic present with the face of the patient, or *patiens*: someone suffering a loss of power, feeling as if in a reclined position, flattened by life. They arrive with the experience of a broken body and with altered self-respect and life plans.[6] This is the face with whom we explore the malady stories. It is the face with whom we journey through the illness experience trajectory. Starting from that moment of uncertainty when the patient notices a change from "normal," we follow along through a

TABLE 5.2 Characteristics of Four Patient Faces

Face of Patient	Characteristics
Patient	Uncertainty Disruption or crisis Striving to regain self and seeking help Regaining wellness
Techno-Consumer	Growth fetish Individualism Entitlement Ruled by desire Prone to litigation Transactional relationships
Person	Particular history Particular family Particular genetics Particular communities/cultures Particular heroic (mythic) narratives
Human Animal	Storytelling-dependent brainy bipeds Locally, coevolved biology Milky way (breastfeeding and pair bonding) Tool-making collectors/hunters Tribalists Fire-making chanters

detectable disruption or crisis where change motivates them to connect with the clinic ensemble. Their efforts, with our help, strive to regain their overall sense of self and, hopefully, finally regain wellness.[7] Along the way on the health and malady journey, we meet the other three faces.

The second face, the techno-consumer, is new to the scene, arriving in the late 20th century with the accelerated appearance of new technologies and the rise of corporate globalization and consumerism. This face expects transactional relationships. This patient-as-consumer shops for care, cell phone in hand, and is, increasingly, captured within a virtual, technological habitat where satisfaction is framed by the marketplace. Expect to see this face on patients with less serious illness hoping for a rapid return to health or on those who, while on the path to recovery, become frustrated with the financial burdens of care and/or the work of rehabilitation. The techno-consumer face is animated by a forceful capitalist ethic that highlights individualism, entitlement, and a belief in progress through technology. This face, prone to litigation, emphasizes the gap between satisfaction and fulfillment. Happiness is defined by what we own and how we appear, often believing it needs some type of enhancement to feel "normal."[8-13] The accompanying transactional relationships are more impersonal, competitive, superficial, and often virtual. Nonetheless, these techno-consumer forces assume a role in informing and shaping the healing process. Pay heed. Tread carefully. Often, this face can be shifted to another by the questions you ask. Are the headaches interfering with your work? How is your family? How did it feel when your partner ignored your distress? These questions serve to shift attention from the techno-consumer face to the patient, person, and human animal faces.

The person represents a third face. The person face is a unique combination of particularities, a repertoire of context-dependent, socially constructed identities composed of genes, history, family, cultures, places, and stories. The person face underlies the whole person health story. The generalist healer greatly benefits from an acquaintance with these particulars of the third face.[14]

We each bear the face of the human animal, our coevolved mammalian, primate, human biology wired for culture, storytelling, and spirituality.[15-17] We are family-forming brainy bipeds with symbolic language and a long dependency requiring intimate emotional and physical support and need for birth assistance. As tool-making scavengers and collectors, we cherish technology. We are nomads, restless and acquisitive, and we are homebodies, tribalists seeking companionship and a sense of fairness. We have the gift of ecological intelligence for navigating a complex food resource labyrinth and the social and emotional intelligence for navigating the complex political labyrinth of group living. And we experience transcendental consciousness with a deep awareness of spirituality. These features of the human animal face are shared within our species and can help us find common ground. Recall the Elephant and the Rider of Changing Behavior (see Figure 2.4).

When you see your next patient, notice which face(s) they present and consider adjusting your style and approach accordingly.

Clinic, Community, and Healing Landscapes

As a family practice resident, my focus was, appropriately, on what was happening in the clinic within the clinical encounter, the two circles in the middle of the Ecological Clinical Map (see Figure 2.5). But after several years practicing the generalist's craft in a very busy community practice, I realized that while the clinic is where change toward health is initiated and/or recharged, the healing emerges out in the community. What a shift in perspective and purpose! My work changed from healing in the encounter to preparing and equipping the patient to leave the encounter and reenter their life space ready to change behavior and see the world differently in such a way that healing and health were more likely to emerge. I was not so much a healer as a facilitator of healing. This shift in my understanding of the purpose of the generalist's craft led to the concept of emergent healing landscapes.[4]

An *emergent healing landscape* is a life space, the terrain and the particular places and living beings with whom a patient coevolves and from which healing emerges. Thus, there is a coevolutionary healing landscape, places, living beings, types of relationships, and paths that are possible sources for healing to emerge. Healing is a community event, a relational process, and includes family, friends, schools, bars, hair salons, and workplaces along with clinicians and their ensembles. The idea of optimal healing environments helps us appreciate some of the important features of a healing landscape.[18] Creating an optimal healing environment begins with your clinic. Table 5.3 identifies several critical aspects of an optimal healing environment, including assessment questions to evaluate how well your clinic is providing an optimal healing environment for both colleagues and patients. Consider asking your patient these questions about their local community and how well it supports them on their way back to the River of Health.

Conventional physician-centeredness and an encounter focus may act as unintentional barriers to healing. Examples include preventing team formation, impeding staff empowerment, impairing practice reflectivity, and increasing competing demands. These can deflect the importance of family and community and build resentment in the physician, resulting in cynicism such that the patient becomes a burden or enemy. Practicing the generalist's craft shifts the focus from healing in the encounter and practice to healing within each patient's healing landscape. Facilitating the emergence of this landscape can occur from any entry point and not just the practice. Think about who else in the community can help the patient in the healing process.

Practices can change to facilitate being mindful of each patient's healing landscape. This was a goal when the word *family* was adopted into the field of *family medicine*. Likewise, using the practice as a means of improving healing landscapes through the community was a hope of community-oriented primary care[19] and the creation of communities of solution.[20] The principles and processes set out for doing community-oriented primary care can expedite your clinic's support of healing landscapes. Community-oriented primary care requires a primary care practice, a defined population/community/neighborhood, and the community-oriented primary care process. Table 5.4 summarizes the features of the community-oriented primary care process.[21,22]

TABLE 5.3 **Optimal Healing Environments**

The Environments	The Constructs	Assessment Questions
Internal	Healing intention	Does the clinic have regular and explicit ways to support and affirm healing intention?
	Personal wholeness	Does the clinic ensure that everyone can show up as their authentic selves?
Interpersonal	Healing relationships	Does the clinic provide time and space for developing healing relationships?
	Healing organizations	Do the clinic organization's policies, operations, and budget support the health of all present?
Behavioral	Healthy lifestyles	Does the clinic support each person's ability to live a healthy lifestyle?
	Integrative care	Does the clinic promote the integrative use of multidisciplinary and culturally responsive approaches to health care?
External	Healing spaces	Are the clinical spaces beneficial to health and healing?
	Ecological resilience	Do the clinic's operations foster ecological sustainability?

TABLE 5.4 Features of the Community-Oriented Primary Care Process

Feature	Description
Involve community	Community advisory group
	Community memorandum(s) of agreement
	Community decision-making structure
	Consensus-building techniques
	Group facilitation
	Community visioning process
Define and characterize community	Define the community of outreach
	Community strengths and community resource list
	Community map
Identify community health problems	Community health profile
	Community symptoms and explanations
	Prioritized concerns
Develop intervention(s) Modify practice services to address priority health issues	Relationship mapping
	Community action planning
	Clinical interventions
	Community education
	Outreach programs/groups
	Collaborations with community-based programs
	Advocacy
Monitor impact(s) of intervention(s)	Participatory mixed methods evaluation

The healing landscape concept maintains the patient focus of practices but broadens the vision. The Ecological Clinical Map suggests extending that vision out from community to the bioregion. A bioregion is a life place whose boundaries are defined by multiple factors: biotic shift, watershed, landforms, cultural and historical considerations, and an ephemeral but felt presence of a region's spirit.[23] Table 5.5 elaborates on these distinguishing features.[24]

Thinking in terms of bioregions has helped many locales reimagine how they address issues related to sustainability and climate change through

TABLE 5.5 — Features of Bioregion

Features	Description
Watershed	The drainage area of the main river in the region
Biotic Shift	15%-25% change in plant/animal species (and often climate and soils)
Landform	Distinguishing ranges, plateaus, valleys
Cultural/Historical	Indigenous boundaries; long-standing historical/cultural traditions
Spirit Presence	An experienced distinguishing presence, psychological influence
Self-sustaining	Sufficient range and diversity to sustain current life internally

regional empowerment, especially in rural areas. These activities stimulate the development of regional foodways, economies, and habitats. Bioregional thinking translates, at the individual level, as *ecological identity*.[25] Our ecological identity refers to how we connect and identify with the natural world, the world around us. Table 5.6 offers four questions to help us formulate and articulate our ecological identity.

For generalist healers in primary care, a bioregional perspective not only offers insights into how to help patients reconnect with their place and habitat but also proposes a viewpoint for paying attention to emerging sources of health problems, such as new viruses and environmental contaminants.

Healing is about making good ripples. A healing landscape is a learning landscape, a terrain where hope flourishes over time. How do we cocreate

TABLE 5.6 — Ecological Identity

Where do the things I consume come from?
What do I know about the place where I live?
How am I connected to the earth and other living beings?
What is my purpose and responsibility as a human being?

multiple optimal healing places such that a patient's landscape becomes an ecology of hope? May that question be a source of inspiration.

Clinical Hand Add-Ons

The Swinging Cultural Ape

What do hemorrhoids, back pain, choking, and antibiotic resistance have in common? They all represent consequences of evolution. I uncovered the connection after some patients asked me why humans seem more prone to hemorrhoids, back pain, and choking than other animals and why antibiotic resistance seems to be getting worse. We can thank walking upright, our bipedalism, for back pain, hemorrhoids, and varicose veins, and selective pressures for language resulting in the positioning of our larynx and, hence, our propensity for choking. We have ourselves and our dominant culture of economic growth to blame for antibiotic resistance due to our excessive and often inappropriate use of antibiotics in both humans and other domesticated animals. Evolution matters when it comes to health—thus the swinging cultural ape (see Figure 5.2). Paying attention to biocultural evolution helps the generalist expand their sensemaking horizon. Let us look more closely at why evolution and bioculture matter to generalist clinicians.[26-28]

The Ecological Clinical Map tool extends our vision to include noticing the earth as a living system within our universe. Health and disease emerge from the dynamics of the living earth system. Figure 5.3 illustrates some of the key drivers of our life story.

The primary subsystems of our living earth include the air, water, and land (atmosphere, hydrosphere, lithosphere) systems, life systems, and climate systems. These three interdependent systems support and challenge each other.

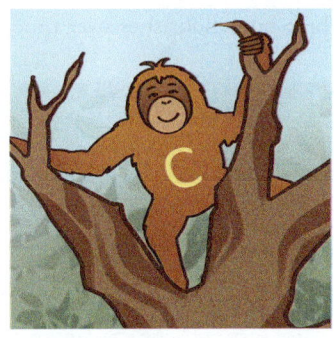

FIGURE 5.2. The Swinging Cultural Ape.

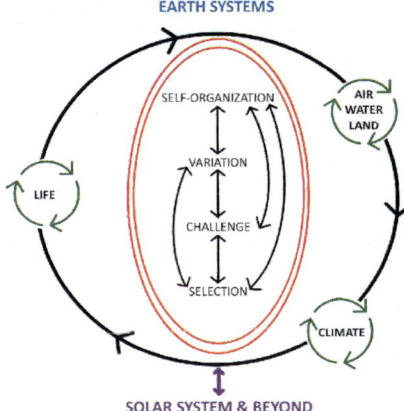

FIGURE 5.3. Drivers of Life Story.

Self-organization processes stabilize these system assemblies of life/climate/air, water, and land, where variation is continually generated. Meanwhile, challenges from subsystem changes and/or from external sources (e.g., asteroids) reveal that some self-organized variations are more adaptive than others. Selection then results in some thriving more than others, thus changing the landscape and the continuation of evolution. All of this is happening at every scale, from atom to planet, in relationship to everything else. The great ongoing story of our living earth! The nesting dolls of synergy and symbiosis! The underlying algorithm for our human narrative.

Genes, nervous system, society, and culture are all information-storage and transmission devices, life's answer to the second law of thermodynamics. Life uses information to thwart entropy. To succeed, the information must be about the habitat, and it must be mostly right. What are the ways in which life transmits new information or learning? How do change and variation get transferred to the next seven generations? Table 5.7 highlights six of the ways life accomplishes this work.[29-32]

Genetics and epigenetics appear to function in all living beings. Endosymbiosis operates mostly in the microbial world, whereas the different mechanisms of natural cooperation act in the animal and plant kingdoms. The five types of natural cooperation use genetic, epigenetic, behavioral, and symbolic inheritance mechanisms to transmit any changes to future generations. Most animals have behavioral inheritance. Symbolic inheritance is a human activity, although there is possible evidence for its existence in a few other mammals. This table is a reminder that heritable change and variation involve much more than genes and natural selection. Life is wonderfully complex.

TABLE 5.7 Mechanisms of Heritable Change and Variation

Mechanism	Description
Genetics	Darwinian natural selection and punctuated equilibrium
Epigenetics	Heritable changes in gene expression without altering nucleotide sequence
Endosymbiosis	How prokaryotes became eukaryotes; one organism lives inside another
Natural Cooperation	
Kin Selection	Altruism for genetic relatives
Direct Reciprocity	Repeated encounters between the same two individuals
Indirect Reciprocity	Based on reputation: a helpful organism is more likely to receive help
Network Reciprocity	Clusters of cooperators outcompete defectors
Group Selection	Competition between groups, not just individuals
Behavioral Inheritance	Imitation, social learning
Symbolic Inheritance	Set of ideas and understandings expressed symbolically (culture)

Humans, as a single species, share many common features from our evolutionary past, but there is regional biologic and cultural variation grounded in geography, climate, and food patterns. Migration and cultural change often generate health concerns stemming from existing outside of our earlier coevolutionary context. Salt sensitivity as an aggravator of hypertension in certain subpopulations[33] and a heightened risk of diabetes among several North American southwest and Alaskan Indigenous people who adopt a processed food diet[34] are examples. We are one species but not a standard package. Pay attention to migration histories and cultural changes.

Table 5.8 summarizes biocultural and evolutionary themes that potentially matter to generalist clinicians in our daily work. Included in the table are some questions to consider as you move through Clinical Discovery and Evaluation and Sensemaking.

The first theme, *interdependence*, shouts for attention from the treetops as a warning to not get lost in the weeds of reductionism. Everything is

TABLE 5.8 Why Bioculture and Evolution Matter to Clinicians

What Matters	Description	Attitude	Questions
Interdependence Nature principle Ripples Reciprocity	Everything is interconnected and interdependent and involved in exchanges—webs, cycles, and nests.	Gratitude, generosity, and responsibility	Where are interconnections? What are the ripples?
Precautionary	In the presence of scientific uncertainty, better safe than sorry.	Burden of proof on safety assurance	What are the potential harms? Is it safe?
Triune brain	Nesting of reptile, mammal, and human (culture) Culture eats strategy for breakfast.	Elephant and the Rider Importance of culture	What are the Elephant's motivations? How is culture playing a part?
Diversity and Variation	In a world of ubiquitous change, life thrives through variation and diversity.	Inclusiveness	What variations and outliers are there?
Contingency	Surprise happens unpredictably and can result in many changes.	Humility	What unique circumstances might be in play?

(continued)

TABLE 5.8 *Continued*

Development	Birth, growth, aging, and death are part of being alive.	Wonder Appreciation of the past	What is the effect of age?
Time	Vast: Earth >4.5 billion years old	Seven-generation thinking (sensible scale for our time)	What is the natural history? How long has this been around?
Change	Nothing stays the same.	Adaptability	What's the evolution story?
Scale	Different properties emerge at each scale.	Perspective-taking	How does it affect other system scales?

connected, nothing separate (see Figure 5.3). Think about the microbiome that intimately shares our body. A derivative of interdependence, the nature principle claims that sensitivity and connection to nature is essential for human health.[35] Similarly, the biophilia hypothesis proposes that humans have an innate tendency to seek connection with nature and other living beings.[36] Because of interdependence, the *precautionary* principle[37] guides the actions of generalists. Potential harms are as important as potential benefits, with an emphasis on "better safe than sorry."

Our *triune* brain serves as a useful metaphor reminding us how nonrational humans are in their decision-making and behavior. Recall the Elephant and the Rider of Changing Behavior. Table 5.9 lists a few rules of thumb from evolutionary psychology[38] that may be helpful when working with patients. The themes of diversity and variation, contingency, development, time, change, and scale were all discussed in Module 3.

Helicobacter pylori is a small, curved, microaerophilic, gram-negative, rod-shaped bacterium. It also serves as a good example of the importance of biocultural evolution for generalist healers that can provide guidance on how to use the questions in Table 5.8.[39,40] A 35-year-old man comes to see you concerned about persistent dyspepsia. He recently visited an urgent care center and tested positive for *H. pylori*. How do you think about this situation? If you search the evidence guidelines, the answer seems clear: attempt eradication of the *H. pylori* using either triple therapy with two antibiotics and a proton pump inhibitor or quadruple therapy with the addition of bismuth. *H. pylori*, in this specialist literature, is considered an infection that initiates gastritis and is the causative agent for peptic ulcer disease. On rare occasions, the gastritis becomes cancerous. Through this lens, the goal surely is eradication of the *H. pylori*.

TABLE 5.9 Behavior Rules of Thumb From Evolutionary Psychology

Emotions usually precede and guide reason.

Loss aversion: We avoid risk when feeling secure, but fight frantically when threatened.

Confidence is usually favored over realism.

Classification placed before calculus—we use categorical thinking.

Social intuition: We seek gossip, practice empathy, use mind reading, and barter.

Looking at this situation through the lens of biocultural evolution changes the conversation.[41] Let us start with the evolution story. *H. pylori* has lived in the human gut since before the first *Homo sapiens* migrated out of northeast Africa over 60,000 years ago. It has coevolved with us throughout our history and is present in every current human population with multiple mutations. Hard to call that an infection. What has changed is that the prevalence of *H. pylori* is down from 90% to 10% among children in industrialized nations like the United States, a phenomenon partly related to improved sanitation. When the initial arrival of *H. pylori* to the stomach is postponed to adulthood, the mature immune system triggers a more aggressive response.[42] Prior to the 19th century and public sanitation, peptic ulcer disease was rare despite the high presence of *H. pylori*.

Notice the interconnections between bacteria, age, immune system, and culture, and the resultant ripples. That is not all. The reason for needing triple and quadruple therapy with antibiotics is because *H. pylori* quickly develops resistance to antibiotics, making eradication problematic and not harmless. Is it safe to eradicate a bacteria that coevolved with us for all of our existence? No definitive answer yet, but being a host to *H. pylori* is associated with a lower incidence of asthma, other autoimmune disorders, and esophageal cancer. The rise in autoimmune disease in industrialized countries is inversely related to the fall in *H. pylori* prevalence in those same countries. This information raises the flag of precaution. *H. pylori* is necessary for a person to have peptic ulcer disease—but with a power law caveat. Only 10% to 20% of those with the bacterium in the United States will ever develop a peptic ulcer. Should we focus more attention on virulence factors, food interactions (fiber and probiotics reduce virulence and sugar increases), and other host-and-habitat influences?

Back to our 35-year-old patient with dyspepsia and a gut microbiome that includes *H. pylori*. In the absence of red flags for peptic ulcer disease or gastric cancer, and in the presence of the above biocultural evolutionary story, my initial advice would not include antibiotics. Fortunately, the swinging cultural ape has several limbs to explore on the Naming and Caring Tree on which to seek alternatives.

Relationship-Centered Clinical Method Add-Ons

Understanding the Whole Person

When the volume of care is high and your employer is pushing for greater productivity, it is easy to forgo time for reflection and just keep running on the hamster wheel focusing on the next presenting concern. Please step off for a moment. Remember the ritual of the five guideposts. Remember to Housekeep after each visit. Remember to save time by taking time to set the agenda. Remember, as you use the Relationship-Centered Clinical Method (see Figure 2.7) and explore understanding the whole person, to briefly check in about family and friends. This is when I might pull out my cell phone and glance at a copy of Table 5.10, which represents the work of a family physician, David Schmidt.[43] He discovered great value in convening the family for a visit when he felt stuck in the care of a patient and wondered what situations best warranted that extra time and effort. He reviewed the literature, and this table is the result. Checking it helps me keep alert and present; it takes me off the caged wheel.

At first look, this list may account for nearly all your visits, so the following caveats may help. I don't recommend always convening the family. Convening happens when the patient and I feel stuck in our progress, not when all is going well. The only exceptions are pregnancy, terminal illness, and bereavement; because these are family events, I usually convene the family at least once.

TABLE 5.10 When to Convene the Family

Pregnancy
Failure to thrive
Recurrent childhood poisoning
Preschool behavior problems
School behavior problems
Adolescent maladjustment
Major depression
Chronic illness
Diabetes
Heart disease
Poor adherence
High utilization
Terminal illness
Bereavement

Adapted from Schmidt DD. When is it helpful to convene the family? *J Fam Pract*. 1983;16(5):967-973.

Discovering Clinical Evidence: Heuristics, Clues, and Biases

I once saw a young woman concerned about night sweats and fatigue. Her complete blood count was normal except for a leukocyte count of 12,000. Her past medical history was one of excellent health, and she was active in regional marathon races. Based on my belief of her good health and the limited information, I concluded she had a viral infection and recommended rest, hydration, and time. I was wrong; she had leukemia. This could also have been an early presentation of lupus. I fell victim to premature closure due to confirmation bias. I interpreted the new information in light of my beliefs about the patient neglecting to explicitly seek information to challenge those beliefs. My fast-thinking brain thought it was offering helpful clues but didn't wait for my slower thought processes to catch up and check in.

In Module 3, Unit 4, we briefly visited four heuristics: anchoring, association, availability, and representativeness. They can offer us hunches and clues, and they can lead us astray unless challenged. Table 5.11 names and defines several of the more common heuristics, clues, and biases impacting our generalist's craft in primary care.[44-55] Heuristics, or rules of thumb, are cognitive shortcuts used by our fast-thinking brains to make quick decisions. Biases, on the other hand, are predispositions that favor a given conclusion. Biases often inform heuristics. Table 5.11 also identifies critical questions to ask yourself to ensure the heuristic or bias isn't leading you astray and down the path of premature closure. This is another useful table to have available at the point of care.

Organizing the Health Story

The standard or transactional medical care package consists of identifying the problem, taking a history, doing a brief exam, presenting a diagnosis, and prescribing a treatment. When exhausted, distressed, and not mindful, I have regressed and tried it. But, upon reflection afterward, I quickly realize it is almost never that simple, and both the patient and I are usually dissatisfied. The generalist's craft of relationship-centered care reminds us to shift into story mode and practice narrative-based primary care.[56,57] In the middle of the Relationship-Centered Clinical Method (see Figure 2.7), under Clinical Discovery and Sensemaking, sits a little box labeled *story building*. This section shares some concepts and tools that I have found particularly valuable in helping patients and me build better health stories. Table 5.12 highlights those tools.

Patient stories generally adhere to one of three narrative frames.[58] Restitution narratives move from a place of brokenness to one of restitution,

TABLE 5.11 Heuristics, Clues, and Biases

Heuristics and Clues	Definition	Critical Question(s)
Anchoring	Relying on or affixing decisions to preexisting or first-identified pieces of information	What else have I uncovered that helps make sense of the information?
Association (Illusory correlation)	Tendency to base decisions on previous clinical situations	What's different or unique about this situation?
Attribution	Tendency to make attributions—judgments and assumptions—about why people behave as they do	What's the evidence for attributing internal motivations to others?
Availability	Tendency to think that examples that readily come to mind are representative of the situation	What other examples muddy the situation?
Framing	Deciding based on the way information is presented	Is there another way to present the information?
Order effects	Tendency to better remember the first and/or last information received about the topic	What did I learn in the middle?
Representativeness	Tendency to judge probability of diagnosis by how it resembles clinical data	What doesn't fit about the diagnosis?
Substitution	Tendency to substitute a simpler approach in the face of complexity	Have I preserved all the complexity in the data?

(continued)

TABLE 5.11 Continued

Biases	Definition	Critical Question(s)
Affective	Aversion to that which evokes strong emotion, which leads to avoidance	What information evokes greatest emotion in me?
Commission	Predisposition to action; tendency when overconfident	How might the proposed action be harmful?
Confirmation	Tendency to interpret new information as confirmation of one's current beliefs—a form of overinterpretation and motivated reasoning (lessens cognitive dissonance)	How might this new information change my current beliefs?
False priors (Implicit bias)	Bringing false beliefs into decision-making (e.g., gender bias, stereotyping—often implicit)	What biases, especially racial and gender, underlie the interpretation?
Narrative	Being drawn toward a particular outcome because it has a better story	How might different outcomes change the story?
Optimism	Overestimating the likelihood of positive things while underestimating the likelihood of negative	Have I overlooked any negative data?
Outcome	Preference for what you want to happen rather than what you believe will really happen	What do I want to happen? What do I believe will happen?

Overconfidence (Egocentric)	Overestimating what you know and relying too heavily on your own perspective (self-serving bias)	What do others think? What information am I missing?
Social desirability	Presenting oneself, in a given social context, in a way perceived to be socially acceptable (impression management and self-deception)	What is expected in this social and cultural situation? Am I willing to openly disagree with the patient or colleagues?
Visceral	Excessive emotional investment in your relationship with patient	What would I think if I didn't know this person?

TABLE 5.12 Story Tools

Tool	Description
Narrative Types	Restitution, Quest, Chaos
Time Patterns	Acute, Cyclic, Chronic (diseased self, chronic threat, integrated self)
Plot Themes	Love, Mastery, Loss (prosperity, security, meaning)
Plot Motivators	Self-esteem and intimacy motivate love. Control motivates mastery. Separation motivates loss.
Plot Complicators	Money, Escape, Sex, Children, Comorbidity
Plot Trajectories	Heroic, Sad, Tragic, Comic
Characters and Settings	People, Pets, and Places
Metaphors	Rebirth, battle, journey, machine, disruption, dying, health-mindedness, survivor
Images	Uncertainty, anxiety, anger, helplessness, depression, isolation, competence
Emplotment	Body as symbol

a return to a prior better state. You find these in clinical routines and some maintenance ceremonies. Chaos narratives contain almost no narrative. The plot is jumbled and confusing. These are new dramas, transition ceremonies. Quest narratives come in many forms, and all of them move from a prior normal state interrupted by affliction, followed by a quest to some new state. These are the dramas of clinical care.

As in all stories, time plays an important part with several possible patterns. The timing of the malady can be acute, meaning symptomatic, temporary, and potentially curable, as in pneumonia, or it might be cyclic, signifying symptomatic and recurrent, as with asthma. A third time pattern, chronic, refers to malady that has become an ongoing part of the self, such as chronic obstructive lung disease. The chronic pattern exhibits several variations. In the diseased self, the malady becomes central to self-identity. Another variation is that of chronic threat, where the affliction is seen as a constant threat requiring unceasing vigilance. Integrated self is a more helpful version of the chronic time pattern for returning to the River of Health. Integrated self is where the malady joins the self and becomes a part to be cared for, but life and the other parts of self usually come first. One of my goals with patients in a chronic quest narrative is to help them rewrite their story toward one of integrated self.

Health and malady stories build upon the three common human themes of love, mastery, and loss motivated by concerns about self-esteem and intimacy for love, control for mastery, and separation for loss. These plot drivers become complicated by issues of money, escape, sex, children, and comorbidity. Thinking stories reminds us of these matters of plot themes, motivators, and complicators that weave through and profoundly affect the malady and its care.

In addition, the metaphors and images mentioned in Table 5.12 alert us to the language of affliction used by the patient. Emplotment is the narrative term for story building.[59] It refers to assembling information into a coherent narrative with a meaningful plot that is embodied by the patient. This information is assembled by exploring the patient's stories and understanding them as a whole person, from your Clinical Discovery and Evaluation work, and from what you learned at the Round Table of Evidence. These are health narratives. Focus them on the body and what it does. Use the body's symbolic referents such as the back for support, heart for life, and spasm for trapped. Build the story together with the patient and connect it to the patient's goals.

A group of family physicians developed a clever prompt, MENCH, to remind generalist healers in primary care of the many important stories available to assist us and help our patients find their way back toward the River of Health.[60,61] Table 5.13 highlights the different stories.

TABLE 5.13 **MENCH: The Multiple Stories of the Generalist Craft**

Story	Description
M: Mindful	Clinician story—reflexivity
E: Evidentiary	Evidence, pathophysiology, knowledge story
N: Narrative	Patient and family story
C: Centered	Context and place story
H: Health care	Healing and craft story

Patient (and Clinician) Denial—or Is It?

Thinking of Erna still makes me sweat. I first met Erna when she was 40 and I was just a few years out of residency. A recent immigrant from Jamaica, Erna struggled with asthma, high blood pressure, migraine headaches, and more. She would always tell me everything was "Just fine, Doc." But it wasn't. I was certain she was withholding important information; she was in denial. Or was she? So, around our fifth visit, I pushed harder—so hard this resourceful, stoic woman broke into tears. But still no new information. The night after that visit, I was on call for our practice and was summoned to the hospital emergency department to see Erna, who was having a hypertensive emergency and in status asthmaticus. Several hours later, breathing more comfortably and her blood pressure stabilizing, Erna raised her head, met my eyes, and forcefully stated in her heavy Jamaican accent, "You pushed too hard, Doc." I did a lot of reflection on my actions that day. Indeed, I had pushed too hard. I have learned more about what we label denial, its many forms, its protective importance, its dangers, and when and how to more appropriately respond and ensure a sense of safety when I do. Erna was not in denial but protecting herself from past trauma until it was safe enough to surface that history.

How symptoms are formed and the illness narrative given meaning are complicated by our human tendency toward denial, wanting and often needing, mostly unconsciously, to maintain things as we would like, not as they are.[62,63] We all have some. But the issues are more thorny than the word suggests. *Denial* carries negative connotations hinting at deceit, weakness, hiding, ignorance. Like thorns on a rose bush, denial may prick those who come too close, but they also guard and protect great but fragile beauty that can draw people in and bring them great joy. Maybe a better word than denial for this protecting of information is "safeguarding."

Safeguarding and denial frequently serve to protect us, especially if supporting resources are not adequate. This is particularly common for those who experience developmental trauma. Similarly, safeguarding and denial can work on behalf of avoidance—to avoid fear, shame, mortality, responsibility, change, loss. Don't push your patients into this treacherous territory! Ask for permission before probing into a line of inquiry. Build resources, and a sense of safety,[64] probe gently, and back off if you encounter significant resistance.

Similarly, safeguarding and denial can serve as a form of self-promotion, as a means of putting your best face forward, and is associated with higher self-esteem and social desirability. Use promotional safeguarding and denial to help motivate the Elephant for needed behavior change. Table 5.14 summarizes four aspects of safeguarding and denial.

TABLE 5.14 — Faces of Safeguarding and Denial

Face	Description	Approach
Protection and Avoidance	Protective—esp. if resources aren't adequate or history of developmental trauma Avoiding fear, shame, mortality, responsibility, change, loss Often associated with poor health, dogmatism, body focus	DON'T PUSH! Go slowly
Promotion	Putting your best face forward Associated with high self-esteem and social desirability	Explore what and who matter
Disease	Patients with chronic disease who maintain acute script Fear, uncertainty, anxiety, anger, helplessness, isolation Lack positive images of competence, humor, family, friends	Connect with support groups; explore fears
Health	Patients without disease who maintain script of illness Fear psychic pain of relationship, potential failure Lack positive images; lack sense of coherence	Develop explicit life plans; explore fears

Clinicians know the processes of safeguarding and denial well. Much of the socialization in clinical training concerns inculcating future clinicians with the ability to shelter themselves from experiencing deep emotions in the midst of caring for others in situations of intense suffering and moral ambiguity. This is necessary in order to maintain professional distance and equanimity. What is often not taught is how to differentiate between safeguarding to enable good care from denial, which can impede intuitive insight and even result in disconnection from self. The thriving skills in Module 1 and many of the tools explored in this *Field Guide* are intended to help with this discernment. The same is true for patients.

Of course, denial of disease is not helpful. This is one denial you can push with vigor. Denial of disease can delay seeking care and can complicate treatment adherence. Improving health literacy and building up resources are helpful strategies. Denial of health can often be the most frustrating for the clinician and the patient. These are patients who struggle to own the health they have, the worried well who need support in generating purpose and meaning and rediscovering the joy in living in the River of Health.

Round Table of Evidence Add-Ons

Sensemaking and Mindlines

I have learned some of the most helpful tips about caring for patients when discussing cases with colleagues or participating in Balint groups. Those were the settings where I discovered that reductionist evidence-based guidelines were insufficient for excellent generalist care. I discovered the Round Table of Evidence (see Figure 2.8). What a delightful surprise when I learned about a team of researchers in the United Kingdom who were intensely observing and unpacking how general practitioners gathered and used their clinical knowledge. How did generalist clinicians handle all the inherent complexity, the multiple factors and challenges of primary care clinical problems, and incorporate guideline evidence into their practice? Their answer: *mindlines*. "These are guidelines-in-the-head, in which evidence from a wide range of sources has been melded with tacit knowledge through experience and continual learning to become internalized as a clinician's personal guide to practicing in varied contexts."[65] Table 5.15 lists the sources and contents of the mindlines.[66] Notice the importance of colleagues and multiple kinds of knowledge sources.

TABLE 5.15 Mindlines of General Practice

Sources of Mindlines	Content of Mindlines
Colleagues	Peer values
Patients' views	Soft skills
Experience	Tacit and experiential knowledge
Textbooks	Heuristics
Journals/Magazines	Embedded science

TABLE 5.15	Continued
Teaching/Training	Teachers'/Trainers' norms
Education sessions	Practical skills
Opinion leaders	Role models' behavior
Organizational infrastructure	Institutional culture
Media	Illness scripts
"They say. . ."	Rules of thumb
Reps, e.g., academic detailing	Technical skills
Local guidance	Local norms and routines
Central guidance	Guidelines

The challenge is sifting the wisdom from all these sources and leaving the misleading behind. The exemplars had excellent critical appraisal skills, avoided groupthink, and were open to being challenged by others. "Above all, the common thread appeared to be creating the space and the comfortable climate for respectful critical dialogue even during the everyday chatting and story-swapping we all enjoy. Mindlines, knowledge-in-practice-in-context, collective sensemaking, communities of practice, contextual adroitness, and knowledge transformation may all play an inescapable role in developing good clinical care."[65] That relational space for respectful critical dialogue awaits you at the Round Table of Evidence.

REFERENCES

1. Schön DA. *The Reflective Practitioner: How Professionals Think in Action*. Basic Books; 1983.
2. Schön DA. *Educating the Reflective Practitioner: Toward a New Design for Teaching and Learning in the Professions*. John Wiley & Sons, Inc; 1987.
3. Hawkins AH. *Reconstructing Illness: Studies in Pathography*. Purdue University Press; 1993.
4. Miller WL, Crabtree BF. Healing landscapes: patients, relationships, and creating optimal healing places. *J Altern Complement Med*. 2005;11(suppl 1):S41-S49.
5. Edgoose JYC, Edgoose JM. Finding hope in the face-to-face. *Ann Fam Med*. 2017;15(3):272-274.
6. Brody H. *Stories of Sickness*. 2nd ed. Oxford University Press; 2003.

7. Morse JM, Johnson JL. Toward a theory of illness: the illness constellation model. In: Morse JM, Johnson JL, eds. *The Illness Experience: Dimensions of Suffering*. Sage Publications, Inc; 1991:315-342.
8. Hamilton C. *Growth Fetish*. Pluto Press; 2004.
9. Ritzer G. *The McDonaldization of Society*. Pine Forge Press; 2004.
10. Layard R. *Happiness: Lessons from a New Science*. The Penguin Press; 2005.
11. Elliott C. *Better Than Well: American Medicine Meets the American Dream*. W. W. Norton & Company; 2003.
12. Stivers R. *Shades of Loneliness: Pathologies of a Technological Society*. Rowman & Littlefield Publishers; 2004.
13. Becker G. *Disrupted Lives: How People Create Meaning in a Chaotic World*. University of California Press; 1997.
14. McWhinney IR. 'An acquaintance with particulars…'. *Fam Med*. 1989;21(4):296-298.
15. Fuentes A. *Evolution of Human Behavior*. Oxford University Press; 2009.
16. Condemi S, Savatier F. *A Pocket History of Human Evolution: How We Became Sapiens*. The Experiment, LLC; 2019.
17. Newsom L, Richerson PJ. *A Story of Us: A New Look at Human Evolution*. Oxford University Press; 2021.
18. Sakallaris BR, MacAllister L, Voss M, et al. Optimal healing environments. *Glob Adv Health Med*. 2015;4(3):40-45.
19. Nutting PA, ed. *Community-Oriented Primary Care: From Principle to Practice*. Health Resources and Services Administration; 1987.
20. Griswold KS, Lesko SE, Westfall JM; Folsom Group. Communities of solution: partnerships for population health. *J Am Board Fam Med*. 2013;26(3):232-238.
21. Rhyne R, Cashman S, Kantrowitz M. An introduction to community-oriented primary care (COPC). In: Rhyne R, Bogue R, Kukulka G, et al, eds. *Community-Oriented Primary Care: Health Care for the 21st Century*. American Public Health Association; 1998:1-15.
22. Nutting PA. Community-oriented primary care: an integrated model for practice, research, and education. *Am J Prev Med*. 1986;2(3):140-147.
23. Aberley D, ed. *Boundaries of Home: Mapping for Local Empowerment*. New Society Publishers; 1998.
24. Dodge J. Living by life: some bioregional theory and practice. In: Andruss V, Plant C, Plant J, et al, eds. *Home! A Bioregional Reader*. New Society Publishers; 1990:5-12.
25. Thomashow M. *Ecological Identity: Becoming a Reflective Environmentalist*. The MIT Press; 1995.
26. Lieberman DE. *The Story of the Human Body: Evolution, Health, and Disease*. Pantheon Books; 2013.
27. Trevathan WR, Smith EO, McKenna JJ. *Evolutionary Medicine and Health: New Perspectives*. Oxford University Press; 2008.
28. Helman CG. *Culture, Health and Illness*. 5th ed. Hodder Arnold; 2007.

29. Jablonka E, Lamb MJ. *Evolution in Four Dimensions: Genetic, Epigenetic, Behavioral, and Symbolic Variation in the History of Life*. MIT Press; 2005.
30. Gray MW. Lynn Margulis and the endosymbiont hypothesis: 50 years later. *Mol Biol Cell*. 2017;28(10):1285-1287.
31. Martin WF, Garg S, Zimorski V. Endosymbiotic theories for eukaryote origin. *Philos Trans R Soc Lond B Biol Sci*. 2015;370(1678):20140330.
32. Nowak MA. Five rules for the evolution of cooperation. *Science*. 2006;314(5805):1560-1563.
33. Choi HY, Park HC, Ha SK. Salt sensitivity and hypertension: a paradigm shift from kidney malfunction to vascular endothelial dysfunction. *Electrolyte Blood Press*. 2015;13(1):7-16.
34. McLaughlin S. Traditions and diabetes prevention: a healthy path for Native Americans. *Diabetes Spectr*. 2010;23(4):272-277.
35. Louv R. *The Nature Principle: Reconnecting with Life in a Virtual Age*. Algonquin Books of Chapel Hill; 2011.
36. Gaekwad JS, Sal Moslehian A, Roös PB, et al. A meta-analysis of emotional evidence for the biophilia hypothesis and implications for biophilic design. *Front Psychol*. 2022;13:750245.
37. Kriebel D, Tickner J, Epstein P, et al. The precautionary principle in environmental science. *Environ Health Perspect*. 2001;109(9):871-876.
38. Buss DM. *Evolutionary Psychology: The New Science of the Mind*. 7th ed. Routledge; 2025.
39. Godavarthy PK, Puli C. From antibiotic resistance to antibiotic renaissance: a new era in *Helicobacter pylori* treatment. *Cureus*. 15(3):e36041.
40. Polk DB, Peek RM. *Helicobacter pylori*: gastric cancer and beyond. *Nat Rev Cancer*. 2010;10(6):403-414.
41. Correa P, Piazuelo MB. Evolutionary history of the *Helicobacter pylori* genome: implications for gastric carcinogenesis. *Gut Liver*. 2012;6(1):21-28.
42. Roberts-Thomson IC. Rise and fall of peptic ulceration: a disease of civilization? *J Gastroenterol Hepatol*. 2018;33(7):1321-1326.
43. Schmidt DD. When is it helpful to convene the family? *J Fam Pract*. 1983;16(5):967-973.
44. Kahneman D. *Thinking, Fast and Slow*. Farrar, Straus, and Giroux; 2011.
45. Preisz A. Fast and slow thinking; and the problem of conflating clinical reasoning and ethical deliberation in acute decision-making. *J Paediatr Child Health*. 2019;55(6):621-624.
46. Gorini A, Pravettoni G. An overview on cognitive aspects implicated in medical decisions. *Eur J Intern Med*. 2011;22(6):547-553.
47. Krumpal I. Determinants of social desirability bias in sensitive surveys: a literature review. *Qual Quant*. 2013;47(4):2025-2047.
48. Taleb NN. *The Black Swan: The Impact of the Highly Improbable*. Random House; 2007.
49. FitzGerald C, Hurst S. Implicit bias in healthcare professionals: a systematic review. *BMC Med Ethics*. 2017;18(1):19.

50. Klein JG. Five pitfalls in decisions about diagnosis and prescribing. *BMJ*. 2005;330(7494):781-783.
51. Bansback N, Li LC, Lynd L, et al. Exploiting order effects to improve the quality of decisions. *Patient Educ Couns*. 2014;96(2):197-203.
52. Gopal DP, Chetty U, O'Donnell P, et al. Implicit bias in healthcare: clinical practice, research and decision making. *Future Healthc J*. 2021;8(1):40-48.
53. Hugh TB, Dekker SWA. Hindsight bias and outcome bias in the social construction of medical negligence: a review. *J Law Med*. 2009;16(5):846-857.
54. Callaham ML, Wears RL, Weber EJ, et al. Positive-outcome bias and other limitations in the outcome of research abstracts submitted to a scientific meeting. *JAMA*. 1998;280(3):254-257.
55. Ogdie AR, Reilly JB, Pang WG, et al. Seen through their eyes: residents' reflections on the cognitive and contextual components of diagnostic errors in medicine. *Acad Med*. 2012;87(10):1361-1367.
56. Charon R. *Narrative Medicine: Honoring the Stories of Illness*. Oxford University Press; 2006.
57. Launer J. *Narrative-Based Primary Care: A Practical Guide*. Radcliffe Medical Press, Ltd; 2002.
58. Frank AW. *The Wounded Storyteller: Body, Illness, and Ethics*. 2nd ed. University of Chicago Press; 2013.
59. Mattingly C. The concept of therapeutic "emplotment." *Soc Sci Med*. 1994;38(6):811-822.
60. Borkan J, Reis S, Medalie J. Narratives in family medicine: tales of transformation, points of breakthrough for family physicians. *Fam Syst Health*. 2001;19(2):121-134.
61. Miller WL. Life matters. *Fam Syst Health*. 2001;19(2):135-137.
62. Patierno C, Fava GA, Carrozzino D. Illness denial in medical disorders: a systematic review. *Psychother Psychosom*. 2023;92(4):211-226.
63. Fricchione GL. Clinical implications of illness denial. *Psychother Psychosom*. 2023;92(4):208-210.
64. Lynch JM. *A Whole Person Approach to Wellbeing: Building Sense of Safety*. Routledge; 2020.
65. Gabbay J, le May A. Mindlines: making sense of evidence in practice. *Br J Gen Pract*. 2016;66(649):402-403.
66. Gabbay J, le May A. *Practice-Based Evidence for Healthcare: Clinical Mindlines*. Routledge; 2011.

Postlude

Our Partners in Health

You answered the call with your senses open wide. Inhale deeply. Take it all in. You now possess a precious gift: the ability to cocreate health in concert with your patient using the generalist's craft in primary care. This gift comes with great responsibility to share your power with those most vulnerable and without voice. Fortunately, you never work alone. Everywhere you turn, partners await your invitation to help. These partners in health-making wear the faces of our patients and our colleagues. There are no gates in primary medical care. Everyone is welcome. Together, practicing the generalist's craft, we become a community of healing.

These are challenging times to be a generalist healer, a personal clinician in primary care. The structural and cultural constraints seem all-encompassing. But they are not defining. The generalist's craft is like water; able to slowly erode rock, it finds a way around or through. And like light, it finds the cracks. No matter the setting, the generalist's craft is ready and adaptable. You are able to meet patients where they are, emotionally or geographically. The craft becomes real only when done in partnership with patients, and it grows finer when you share wisdom with colleagues. Health emerges when you exert agency in communion with others. Remember to thank your partners.

Aphorisms and Wisdom

Before sounding the last notes of our clinical jazz improvisation, I want to share a few aphorisms and wisdom from David Loxterkamp, a family physician practicing the generalist's craft in Belfast, Maine, since 1984. Here he shares 14 pithy reflections or aphorisms published in 2013.

> *Health is not a commodity.*
> *Risk factors are not disease.*
> *Aging is not an illness.*
> *Quality is more than metrics.*
> *Doing all we can is not the same as doing what we should.*
> *Time is precious. We spend it on what we value.*
> *Doctors expect too much from data and not enough from conversation.*
> *To fix a problem is easy; to share another's suffering is hard.*
> *The most common condition we treat is unhappiness.*
> *The greatest obstacle to treating patients' unhappiness is our own.*

> *Patients cannot see outside their pain; we cannot see in. Relationship is the bridge between.*
> *Nothing is more patient-centered than the process of change.*
> *Community is the locus of healing, not the hospital or the clinic.*
> *The foundation of medicine is conversation, friendship, and hope.*[1]

These words continue to ring true. More recently in a personal communication, David shared some observations on what he terms the elements favoring healing. They are as follows:

The patient's desire to get better
The patient's belief in you
A trusting relationship built on attention, touch, and kindness
A generalist's appreciation that diagnoses are provisional, outcomes uncertain
The reassurance—sometimes merely the appearance—that things are under control
Our license to ask anything
The active inclusion of family and community in the patient's care

Apply these generously, and health will be nearby. Another source of clinical wisdom is found in the April 12, 2024, issue of *Family Medicine and Community Health*, wherein 100 authors published 99 mini-essays exploring the many dimensions of our generalist's craft in a 12-part series titled, "Storylines of Family Medicine." Many of the essays relate directly to topics in the *Field Guide*.

More Than a Craft

The *Field Guide*'s purpose is to provide practical tools and models in a memorable and helpful way for doing the craft of generalist primary medical care and making healing clinical encounters. I hope, as you apply the tools and models, you rediscover the joy and love that follow. What we do is more than a craft. The craft finds its nourishment in time, place, and relationships. It is always personal and local. May the local space where you practice the generalist's craft be safe, filled with reciprocity, and steeped in a culture of gratitude.

A portal closes. On the other side, the space opens...

REFERENCE

1. Loxterkamp D. *What Matters in Medicine: Lessons From a Life in Primary Care.* The University of Michigan Press; 2013.

PART III

Supplements

SUPPLEMENT 1

Empirical and Theoretical Foundations of the Generalist's Craft

Overview

Congratulations! You are practicing the generalist's craft in primary care! You may be wondering how and why the generalist's craft works and how to make it better. Practice comes first, then the evidence and theory that, in turn, improves practice. We make better sense in retrospect.[1] Supplement 1 shares the evidence behind the craft and seeks to make sense of your experiences by presenting an overview of the empirical and theoretical foundations for this generalist craft work. The explanatory story of the generalist's craft weaves together the *primary medical care* setting and the *patients who seek care* there hoping to find *healing* and a return to *health* through *changing behavior and biology* using the perspective of *generalism*. The resulting dynamic, activated by the generalist's craft, generates *high-value primary care*.

The story begins with a fresh look at the context of care for the generalist's craft, the setting of primary medical care within the larger frame of primary health care. What is it, what are its functions, how does it fit within the larger framework of health care domains, and what features, including the generalist's craft, facilitate its effectiveness? I then consider the people and patients who currently contact primary medical care. How do people seek health care? What are their concerns and backgrounds? How do symptoms arise and get noticed or overlooked? How does understanding developmental trauma inform both illness behavior and care seeking?

Patients come for health and healing, the purpose and process of the generalist's craft in primary care. What is health? How does it happen? How does health relate to disease? What promotes health and what undermines it? You discover that health and healing emerge from lifespans of complex, interdependent dynamic webs of relationships. Moving from a lifeworld of malady (or suffering) to health requires some change in behavior and biology. I briefly showcase the metaphor of the Elephant and the Rider to highlight some of the challenges and opportunities of that change work and how the generalist's craft helps perform it.

Understanding and managing these complex activities require a generalist perspective. I unpack the many layers and meanings of generalism, and how it accommodates the expansiveness and dynamism of health. Along the way, I acknowledge how generalism both differs from and complements the tools and skills of the specialties learned in medical and nursing schools.

The discussion continues with a review of how generalism increases primary medical care's value. I conclude by summarizing the explanatory story of the generalist's craft in primary care.

Primary Medical Care

Primary Health Care

The 1978 Declaration of Alma-Ata from the World Health Organization (WHO) named primary health care as the means for ensuring comprehensive, universal, equitable, and affordable health care for everyone in the world.[2] Primary health care is defined as a multisectoral approach including community participation, public health, primary medical care, and health-related community organizations. "Primary" means, first and foremost, of chief importance and earliest in time. Primary, in terms of community participation, refers to self, friends, family, and the Internet. This primary care is who we contact first when noticing early indications of possible illness. Public health represents a community's front lines of protection against sources of affliction such as poor sanitation, infections, and environmental hazards. In terms of direct medical services, primary medical care comes first. It is the entrance to the larger health care system.

Primary medical care includes the services of physicians, nurse practitioners, midwives, and other supporting medical care professionals. The physicians are usually general practitioners/family physicians but can include general internists and pediatricians. The fourth sector of primary health care are those health-related community organizations offering frontline services such as Planned Parenthood, social workers, food banks, and community health coalitions. Figure S1.1 depicts the domains of primary health care within the larger context of the health care system including secondary, tertiary, and ancillary services. Ancillary services include diagnostics, rehabilitation services, long-term care, home care services, durable medical equipment, and pharmacies that support both primary health care and secondary health care.

Unfortunately, what's clear in the figure has become somewhat muddled in our language; primary medical care has been conflated into primary

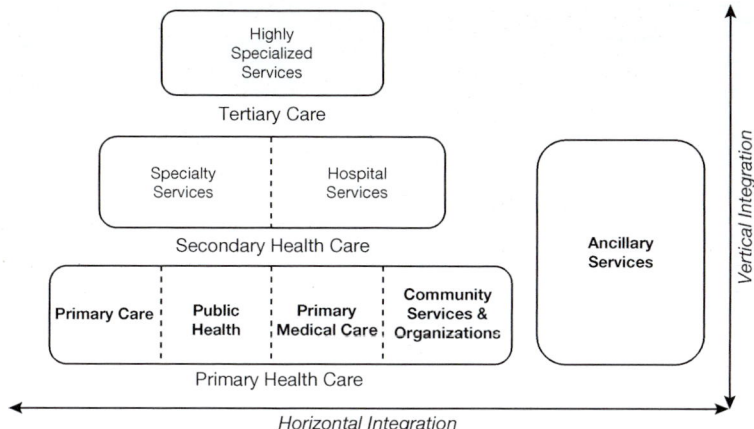

FIGURE S1.1. Domains and Context of Primary Health Care.

care. The same year as the 1978 Declaration of Alma-Ata, the United States' Institute of Medicine adopted "primary care" as shorthand for "primary medical care," with only rare mention of the larger integrated vision of "primary health care."[3] A muddle of confusion began and remains. This was unfortunate as the conflation obscured the primary care of community participation. Now, primary care solely applies to clinicians and their services, which makes invisible the real sources of primary care in the community, specifically family, friends, neighbors, coworkers, and other forms of lay health support and self-care, including virtual means. In this *Field Guide*, we restore the original meaning of primary care from Alma-Ata.

Primary Medical Care: Functions, Facilitators, and Principles

Primary medical care is home to the generalist's craft and specifically refers to general practice–type services delivered to individuals and families at the entrance to the health care delivery system. This includes behavioral health, dental, and eye care services. An important role for primary medical care is serving as an integrator of health care services (see Figure S1.1). Horizontal integration refers to the connections and interdependencies across the four domains of primary health care, including ancillary services. Vertical integration concerns the connections and coordination between the primary, secondary, and tertiary sectors of health care.

Primary medical care has the following four functions: *guiding* and *bridging* with *breadth* and *depth* (see Table S1.1).[4] All four are addressed in the

TABLE S1.1	The Four Functions of Primary Medical Care
Function	**Description**
Guide	Through malady journey toward health
Bridge	Within primary health care
	With specialists, hospital, and other secondary/tertiary care services
	Between landscapes of malady and health
	Between capacity and burden
Breadth	Encompass multiple knowledges
	Be information masters
Depth	Know the particulars of clinical medicine
	Know the particulars of persons, families, and friends
	Know the particulars of neighborhoods

generalist's craft. A patient enters primary medical care seeking *guidance* about their affliction and any necessary assistance *crossing bridges* to what else is needed, and they hope to receive that care for whatever their problem (*breadth*) in a personal, context-specific, and competent manner (*depth*).

These functions are facilitated by what are known as the four Cs of primary medical care, affirmed in the research of Barbara Starfield and her team[5,6]: First Contact access, Continuity, Comprehensiveness, and Coordination.[7] *First contact access* represents the "primary" in primary medical care and facilitates the bridging function. Not everyone feeling ill or struggling with a behavioral problem needs medical intervention. An important bridging role for primary medical care is to identify those situations and return them to the community and prevent excessive medicalization.[8] *Continuity of care* aids the depth function and refers to the relational and personal aspects of primary medical care. Continuity of care generates shared stories; shared experiences creating greater trust; a sense of safety, especially at vulnerable times; and a sense of predictability of what will happen in the relational space. *Comprehensiveness* facilitates the breadth function and highlights the broad and inclusive scope of good primary medical care and the welcoming of all concerns of people of all ages and genders. It helps prevent fragmentation of care. *Coordination* encompasses both the horizontal and vertical integration aspects of primary medical care and enables the guide function. The generalist's craft specifically builds upon these four features through its use of ritual

TABLE S1.2 The Four Cs and the Shared Principles of Primary Medical Care

The Four Cs Facilitators of Primary Medical Care	Shared Principles of Primary Medical Care *Primary Medical Care Is:*
First Contact Access	Accessible
Continuity of Care	Continuous
Comprehensiveness	Comprehensive and equitable
Coordination of Care	Coordinated and integrated
	Person- and family-centered
	Team-based and collaborative
	High value

Source: Starfield, B. *Primary Care: Concept, Evaluation, and Policy.* Oxford University Press; 1992.

Source: Epperly T, Bechtel C, Sweeney R, et al. The shared principles of primary care: a multistakeholder initiative to find a common voice. *Fam Med.* 2019;51(2):179-184.

structure via the fingers of direction and the guiding content of the Clinical Hand and its supporting tools, ensuring a sense of safety, patient engagement, and flexibility to adjust to the issues at hand while addressing what matters most to the patient.

The recently released Shared Principles of Primary Medical Care[9] restates the four Cs and adds "person and family-centered" and "team-based and collaborative," highlighting the deeply relational qualities of primary medical care (see Table S1.2 where the two are side-by-side). The result is "high value," meaning better health, higher quality, and greater equity at lower cost. One of the reasons for this high value becomes evident with a better understanding of the patients who seek and use primary medical care services. Let's explore that next.

Patients Who Seek Primary Medical Care

The Ecology of Medical Care

A series of studies on the ecology of medical care in the United States between 1961 and 2012 showed remarkable consistency in how people, including children,[10] accessed medical care. These studies depicted the number of

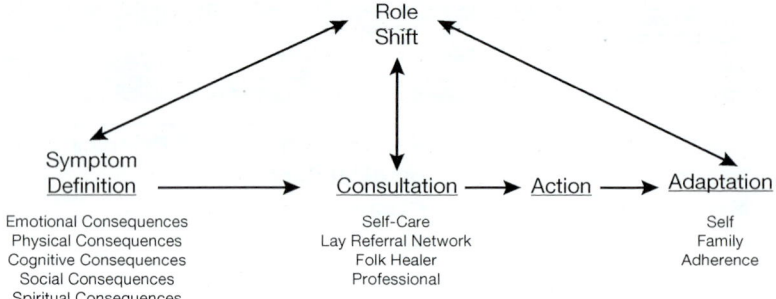

FIGURE S1.2. The Health-Seeking Process. (Modified from Chrisman NJ. The health seeking process: an approach to the natural history of illness. *Cult Med Psychiatry*. 1977;1(4):351-377.)

individuals per 1,000 persons per month who used a medical service.[11-13] The data are presented as a momentary snapshot but represent a journey that takes place over time. That journey from awareness of body change to clinical encounter and healing action is represented as the health-seeking process in Figure S1.2.[14] The figure also indicates the many options along the way, including self-care and consulting the lay referral network and the Internet, which is fancy social science language for checking with friends and family, the primary care of primary health care. During a 1-month period, about 80% of people report symptoms (experience symptom definition) but only 22% of individuals seek professional medical care and around 56% of them (12% of the thousand) access primary medical care. About 46% do self-care and/or consult friends and family (lay referral network) and almost 7% consult a folk healer. Only 8 individuals (less than 1%) out of the 1,000 people are hospitalized. Before exploring more about the 12% accessing primary medical care, let us look more closely at how people become aware of symptoms and decide to seek care.

Health, Symptoms, and Illness Behavior

Why do some people notice the palpitations of atrial fibrillation and others not? Why do some patients seemingly feel every contraction of their intestinal tract and others seem to feel them hardly at all? We can't fully answer these questions, but we have learned much about what influences our awareness of internal bodily behavior, our awareness of what become symptoms.[15-17]

Examine Figure S1.3 illustrating the symptom awareness process. The baseball player on the left has just gone into atrial fibrillation but barely notices, if at all. The person on the right, resting in a darkened and quiet room,

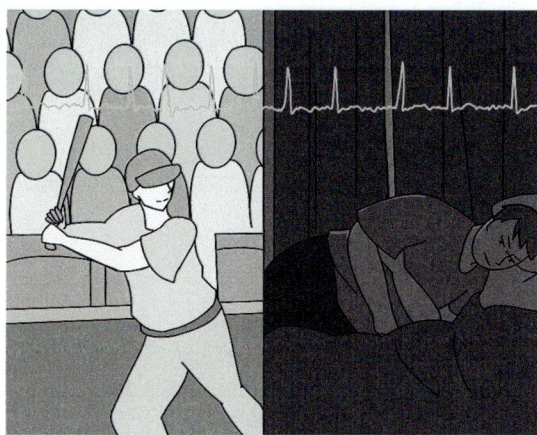

FIGURE S1.3. Symptom Awareness Process.

has also just converted to atrial fibrillation and immediately notices palpitations and feels distressed. The contexts reveal part of the explanation for the differences in symptom awareness. Let us assume the strength of the body signal indicating atrial fibrillation is the same in the two situations. Since it is the same person, we can presume cultural (cultural expectations and symbolic associations) and personal (past illness prototypes, childhood illness memories, self-identity such as stoic or expressive, etc.) factors are the same. What differs are the amount of conscious body attention and external information being processed. The baseball player focuses all attention on the pitcher and the ball amid a distracting environment of a cheering crowd and teammates. The reposing person, immersed in quiet, hears the heartbeat in his ear where it rests on the pillow. He immediately recognizes irregularity and feels palpitations. All of this is quickly processed through the emotional limbic brain, cortical locator, and cognitive processor, with a quick check on social/cultural context and spiritual significance. I call this *five-limb processing and encoding*. (Notice their alignment with the five limbs of the Naming and Caring Tree.) In summary, awareness of an internal physiologic change is a function of the ratio of internal to external signals.

Awareness of body change does not necessarily mean a symptom. The feeling of mild cramping in the lower abdomen might only be physiologic intestinal contractions triggered by the gastrocolic reflex following a satisfying meal. To become a symptom requires further interpretation and formative processes. The three-step process of symptom formation is outlined in Table S1.3.[15-17] The process begins with recognition of an internal bodily

| TABLE S1.3 | **Symptom Formation Process** |

Awareness of Body Change
Awareness of body change is a function of internal signals/ external signals (f(I/E))

Equation 1
$BA = (1/EI)(Cf)(Pf)$
where BA is the strength of conscious Body Attentiveness (values from 0.1 to 4)
EI is amount of External Information (values from 1 to 10)
Decreases with boredom, relaxation
Increases with surprise, social situations
Cf is amount of Cultural factors influence (values from 1 to 2)
Influenced by cultural expectations, symbols
Pf is amount of Personal factors influence (values from 1 to 2)
Decreases with denial/safeguarding, suppression
Increases with developmental trauma, negative affect

Equation 2
$ABC = (BS)(BA)$
where ABC is Awareness of Body Change (values from 0.1 to 20)
BS is strength of Body Signals (values from 1 to 5)
Increases with internal change, magnitude of signal
Threshold for when likely to notice body change is ABC value >1-2

Interpretation of Body Change
Is the body change related to normal physiology? If so, ignore.
Is the body change a symptom related to a disease process (expression of bodily problem requiring medical attention)? If so, seek care or temporarily deny and rationalize.
Or is this something else? If everyday explanation, correct issue. If uncertain, wait, observe, and/or test.

Symptom Formation
Symptom is bounded, contextualized, and given meaning (will become basis for parameters of history of present illness)
Five-limb encoding (from Naming and Caring Tree)

change as described earlier. The values associated with the different variables in the table are rough estimates that allow you to experiment with the model and better appreciate the variability in symptom awareness.

This awareness then needs interpretation, which includes both an explanation and a possible response. Is it normal bodily function, an indicator of pathophysiology, or something else? Knowledge, past experiences, current situation, cultural expectations, and more influence the explanatory interpretation. The response depends upon the explanation. If the belly rumbling is deemed normal, then it can be ignored, and you smile. On the other hand, if you decide the abdominal discomfort is an early indicator of possible colon cancer, you groan and contact your primary care clinician. If that is too scary to think about, you suppress your fear and choose to delay checking it out. The abdominal discomfort happened shortly after an unusually spicy meal, so you conclude the spices triggered the cramps and vow to stick with less spicy foods in the future. Of course, you might be uncertain about what is going on and therefore elect to wait and observe before taking some other action.

Once you decide the experienced change is a symptom worthy of care seeking or consultation, the body takes note, begins processing it as such, and stores that information in cellular and neurologic memory. That processing, or five-limb encoding, includes associating the symptom with other body experiences, bounding and contextualizing it, then giving it meaning. The symptom gets linked to the current emotional state, localized to a physical body area with imagined cognitive explanations, and informed by the opinions of others, including its impact on social roles and relationships. Finally, the symptom often heightens the sense of mortality. Thus, every symptom has at least five sets of consequences that the body never forgets. Once a symptom is identified as such, body history is being written. That body history comes with the patient to the clinical encounter and will call upon your generalist's craft and your specific skill at swinging on the limbs of the tree on the Palm of Hope on the Clinical Hand to coax it out while doing clinical discovery and evaluation.

The original question of this section was, "Who connects with primary medical care?" At any given moment, it could be anyone experiencing most anything. That is the surprise factor in primary medical care. Most frequently, however, a person who connects with primary medical care is more likely to be someone with multiple concerns, often socially isolated with limited resources, with a history of developmental trauma. Time to examine in more detail who those 12% are that access primary medical care and benefit from the generalist's craft.

Frequent Attenders and Power Laws

Our patients—the population of people who choose to connect with primary medical care in any given neighborhood—are neither the entire population of that community nor a representative sample of that community. Instead, we witness more examples of power laws and the 80/20 Pareto distribution.[18] Many members of the community rarely or never connect with primary medical care, whereas a few account for most visits. Ten percent of patients, the frequent attenders, account for 50% of visits.[19] Frequent attenders are much more likely to be socially isolated,[20] and at least a quarter of these frequent attenders are children brought to us by parents or caregivers.[21] Frequent attenders, often referred to as "frequent symptom reporters" or "heartsink" patients, are often lonely, sad, anxious, and/or angry individuals with multiple chronic, recurrent problems, accompanied by family and interpersonal stress and inadequate personal resources.[22] They come to us with the experience of being "flattened by life" with complicated, painful, poorly understood stories of their illness, of themselves, and of their families, struggling to find agency and belonging. They want a deeper wisdom, not just medical information, and are often in denial or safeguarding (hiding or protecting from some part of their past or future). Attending to them requires use of the generalist's craft and especially our use of the Relationship-Centered Clinical Method.

Primary medical care clinicians chronicle what they see in their clinics in the form of diagnoses as the reason for visit (RFV). Patients, on the other hand, are more likely to report symptoms. The 10 most common clinician-reported RFVs were upper respiratory tract infection, hypertension, routine health maintenance, arthritis, diabetes, depression or anxiety, pneumonia, acute otitis media, back pain, and dermatitis. The 10 most common patient-reported RFVs were symptomatic conditions including cough, back pain, abdominal symptoms, pharyngitis, dermatitis, fever, headache, leg symptoms, unspecified respiratory concerns, and fatigue.[23] Love the variety! Again, this calls for applying the generalist's craft. Table S1.4 summarizes the above information regarding who connects with primary medical care. Notice how frequently developmental trauma appears in this table.

Developmental Trauma and Trauma-Informed Care

Developmental trauma accounts for or plays a significant role in over half of people coming to primary medical care, and perhaps four out of five people coming most often.[24] Developmental trauma damages health in many ways. Early life adversity, mitigated by protective factors and aggravated by predisposed vulnerability, is scarring for life. It generates toxic stress through chronic dysregulation of neurologic, endocrine, and immune systems, resulting in

TABLE S1.4 — Who Connects With Primary Medical Care

Patient Feature	Background
Frequent Attender	Socially isolated and social insecurity
	Often children with underlying family issues
	Chronic illness
	History of family conflict/abuse
Medically Unexplained Symptoms	Overlap with Frequent Attender
Developmental Trauma History	Common with Frequent Attenders
	Common with Medically Unexplained Symptoms
	Excess physiologic activity
Acute Concerns	Often associated with behavioral health concerns
Chronic Concerns	Often multiple
	Often associated with developmental trauma history
	Associated behavioral health concerns
Health Maintenance	Often associated with key life cycle moments
	Prevention and health promotion
Administrative Issues	Sanctioning sick role
	Attesting health status (insurance, sports, etc.)

health problems often involving epigenetics that can carry on to future generations.[25] Many chronic illnesses develop from the unhealthy soil of developmental trauma. The two most common sources of developmental trauma are *adverse childhood experiences* and *adverse community environments*, often referred to as the "pair of ACES." The former includes maternal depression, emotional and sexual abuse, substance use, domestic violence, physical and emotional neglect, divorce, mental illness, incarceration, and homelessness. Poverty, discrimination, community disruption, violence, poor housing quality and affordability, and lack of opportunity, economic mobility, and social capital are examples of adverse community environments.[26]

Go back a few pages and carefully review Table S1.4. A history of developmental trauma informs nearly every category. It is omnipresent in the primary medical care clinic. Thus, the care we offer needs to be trauma-informed such that everyone on the clinic team or ensemble takes the individual's experience of trauma into account, and this occurs at clinical and organizational levels. Instead of a clinician mindset pondering, "What's wrong with you?" shift to wondering "What happened to you?" Table S1.5 identifies some key principles of a trauma-informed approach.[27] In the primary medical care setting, it becomes especially important to build a foundation of trauma-informed values, partnerships in the community, clinic champions, and ongoing monitoring and evaluation.[28]

Table S1.6 summarizes an approach to trauma-informed primary medical care at the practice level using the six Rs.[29]

Our community neighbors usually come to connect with us when troubled and/or pursuing better health. It is those most vulnerable who seek us

TABLE S1.5 Key Principles of Trauma-Informed Approach

Principle	Description
Safety	For patients and staff
	Freedom from threat or harm
	Prevention of further retraumatization
Trustworthiness and Transparency	Of policies and procedures
	Build trust among staff, patients, and wider community
Collaboration and Mutuality	Recognize the value of everyone's experiences and strengths
	Use to improve care
Empowerment and Choice	Share power
	Involve patients in decision-making
	Ensure patients' voice in practice
Inclusiveness	Cultural and gender issues paid attention to
	Historical issues paid attention to, e.g., race

Adapted from Fallot R, Harris M. *Trauma-Informed Services: A Self-Assessment and Planning Protocol*. Community Connections; 2006.

TABLE S1.6	Trauma-Informed Primary Medical Care at the Practice Level
Action	**Description**
Review	Educate team about trauma and health; hold regular meetings
Recognize	Collect trauma history; screen
Realize	Understand health effects of trauma; educate patients
Respond	Prioritize patient-centered communication; shared decision-making; connect to community-based programs
	Shift mindset from "What's wrong with you?" to "What happened to you?"
Respect	Prioritize emotional safety; avoid triggers; maintain calm and participatory safe space
Resilience	Emphasize strengths and positive aspects of patients

Adapted from Roberts SJ, Chandler GE, Kalmakis K. A model for trauma-informed primary care. *J Am Assoc Nurse Pract*. 2019;31(2):139-144.

most often. These patients demonstrate why the generalist healer addresses the emotional, physical, cognitive, social, spiritual, and contextual dimensions in their care.[30] As clinicians, we both witness[31] and act.[32] That action involves using the generalist's craft to promote healing and generate better health. What do I mean by health and healing?

Health and Healing

Introduction

The goal of primary medical care is health, and health is the purpose for the generalist's craft. Understanding the meaning and lived experience of health becomes foundational for appreciating how and why the generalist's craft works. Thus, what follows is a brief but deep dive into the definition of health and what supports and hinders it. I will begin by exploring the relationship between health and disease and how the concept of health has evolved over the past 75 years. This is followed by a detour into complexity theory and how it informs our considerations of health. The conceptual history and insights from complexity theory are then combined into a working definition of health as membership and imagined as the guiding metaphor, River of Health. After a quick overview of the drivers of health, I'll explore how healing happens, the role of healing relationships, and close with the guiding metaphor, the Spiral of Healing, which supports the generalist's craft.

Health as Concept

A common misunderstanding views health and disease as a dualism, an either/or. If you are healthy, you are free of disease and if you have a disease, you are unhealthy. Through this lens, the purpose of all doctoring is the elimination of disease. A review of the history of healing and medicine quickly reveals that this is too simplistic.[33] The boundaries between health and disease have always been blurry and overlapping. But it took the developing early- to mid-20th-century scientific comprehension of disease as an abnormal or harmful condition that adversely affects the structure or function of the body to help clarify the distinctions. That same time period also saw the emergence of medical specialties focused on the diagnosis and management of disease and medical generalists doing primary care and emphasizing the promotion of health. In 1948, the WHO declared a new definition for health as "a *state* of *complete* physical, mental and social well-being and *not merely the absence of disease* or infirmity" (emphasis mine).[34] This definition highlights three features important for our understanding: (1) health as a "state" maintained in the face of uncertainty and disruption; (2) health as a holistic ("complete") understanding of the body with multiple components[35]; and (3) health as more than "the absence of disease." Several decades later, WHO and others added the ability to lead a productive life as well as a spiritual dimension to their articulations of health.[35]

Additional perspectives on health arise from patient advocates and the world of general practice. From a lay perspective, the definition of health includes holism and two additional dimensions: (1) health as relative, that is, *How do I perceive myself relative to my particular culture and situations?*; and (2) health as personal and functional, that is, *How do my particular abilities act in the world?*[36] Family physician and epidemiologist Kurt Stange defines health as the "ability to develop meaningful relationships and pursue a transcendent purpose in a finite life."[37] Notice the addition of "meaningful relationships" and a lifespan viewpoint. Michael Fine, another family physician, and writer James Peters suggest health is the ability to function in relationships appropriate to one's culture and place in the life cycle.[38] They reinforce the centrality of relationships and again include the importance of a developmental or life course perspective.[39] These insights receive even more support from medical sociologist Aaron Antonovsky, who introduced the concept of health as a "sense of coherence," where life is manageable and comprehensible, with sufficient resources available.[40-42] Our understanding of health is becoming more expansive and complex.

Health in Complexity Theory

The world of complexity science brings more insights into our search for a deeper appreciation of health.[43-45] From a complexity perspective, people are complex adaptive systems highly influenced and sensitive to their contexts.[46-48] As complex systems, individuals are self-organized, emergent, and nonlinear. They coevolve, exhibit power law dynamics,[49] yet often operate according to deceptively simple rules (see Table S1.7 to clarify all this jargon).

Health is conceptualized as an emergent property with dimensionalities of *robustness*, *resilience*, and *antifragility* relative to any particular vibrant

TABLE S1.7 Properties of Complex Adaptive Systems

Property	Definition
Self-Organization	Bounded spontaneous development of order and behaviors within a basin of attractors, a habitat characterized by local interactions and multiple feedback loops A person is a self-organizing, complex, adaptive system!
Emergence	Process by which nonlinear interactions result in new patterns of behavior. The pattern that evolves is greater than the sum of its parts and cannot be understood by understanding the individual parts Health is emergent!
Nonlinear	Multiple feedback loops with different time frames result in unpredictability yet within bounds influenced by multiple interdependent factors People are more than machines!

(continued)

TABLE S1.7	*Continued*
Coevolution	Process of mutual change (adaptation) of a complex adaptive system and the habitat in which it exists
	No person is fully autonomous or alone; our life and health are dependent on relationships
	Everything changes in response to everything else within a habitat: interdependence rules!
Power Law Dynamics	A relative change in one quantity gives rise to a proportional relative change in the other quantity. Power laws are common in complex systems (think 80/20). For example, a power law of heart rate variability (high tail of lower HRV) predicts mortality in older adults.[50]
	With power laws, there are no normal distributions, so averages are meaningless!
Simple Rules	Self-organization and emergence are often the result of applying a few simple rules (the simplicity within the complexity), for example, the flocking behavior of starlings.[51]

setting with some degree of uncertainty and periodic disruptions. In other words, a setting like everyday life.[52] *Robustness* refers to the ability to maintain, cope, and withstand disruption, reflecting how resistant a living being is to exogenous influence—such as the ability of a rugged oak tree to withstand strong winds, or the ability of a person to repel infection. *Resilience*, on the other hand, indicates the ability to recover or bounce back after disruption and performance degradation—think of a palm tree resuming its uprightness after being deeply bent by high winds, or a person quickly returning to vigorous health after a serious illness. *Antifragility* refers to performance gains when exposed to adversity, the ability to get even better after a disruptive event, such as when a person takes advantage of the rehabilitation process to become a competitive athlete following multiple fractures from a car accident.

The properties of a complex adaptive system ensure much communication and cross-talk and many reverberating ripples across the system/organism such as a human body in its habitat. As such, any change in one part of a complex adaptive system will have ripple effects through the other parts. One agent's actions can change the context for many other agents. Expect the unexpected, especially when the scale becomes very large as at a national level, or very small as at the molecular level. An example of ripples from social network theory are the notions of three degrees of influence (our influence most likely extends out to a friend of a friend)[53] and of six degrees of separation (we are all connected within five to six social connections).[54]

The implications of complexity theory for understanding what we mean by "health" resonate deeply. Health emerges from within the spiraling whirlwind of complexity. Health is NOT harmony, perfection, wholeness, or the absence of disease. The health of a person embodies a dynamic state of creative tensions between conflicting values and goals of the human condition continually enacted over time. *Health is not harmony* because some form of stress and disruption continuously manifest somewhere, both within our physiologic systems and in our external world. When healthy, those disruptions do not prevent our meaningful participation in living. *Health is not perfection* because time and change never stop; an ideal state is never achieved. *Health is not wholeness* because of the paradox that we appear to exist as individuals, but only exist because of supporting interdependences with others. Like a Möbius strip, we are simultaneously bounded but with only one side: health as agency and belonging.[55] This turbulent space between individual and community is where generalist primary care healing thrives. We help make the populations within a community healthier by focusing on individual, personal health in context, by acting and thinking locally.

Health is not the absence of disease because disease and death are essential parts of life and often coexist with health. This means the optimal management of diseases in a person, although a very helpful goal, does not necessarily result in health. On the other hand, a person can be ill and unhealthy without having a disease. Health is much more complex, and it calls for the complementarity of specialism and generalism. Medical specialties purposefully focus on disease, whereas health is the goal for medical generalists.

Health as Membership

Table S1.8 outlines key features of health, which Wendell Berry condenses with the assertion, "health is membership."[56] **That is the goal for the generalist healer: to help people return and maintain their membership.** Table S1.8 also serves as our working understanding of health for the *Field Guide*.

TABLE S1.8 Definitional Features of Health

Domain	Feature
Policy Perspective	Dynamic state
	Multiple components
	• Emotional
	• Physical
	• Cognitive
	• Social
	• Spiritual
	MORE than absence of disease
Lay Perspective	Holistic
	Relative to culture/situation/development/lifespan
	Personal and functional (agency)
Other	Meaningful
	Relational and interdependent
	Sense of coherence
	Complex and emergent
	• Robust
	• Resilient
	• Antifragile

As generalist clinicians, we are agents of complex interdependencies and diplomats of the space between agency and community, that space of complex interdependence.[57] No person is an island, thus the personal is always relational. Several new terms have emerged to signal this more expansive and complex understanding, "Whole Health" and "One Health." "Whole Health" represents "the physical, behavioral, spiritual, and socioeconomic wellbeing as defined by individuals, families, and communities"[58] and is consistent with the content of Table S1.8. The concept of "One Health" extends the definition to include land and animal relations and expresses this as an "integrated, unifying approach that aims to sustainably balance and optimize the health of people, animals, and ecosystems. It recognizes that the health of humans, domestic and wild animals, plants, and the wider environment (including ecosystems) are closely linked and interdependent."[59] Whole health becomes incorporated within the primary medical care setting through the construct of "Whole-Person Care." In a recent review, whole-person care is identified with six themes: multidimensional and integrated approach; importance of therapeutic relationships; acknowledgment of doctors' humanity; recognition of personhood of each patient; health understood as more than absence of disease; and employment of a range of treatment modalities.[60] These resonate exquisitely with the generalist's craft in primary medical care as we help patients return to the River of Health as whole persons.

River of Health

The reviews of health as a concept, as complex, and as membership are encapsulated in this *Field Guide* in the metaphor of the River of Health, described in detail in Module 2 (see Figure S1.4 for a reminder). Healthy people thrive and live together within the River of Health; it is their place of membership and a zone of complexity flowing through time. While in the river, people feel well and experience meaningful agency and a sense of purpose and belonging. When maladies (disease, illness, and sickness) afflict them, they leave the River of Health and become patients on the banks of the river. Hopefully, they seek and find help from generalist healers, then return to the waters of health.

Drivers of Health

Now we explore how healing happens, beginning with the drivers of health. Table S1.9 summarizes the current literature on the drivers of health.[61-63] These are the agents and forces that sustain and promote health and/or impair it. Better health and the ability to heal build on top of a foundation upon which basic needs are met without unnecessary suffering and premature death. These needs include the absence of excessive violent conflict and/or poverty,

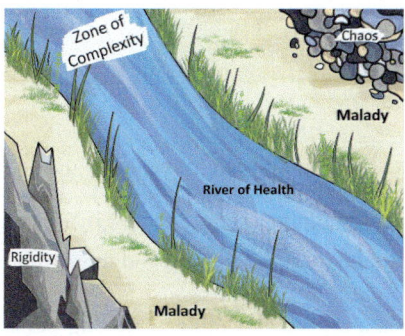

FIGURE S1.4. River of Health.

TABLE S1.9 — Drivers of Health (Longevity and Quality of Life)

Type of Driver of Health	Drivers of Health	Relative % Effect
Basic Needs and Safety Factors	Absence of war Absence of poverty Absence of epidemics Minimal developmental trauma	Baseline
Body Factors	Genes and epigenetics Physiology	20%–30%
Behavioral Factors	Food, activity, and sleep Absence of tobacco and substance use Moderation in alcohol use Sexual activity	30%–40%
Habitat Factors	Air and water quality Housing and transit Healthy ecology	10%
Clinical Care Factors	Access Quality of care	10%–20%
Policy and Livelihood Factors	Education Social status and finances Racial identity and equity Family and social support and engagement Work life Community safety Faith and meaning	20%–30%

sufficient food and shelter, avoidance of rampant deadly infectious disease, and limited developmental trauma. Unfortunately, these situations continue to exist for far too many people, reminding us of critical policy and political change that is essential if all of us are to spend more of our lives in the River of Health.

Mercifully, life is a miracle. Health and healing can still happen despite painful beginnings and adverse baseline circumstances, especially if the other drivers of health—the body, behavioral, habitat, and livelihood factors and appropriate clinical care—are present. Enhancing the drivers of health offers a significant means for maintaining and restoring health. These drivers influence a particular individual's bandwidth of health, their degree of robustness, resilience, and antifragility. In short, they determine both how well they can resist leaving the River of Health and moving into the world of malady and how easily they can return to the River of Health.

How Healing Happens

The way to the goal of health is healing: the process of maintaining, restoring, and enhancing health. Healing happens through three major means: activating the meaning response, generating communal healing support, and implementing specific targeted treatments (see Table S1.10).

The relative percentage effect numbers in the table may surprise you. All the *specific targeted treatments*—the drugs, surgeries, radiation, etc.—you learned in medical school are only responsible for about 20% to 30% of healing. The meaning response and communal healing support are responsible for the

TABLE S1.10   Three Ways for Healing

Healing Approach	Mechanisms of Action	Relative % Effect
Meaning Response (Placebo Effect)	Mitigate generalized adaptation syndrome[64,65] (stress response) Activate neuro-psycho-endocrine-immune pathways	40%-50%
Communal Healing Support	Mitigate generalized adaptation syndrome[64,65] (stress response) Activate neuro-psycho-endocrine-immune pathways	30%-40%
Specific Targeted Treatments	Alleviate targeted pathology and pathophysiologic mechanisms	20%-30%

other 70% to 80%. It is how we survived as a species. We do live longer and with a greater quality of life today because of the reliability of the medical (allopathic and osteopathic)-specific targeted treatments. But the effect of those medical treatments is limited and often harmful in the absence of the other 70% to 80%. There is great synergy when all three ways are engaged, a tactic encouraged by the generalist's craft.

The *meaning response*, also named the placebo effect or placebo response in the literature, is used in randomized clinical trials (RCTs) because of its powerful, although unreliable, effect.[66,67] When comparing across RCTs of the same drug, the placebo arm of a trial can range from 10% to 80% effectiveness.[68] The key factors that provoke and strengthen the meaning response are belief and expectation, meaningful social learning, and reinforcement of past conditioning.[69,70] Essentially, these are aspects of the way the treatment is delivered, specifically the expectancy of the patient, the setting, and the ritual. Jerome Frank identified the following three basic features of successful psychotherapy: (1) an emotionally charged relationship; (2) a healing setting; and (3) a rationale or myth explaining the symptoms and the process for resolving them.[71] Notice the overlap between what encourages the meaning response and what boosts successful psychotherapy. Wayne Jonas, a family physician, integrated these findings into three common factors for inducing healing (see Table S1.11).[72] Notice that all three are active when using the generalist's craft.

Healing Relationships

Healing happens during the activities of living and the *communal healing support* available there. For humans, it is often beneficial to have others involved in the form of healing relationships. Table S1.12 identifies three key processes that foster healing relationships: (1) valuing, or creating a nonjudgmental emotional bond, which builds trust; (2) appreciating power, or consciously managing clinician power in ways that most benefit the patient, which inspires hope; and (3) abiding, or displaying a commitment to caring for patients over time, which imbues the patient with a sense of being known. Certain clinician competencies facilitate these processes, including self-confidence; emotional self-management; and mindfulness and knowledge.[73] All of these are encouraged when using the generalist's craft.

A follow-up study to the one summarized in Table S1.12 led to a Healing Journey Model. This model demonstrates a process through which wounded and suffering individuals begin a journey where, through persistence, they can develop a sense of safety and trust that allows them to build helping relationships and acquire resources such as reframing, responsibility, and positivity.

TABLE S1.11	Three Common Factors Inducing Healing
Factor	**Description**
Rituals	Help the person have meaningful experience—activate and address beliefs and expectations
	Enhanced if person is emotionally charged with high expectancy
Support	Whole person in their life space and relationships
	Meaningful social learning
	In safe clinical setting
	Galvanize drivers of health
Regular Stimulation	Stimulation of biological response through activity, medication, surgery, needles, manipulation, etc.
	Stimulation of immunity and reduction of generalized stress response—actuate conditioning

TABLE S1.12	Significant Aspects of Healing Relationships	
Key Processes	**Relational Outcomes**	**Clinician Competencies**
Valuing	Trust	Self-confidence
Appreciating Power	Hope	Emotional Self-management
Abiding	Sense of Being Known	Mindfulness
		Knowledge

Adapted from Scott JG, Cohen D, Dicicco-Bloom B, et al. Understanding healing relationships in primary care. *Ann Fam Med*. 2008;6(4):315-322.

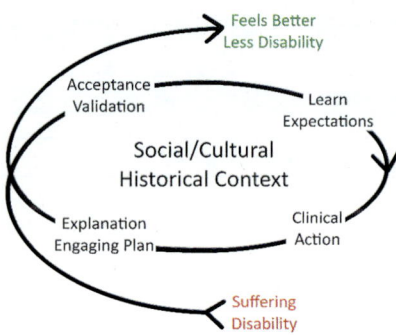

FIGURE S1.5. Spiral of Healing. (Adapted from Coulehan JL. Chiropractic and the clinical art. *Soc Sci Med*. 1985;21(4):383-390.)

Over time, these resources foster hope, self-acceptance, and the desire to help others, leading to the emergence of healing.[74] They have traveled the Spiral of Healing.

Spiral of Healing

Our explorations of health, healing, and healing relationships as the purpose, ways, and means for enacting the generalist's craft in primary care come together in the *Field Guide* as the Spiral of Healing, recalled in Figure S1.5.[75] The Spiral of Healing incorporates the ways and factors for healing and healing relationships.

Healing involves a repeated four-step cycle, a spiral over time. Suffering improves when patients' experiences are accepted and validated, their expectations are recognized, clinical action is taken, and an explanation with an engaging plan is shared and embraced that acknowledges the social/cultural and historical context. The Spiral of Healing acts as the cauldron for the magic of the generalist's craft where patient and clinician cocreate a relationship oriented to making a right and good healing action for the particular patient in their particular circumstances.[76] (See Module 2 for a more in-depth discussion.) That healing action always involves some change in behavior.

Changing Human Behavior

Since the Enlightenment, many of us wish to believe that humans behave based upon rational thinking. As a result, lots of us keep advocating for more education as a solution to problematic behaviors. But that rarely works. We now know better. Education may be necessary but is insufficient to effect change. Educational solutions rarely work because the assumption about rationality is wrong. Human behavior is more complicated than rational. Physicians, deeply socialized in the ethos of science and the Enlightenment, are especially prone to this mistake and often scratch their heads in disbelief when patients do not follow our well-reasoned advice or refuse vaccines. Not a surprise. Explicitly acting on pathophysiologic processes through surgery, pharmacology, and other modalities has dramatically expanded, making more reliable our abilities to help people on their healing journey. But they only work if people take the medicines, receive the vaccinations, and change their behavior. Change behavior and change biology. Most human behavior and decisions arise from our older, fast-thinking, emotionally charged part of the brain, with our newer but slower-thinking analytic, rational cortex circuits providing after-the-fact explanations or rationalizations.[77] For generalist healers, this means learning to motivate the fast-thinking part of the brain in each of our patients. The generalist's craft is designed to do just that.

Quite helpful is the analogy of the Elephant and the Rider from the work of Jonathan Haidt.[78,79] The Elephant represents the ancient, fast-thinking, usually subconscious, emotionally charged brain built on perception and heuristics. The Rider signifies our more recent, slow-thinking, cortical, rational brain. The Rider, although rather small, thinks it is in charge, but it is not. The Rider mostly rationalizes the actions/decisions already done by the very large Elephant. For the Spiral of Healing to work, a person needs to change a current behavior or develop a new one. As healers, we seek to facilitate that change. Figure S1.6 (see also Figure 2.4) illustrates a path toward change (see Module 2 for more details).[79,80]

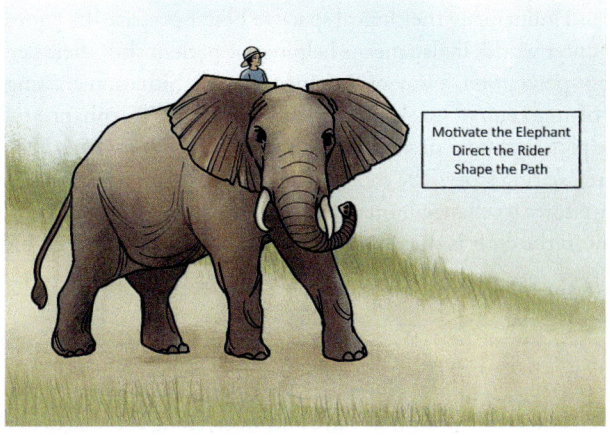

FIGURE S1.6. The Elephant and the Rider of Changing Behavior.

Notice that the Elephant in the figure is looking at you. Make eye contact with your patient's Elephant, the emotionally charged part of their brain. The first step toward changing resistant human behavior entails motivating the Elephant. That is who you connect and communicate with. Learning to connect with the Elephant compels you to appreciate any history of developmental trauma. A key to behavior change is helping your patient convert their fear into a motivating desire they value. The stories we hear and those we tell ourselves speak directly to the Elephant.[81] Change the stories, and perception shifts, and behavior changes.[82,83] Much of our work as generalist healers in primary care involves motivating the Elephant and helping patients reveal, revisit, and revise their stories. Using the techniques of motivational interviewing helps in this effort.[84]

The second step for changing human behavior directs the Rider and helps the Rider support the Elephant. Notice how the Rider is looking away from you, lost in thought. Now get the Rider's attention. Speak directly to the Rider so they can provide the Elephant with a sense of satisfaction for the decisions already motivated. Step three is shaping the path in the direction of health, which keeps the Rider and the Elephant aligned. You assist the Rider in shaping the desires, now motivating the Elephant to take interest in the goals. You provide explanations and knowledge to the Rider that support the Elephant's awakened aspiration to shift its attention from the grass and begin moving toward the River of Health.

It is important to remember that the actual work of healing occurs after the patient leaves the clinical encounter. The time in the presence of the generalist healer is when that healing work becomes crafted. In many ways, much of the work of the generalist's craft comprises situation crafting. This includes forming and influencing the clinical space to better prepare the patient for the postencounter world. It also means helping the patient shift their perspectives and change perception, a way of shaping the path. Situation crafting, like the priming of marketers,[85] seeks to rouse and alert the Elephant and then to shape the path with new desired expectations, perceptions, and the possibility for a more exciting story. The tools and strategies of the generalist's craft help us in our efforts to change human behavior toward better health. The secret ingredient in the craft is the "generalist way." Understanding that comes next.

Generalism

Generalist Ways

Generalist healers in primary care live and work along the shores of the River of Health, while the masters of disease care apply their specialist skills on the hills above the river. **Successful understanding and management of the expansiveness, dynamism, and complexity of health require a trained generalist approach.** Generalism and specialism are not two sides of the same coin. Specialism, in the health care context, refers to a specific means of knowing and doing that focuses on a particular domain of diseases using a science of reductionism. For example, internal medicine is the specialty dedicated to the diseases of adults. Cardiology specializes even further by concentrating only on diseases of the cardiovascular system, and electrophysiologists focus only on diseases of the heart conduction fibers and pathways related to its electrophysiology.

If there is an opposite to a specialist, a good candidate is a *jack-of-all-trades*, a person of many skills in many areas or trades. This was a compliment of the highest regard in the days before iron and steam. The addition of "and master of none" first appears in a 1741 book bemoaning the lack of standards in the world of pharmacy or apothecaries. In it, Charles Lucas comments that too many pharmacists are "a Jack of all trades, and in truth, master of none. . ."[86] This derogatory addition came with the rise of industrialism and specialism.

Generalism refers to something much more. Generalism is a holism representing a way of being, knowing, perceiving, doing, and belonging in the world. In health care, generalism approaches health in all its complex, relational, and dynamic context (see Table S1.13).[87]

TABLE S1.13 The Generalist Ways

The Way	Description
Way of Being	Open stance, receptive to diverse perspectives, humble
Way of Knowing	Broad knowledge of self, others, systems, and natural world and its interconnectedness; grounding in multiple knowledges and experiences
Way of Perceiving	Scanning and prioritizing; focusing on particulars while keeping horizon in view
Way of Doing	Engaging with most important parts in context; iterating between breadth and depth, action and reflection, parts and whole
Way of Belonging	Connecting and relating to self, others, systems, and natural world

Ian McWhinney noted that personal or generalist clinicians' "commitment is to people more than to a body of knowledge or a branch of technology."[88] A better medicine combines both generalists and specialists. The generalist and their medicine of relations do the heavy lifting in primary medical care while recognizing those who would benefit most from targeted specialized care.

Generalist as Jack-of-All-Trades, Polymath, Eclectic, and *Phronimos*

Understanding and explaining generalism in our highly specialized world is quite difficult. In many ways it encompasses four related but different notions: the jack-of-all-trades, the polymath, the eclectic, and the *phronimos*, or one with prudence and moral virtue. As previously mentioned, the *jack-of-all-trades* is a person of many everyday skills, sort of the ultimate handyperson. The *polymath* is someone with broad and comprehensive knowledge about many different subjects. Leonardo da Vinci exemplifies a polymath through his work as a painter, architect, scientist, engineer, and draftsman. *Eclectics* practice drawing upon a wide and diverse range of sources to address an issue without adherence to a particular philosophy, ideology, or theory.[89] A *phronimos* is one who enacts practical wisdom and applies general rules for right conduct or practice to the particular circumstances of a given situation resulting in action that promotes flourishing.[90,91] Phronesis or practical wisdom is an indispensable virtue for the generalist practitioner, a guide to right practice, a right way of acting at any given moment, in any particular situation.

Generalists manifest all four of these understandings. Like a *jack-of-all-trades*, we help with the everyday afflictions of life across the life cycle from birth to death. We suggest home remedies, write prescriptions, give advice to a struggling parent, provide ingrown toenail care, and offer comfort at the end of life. Endlessly curious, we are also *polymaths* exploring and learning the languages of the many medical specialties; deepening our understanding of the human experience in novels, short stories, poems, music, and art; and branching out into the other sciences and humanities. When confronted with problems, we reach out, as *eclectics*, across disciplines and perspectives, for ideas and skills that might apply; perspective-getting becomes more important than perspective-taking. We sit at the Round Table of Evidence. And we practice *phronesis* by applying our wisdom, our broad knowledge and experience to each particular situation. Generalists sample widely; we have range, take detours, experiment relentlessly, and gain a breadth of experiences. We especially focus on becoming omnicompetent in open skills, those skills that bridge types of knowledge, such as how to hunt for and connect contextual clues and create a broad range of strategies.[92]

Generalism, as a way toward health, recognizes the world as inherently filled with uncertainty. Diagnostic tests are often ambiguous; patients' stories are frequently incomplete, and not everyone has a clearly identifiable disease diagnosis. This partly explains why diagnosis, although an important construct, is not a primary goal for generalist clinicians. On the other hand, diagnosis is especially important for specialists because their knowledge and skills are mostly disease-based. This difference became quite evident when general practice attempted to fit its experience into the International Classification of Diseases (ICD) that first appeared in 1949.[93] Ten revisions later, ICD-10 still does not work well for primary medical care, and international general practice continues to create its own classification, the International Classification of Primary Care (ICPC). The ICPC is based more on episodes of care, reasons for encounter from the patient perspective, assessment from the clinician's perspective, and the decision, action, or plan of care.[94,95]

Principles of Generalism

Time to pause and summarize the understanding of generalism being presented. Generalism is a holistic and inclusive way of being, knowing, perceiving, doing, and belonging. A generalist healer is a jack(or jill)-of-all-trades, polymath, eclectic, and *phronimos* who applies practical wisdom using a relational process and operating within sensible scales in a world of uncertainty and complexity. Generalist healers are also more attentive to health than diagnosis. For the purposes of this *Field Guide*, I have organized this understanding of generalism using a set of principles of the generalist's craft developed by Johanna Lynch (see Table S1.14)—a way or approach for practicing the generalist's craft in primary care.[96-98] Generalist practitioners of the healing craft are recognized by their broad, inclusive, and whole-person scope. They use integrative practical wisdom and a relational process that is focused by a healing orientation. This generalist's craft is practiced in a setting where the practitioner courageously ensures and protects the sense of safety in the clinical space so that what is necessary to move toward health can be shared. The tools and strategies of the generalist's craft presented in this *Field Guide* have all been tested through the prism of these principles.

Another helpful depiction of clinical generalism visualizes two axes of *integrated* and *interpretive* care. The first, degree of integration, is one end of a systems axis that goes from single-problem, easily accessed care (think routine visit) to complex, integrated care involving coordination across multiple access points and teams (think drama visit). The second, degree of interpretation, is an individual care axis going from standardized, replicable, evidence-informed to highly individualized interpretive care.[99] On any given

TABLE S1.14	**Principles of the Generalist's Craft in Primary Care**

Whole-Person Scope
    Integrate biology and biography
    Inclusive—breadth, depth, awareness over time
    Scan horizon and attend to particulars
    Family and neighborhood context
    Developmental
    Integrate behavioral health
    Generalist Wheel of Inquiry (see Figure S1.7)

Relational Process
    Collaborative understanding and shared language
    Participatory cocreation

Integrative Practical Wisdom
    Address complex problems
    Coherent interpretation of diverse knowledge
    Attentive to capacity and burden
    Focus on pragmatic outcomes
    Apply Windmill Sails of Generalism (see Figure S1.8).

Healing Orientation
    Establish priorities for gathering knowledge
    Facilitate relief, repair, and meaning
    Emergent attitude to provisional knowledge
    Reflexive position of embedded practitioner

Sense of Safety
    Safe for patients and for clinical colleagues to explore and grow

day, the generalist clinician is likely to experience care situations across the four quadrants of the two intersecting axes. You may see a patient with a simple sore throat and use an evidence-informed pharyngitis protocol to organize the treatment recommendations, only to have that patient followed by another with a sore throat but with multiple chronic conditions requiring interpretive judgment to determine an individualized treatment plan. That same day, a third patient, also with multiple chronic conditions, arrives with concerns about multiple episodes of dizziness resulting in several falls—this time, a highly individualized management strategy emerges. A fourth patient, an overweight young adult with type 2 diabetes, presents with palpitations

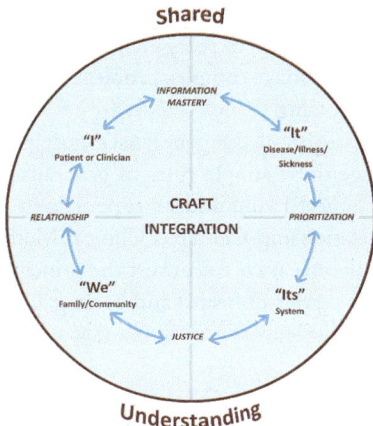

FIGURE S1.7. The Generalist Wheel of Inquiry.

from new-onset atrial fibrillation, and you, the generalist healer, use stroke-risk algorithms to help determine the need for anticoagulation. These four patients unveil the two axes of generalist care and the range of their manifestations.

Notice that Table S1.14 includes two of the figures used in the *Field Guide*. The Generalist Wheel of Inquiry (see Figures S1.7 and 3.24) represents the broad, whole-person scope of generalism and identifies the ways of knowing needed by generalist healers (see Module 3, Unit 5, for more detail). It also constitutes the central part of the Round Table of Evidence.

In the *Field Guide*, I invoke the metaphor of the Windmill Sails of Generalism (see Figures S1.8 and 2.3) to help us enact integrative practical

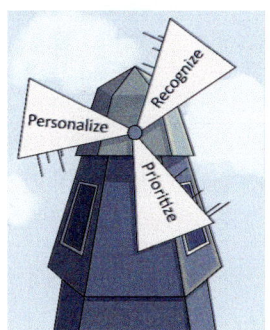

FIGURE S1.8. Windmill Sails of Generalism.

wisdom while doing the generalist's craft in primary care. When we remember to attend to the simple rules of recognizing, prioritizing, and personalizing, we are better able to manage complex problems and find our way through the multiple ways of knowing.

The tools and strategies of the generalist's craft presented in this *Field Guide* explicitly engage these simple rules of generalism (see Module 2 for more details). The Clinical Hand and its supporting tools—the Ecological Clinical Map, the Relationship-Centered Clinical Method, and the Round Table of Evidence—all offer ways to convert the principles of the generalist's craft into action in the service of health and healing. Using them brings generalism to life.

Montreal Statement on Generalist Practice

In 2018, a community of international researchers in general practice generated the Montreal statement on Generalist Practice, which seeks to both define and recognize better practice in doing expert generalist care. Their statement is summarized in Table S1.15.[100]

Ten years earlier, another group of international general practitioners outlined the promise and high value of generalism for achieving a vision of health for all through a more effective and supported primary health care.[101] Generalism not only informs all the tools of the generalist's craft, but is the often forgotten driver of high-value primary medical care.

TABLE S1.15 Montreal Statement on Generalist Practice

Defining Best Practice: Describing Quality Generalist Practice	Recognizing Best Practice: What You'd Expect to See When Delivering Expert Generalist Care
The Goals of Care Best care optimizes a person's health-related ability to continue their daily life.	Individual tailored care is endorsed. Individual goal-related care is emphasized Individual health-related capacity for daily living is enhanced, resulting in better health literacy and minimized illness burden

TABLE S1.15 *Continued*

The Data Used in Practice

Best care is informed by scientific evidence, patient accounts, and professional experience in the patient's particular context.

Scientific evidence is not "top of an evidence hierarchy" but a source of a wide range of data, information, and knowledge.

Contact time with patients is designed to support the use of an appropriate range of evidences.

The Tasks of Clinical Practice

Integrate data, information, and knowledge.

Construct a unique individual interpretation of the illness experience.

Safety Net that interpretation.

Empower the patient to own the decision process.

Assessment of Quality of Care/Practice

Quality is described with reference to the context of decision-making.

Context and care have enhanced health-related capacity for daily living.

Generalist Practice Is Enabled by:

Informational continuity

Scientific data readily accessible

Patient-centered consultation spaces

Professional-centered workspaces for use outside of consultation to create and maintain "mindlines" or "knowledge-in-practice-in-context."

Clinicians are trained in skills for using data to construct new context-sensitive knowledge about the individuals they encounter, and they are confident in those skills

Clinicians and patients perceive they have adequate resources, including prioritization of workload

Process of care is described with reference to context

Feedback and monitoring processes assess both context of and outcomes from care from a person-centered perspective

Services support longitudinality of care

Clinicians and patients are supported to judge quality of care based on impact of decisions over time

Adapted from Reeve J, Beaulieu MD, Freeman T, et al. Revitalizing generalist practice: the Montreal Statement. *Ann Fam Med*. 2018;16(4):371.

High-Value Primary Medical Care and Generalism

High-value primary medical care requires a generalist approach. The effective implementation of the simple rules of generalism—recognizing, prioritizing, and personalizing care—is the mechanism that produces high-value medical care. At the same time, without a strong generalism standing beside effective specialties, in constructive collaboration, there is no achieving the health care system quadruple aims of better health, better care, better cost, and greater equity. Critical to the evidence underlying that assertion is that 40% to 50% of the clinician workforce should be in primary medical care.[102] Table S1.16 summarizes the equation for high-value primary medical care.[103]

The generalist's craft enacts this equation. Three additional features, along with the generalist framework, are needed for high-value care. These other three include clinician, primary, and relational/personal and are characterized in Table S1.17. Primary medical care models that don't include all four features are less likely to be of high value.[104]

The presence of the four features from Table S1.17 is measured using the Person-Centered Primary Care Measure (PCPCM). Table S1.18 shows how all the components of high-value primary medical care are measured using the PCPCM tool.[105]

TABLE S1.16 High-Value Primary Medical Care

When the following are enacted...	40%-50% of clinical workforce are primary medical care (and 50%-60% of clinical workforce are specialists)
	The four functions of primary medical care
	The four Cs of primary medical care
	The simple rules of generalist care
	Using a health perspective
These outcomes happen...	Better population health
	Better care experience
	Lower cost
	Greater equity
	Healthier workforce

TABLE S1.17 Features of High-Value Primary Medical Care

Feature	Description
Clinician	• Professionalism • Clinical competence
Primary	• Entranceway to health care system—first contact access • Coordination of care
Relational/Personal	• Sustained partnership—continuity of care • Knows a person in the family/community and the ecological context • Advocacy • Goal-oriented

Generalist	• Whole-person scope
	  ◦ Integrates biology and biography
	  ◦ Inclusive—breadth, depth, awareness over time
	  ◦ Scans horizon and attends to particulars
	  ◦ Family and neighborhood context
	  ◦ Developmental
	• Relational process
	  ◦ Collaborative understanding and shared language
	  ◦ Participatory cocreation
	• Integrative practical wisdom
	  ◦ Addresses complex problems
	  ◦ Coherent interpretation of diverse knowledge
	  ◦ Attentive to capacity and burden
	  ◦ Focuses on pragmatic outcomes
	  ◦ Applies simple rules of generalism
	• Healing orientation
	  ◦ Establishes priorities for gathering knowledge
	  ◦ Facilitates relief, repair, and meaning
	• Sense of safety
	  ◦ Safe for patients and for clinical colleagues to explore and grow

TABLE S1.18 Person-Centered Primary Care Measure

Items	Feature
My practice makes it easy for me to get care.	Primary
My practice is able to provide most of my care.	Generalist
In caring for me, my doctor considers all the factors that affect my health.	Generalist
My practice coordinates the care I get from multiple places.	Primary
My doctor or practice knows me as a person.	Relational and Generalist
My doctor and I have been through a lot together.	Relational
My doctor or practice stands up for me.	Relational
The care I get takes into account knowledge of my family.	Relational and Generalist
The care I get in this practice is informed by knowledge of my community.	Relational and Generalist
Over time, my practice helps me to stay healthy.	Generalist
Over time, my practice helps me to meet my goals.	Relational and Generalist

We began this supplement by exploring the primary care medical setting and the patients who come there seeking health. We delved into the meaning of health and reviewed the processes for healing and changing behavior. Then, we highlighted the distinguishing features and principles of generalism, and we just finished clarifying the key characteristics of the high-value primary medical care setting in which the generalist's craft is practiced and how to measure them. Time to wrap up.

Summary

The generalist's craft in primary care and the tools and strategies shared in the *Field Guide* find their roots and value in the empirical and theoretical foundations explored in this supplement. The craft's purpose is to help make health in all its complexity and wonder, to ensure that everyone spends as much of their life as possible in the River of Health. The craft and its tools are purposefully planned to fulfill the requirements of high-value primary medical care no matter what the challenges and constraints of the particular health care system and to address the needs of those who visit generalist healers in primary care, especially those with a history of developmental trauma. The craft is intentionally designed to activate the processes and mechanisms of healing, to change physiology for a better life together. Implementing the generalist way and the simple rules of generalism are built into the generalist's craft presented here. Finally, the generalist's craft shared in the *Field Guide* restores the joy of this remarkable calling. Do it and have fun!

REFERENCES

1. Weick KE. The collapse of sensemaking in organizations: the Mann Gulch disaster. *Adm Sci Q.* 1993;38(4):628-652.
2. World Health Organization. *Primary Health Care: Report of the International Conference on Primary Health Care, Alma Ata, USSR, 6-12 September 1978.* World Health Organization; 1978.
3. Institute of Medicine. *A Manpower Policy for Primary Health Care.* National Academies Press; 1978.
4. Stange KC, Jaén CR, Flocke SA, et al. The value of a family physician. *J Fam Pract.* 1998;46(5):363-368.
5. Starfield B, Shi L, Macinko J. Contribution of primary care to health systems and health. *Milbank Q.* 2005;83(3):457-502.
6. Macinko J, Starfield B, Erinosho T. The impact of primary healthcare on population health in low- and middle-income countries. *J Ambulatory Care Manage.* 2009;32(2):150-171.
7. Starfield B. *Primary Care: Concept, Evaluation, and Policy.* Oxford University Press; 1992.
8. Heath I. Divided we fail. *Clin Med.* 2011;11(6):576-586.
9. Epperly T, Bechtel C, Sweeney R, et al. The shared principles of primary care: a multistakeholder initiative to find a common voice. *Fam Med.* 2019; 51(2):179-184.
10. Dovey S, Weitzman M, Fryer G, et al. The ecology of medical care for children in the United States. *Pediatrics.* 2003;111(5 Pt 1):1024-1029.
11. White KL, Williams TF, Greenberg BG. The ecology of medical care. 1961. *Bull N Y Acad Med.* 1996;73(1):187-212.

12. Green LA, Fryer GE, Yawn BP, et al. The ecology of medical care revisited. *N Engl J Med.* 2001;344(26):2021-2025.
13. Johansen ME, Kircher SM, Huerta TR. Reexamining the ecology of medical care. *N Engl J Med.* 2016;374(5):495-496.
14. Chrisman NJ. The health seeking process: an approach to the natural history of illness. *Cult Med Psychiatry.* 1977;1(4):351-377.
15. Pennebaker JW, Skelton JA. Psychological parameters of physical symptoms. *Pers Soc Psychol Bull.* 1978;4(4):524-530.
16. Pennebaker JW. *The Psychology of Physical Symptoms.* Springer-Verlag Publishing; 1982:197.
17. Pennebaker JW. Psychological bases of symptom reporting: perceptual and emotional aspects of chemical sensitivity. *Toxicol Ind Health.* 1994;10(4-5):497-511.
18. Newman M. Power laws, Pareto distributions and Zipf's law. *Contemp Phys.* 2005;46(5):323-351.
19. Vedsted P, Christensen MB. Frequent attenders in general practice care: a literature review with special reference to methodological considerations. *Public Health.* 2005;119(2):118-137.
20. Cruwys T, Wakefield JRH, Sani F, et al. Social isolation predicts frequent attendance in primary care. *Ann Behav Med.* 2018;52(10):817-829.
21. Courtenay MJ, Curwen MP, Dawe D, et al. Frequent attendance in a family practice. *J R Coll Gen Pract.* 1975;24(141):251-261.
22. Westhead JN. Frequent attenders in general practice: medical, psychological and social characteristics. *J R Coll Gen Pract.* 1985;35(276):337-340.
23. Finley CR, Chan DS, Garrison S, et al. What are the most common conditions in primary care? Systematic review. *Can Fam Physician.* 2018;64(11):832-840.
24. Forkey H, Szilagyi M, Kelly ET, et al; Council on Foster Care, Adoption, and Kinship Care, Council on Community Pediatrics, Council on Child Abuse and Neglect, Committee on Psychosocial Aspects of Child and Family Health. Trauma-informed care. *Pediatrics.* 2021;148(2):e2021052580.
25. Bucci M, Marques SS, Oh D, et al. Toxic stress in children and adolescents. *Adv Pediatr.* 2016;63(1):403-428.
26. Ellis WR, Dietz WH. A new framework for addressing adverse childhood and community experiences: the building community resilience model. *Acad Pediatr.* 2017;17(7 suppl):S86-S93.
27. Fallot R, Harris M. *Trauma-Informed Services: A Self-Assessment and Planning Protocol.* Community Connections; 2006.
28. Machtinger EL, Cuca YP, Khanna N, et al. From treatment to healing: the promise of trauma-informed primary care. *Womens Health Issues.* 2015;25(3):193-197.
29. Roberts SJ, Chandler GE, Kalmakis K. A model for trauma-informed primary care. *J Am Assoc Nurse Pract.* 2019;31(2):139-144.
30. Fehrsen GS, Henbest RJ. In search of excellence. Expanding the patient-centred clinical method: a three-stage assessment. *Fam Pract.* 1993;10(1):49-54.

31. Heath I. *The Mystery of General Practice*. Nuffield Provincial Hospital Trust; 1995.
32. Butler CC, Evans M. The "heartsink" patient revisited. The Welsh Philosophy and general practice discussion group. *Br J Gen Pract*. 1999;49(440):230-233.
33. Ackerknecht EH. *A Short History of Medicine*. Rev and Expanded ed. Johns Hopkins University Press; 2016.
34. World Health Organization. *Constitution of the World Health Organization*. World Health Organization; 1946. Accessed September 4, 2025. https://apps.who.int/gb/bd/PDF/bd47/EN/constitution-en.pdf
35. Schramme T. Health as complete well-being: the WHO definition and beyond. *Public Health Ethics*. 2023;16(3):210-218.
36. Svalastog AL, Donev D, Jahren Kristoffersen N, et al. Concepts and definitions of health and health-related values in the knowledge landscapes of the digital society. *Croat Med J*. 2017;58(6):431-435.
37. Stange KC. Power to advocate for health. *Ann Fam Med*. 2010;8(2):100-107.
38. Fine M, Peters JW. *The Nature of Health: How America Lost, and Can Regain, a Basic Human Value*. Radcliffe Publishing; 2007.
39. Halfon N, Hochstein M. Life course health development: an integrated framework for developing health, policy, and research. *Milbank Q*. 2002;80(3):433-479.
40. Antonovsky A. *Unraveling the Mystery of Health—How People Manage Stress and Stay Well*. Jossey-Bass; 1987.
41. Antonovsky A. The structure and properties of the sense of coherence scale. *Soc Sci Med*. 1993;36(6):725-733.
42. Antonovsky A. The salutogenic model as a theory to guide health promotion. *Health Promot Int*. 1996;11(1):11-18.
43. Thurner S, Hanel R, Klimek P. *Introduction to the Theory of Complex Systems*. Oxford University Press; 2018.
44. Mitchell M. *Complexity: A Guided Tour*. Oxford University Press; 2009.
45. Sturmberg JP, Martin CM. Complexity in health: an introduction. In: Sturmberg JP, Martin CM, eds. *Handbook of Systems and Complexity in Health*. Springer; 2013:1-17.
46. Ollhoff J, Walcheski M. *Stepping in Wholes: Introduction to Complex Systems*. Sparrow Media Group, Inc; 2002.
47. Theise N. *Notes on Complexity: A Scientific Theory of Connection, Consciousness, and Being*. Spiegel and Grau; 2023.
48. Sturmberg JP, Topolski S, Lewis S. Health: a systems-and complexity-based definition. In: Sturmberg JP, Martin CM, eds. *Handbook of Systems and Complexity in Health*. Springer; 2013:251-253.
49. Katerndahl D. Power law relationships between health care utilization and symptom assessment among people with panic attacks. *J Eval Clin Pract*. 2010;16(3):421-426.
50. Huikuri HV, Mäkikallio TH, Airaksinen KE, et al. Power-law relationship of heart rate variability as a predictor of mortality in the elderly. *Circulation*. 1998;97(20):2031-2036.

51. Hildenbrandt H, Carere C, Hemelrijk CK. Self-organized aerial displays of thousands of starlings: a model. *Behav Ecol.* 2010;21(6):1349-1359.
52. Munoz A, Billsberry J, Ambrosini V. Resilience, robustness, and antifragility: towards an appreciation of distinct organizational responses to adversity. *Int J Manag Rev.* 2022;24(2):181-187.
53. Christakis NA, Fowler JH. *Connected: The Surprising Power of Our Social Networks and How They Shape Our Lives.* Little, Brown and Company; 2009.
54. Barabasi A-L. *Linked: The New Science of Networks.* Perseus Publishing; 2002.
55. McDaniel SH, Hepworth J, Doherty WJ. *Medical Family Therapy: A Biopsychosocial Approach to Families with Health Problems.* Basic Books; 1992.
56. Berry W. Health is membership. In: Berry W, ed. *Another Turn of the Crank: Essays.* Counterpoint; 1995:86-109.
57. Morizot B. *Ways of Being Alive.* Polity Press; 2022.
58. National Academies of Sciences, Engineering, and Medicine, Health and Medicine Division, Board on Health Care Services, et al, eds. Defining whole health. In: *Achieving Whole Health: A New Approach for Veterans and the Nation.* National Academies Press (US); 2023. Accessed February 23, 2025. https://www.ncbi.nlm.nih.gov/books/NBK591719/
59. Adisasmito WB, Almuhairi S, Behravesh CB, et al. One health: a new definition for a sustainable and healthy future. *PLoS Pathog.* 2022;18(6):e1010537.
60. Thomas H, Mitchell G, Rich J, et al. Definition of whole person care in general practice in the English language literature: a systematic review. *BMJ Open.* 2018;8(12):e023758.
61. Magnan S. *Social Determinants of Health 101 for Health Care: Five Plus Five.* National Academy of Medicine; 2017.
62. McGinnis JM, Williams-Russo P, Knickman JR. The case for more active policy attention to health promotion. *Health Aff (Millwood).* 2002;21(2):78-93.
63. McGovern L, Miller G, Hughes-Cromwick P. The relative contribution of multiple determinants to health. *Health Aff.* Published online August 21, 2014. https://www.healthaffairs.org/do/10.1377/hpb20140821.404487/full/
64. Selye H. A syndrome produced by diverse nocuous agents. *Nature.* 1936;138(3479):32-32.
65. Selye H. *The Stress of Life.* Rev ed. McGraw-Hill; 1984.
66. Guess HA, Kleinman A, Kusek JW, et al, eds. *The Science of the Placebo: Toward an Interdisciplinary Research Agenda.* BMJ Books; 2002.
67. Brody H, Brody D. *The Placebo Response: How You Can Release the Body's Inner Pharmacy for Better Health.* Cliff Street Books; 2000.
68. Moerman DE. *Meaning, Medicine, and "Placebo Effect".* Cambridge University Press; 2002.
69. Petrie KJ, Rief W. Psychobiological mechanisms of placebo and nocebo effects: pathways to improve treatments and reduce side effects. *Annu Rev Psychol.* 2019;70:599-625.
70. Benedetti F. *Placebo Effects: Understanding the Mechanisms in Health and Disease.* Oxford University Press; 2009.

71. Frank JD, Frank JB. *Persuasion and Healing: A Comparative Study of Psychotherapy*. 3rd ed. Johns Hopkins University Press; 1991.
72. Jonas W. *How Healing Works*. Lorena Jones Books; 2018.
73. Scott JG, Cohen D, Dicicco-Bloom B, et al. Understanding healing relationships in primary care. *Ann Fam Med*. 2008;6(4):315-322.
74. Scott JG, Warber SL, Dieppe P, et al. Healing journey: a qualitative analysis of the healing experiences of Americans suffering from trauma and illness. *BMJ Open*. 2017;7(8):e016771.
75. Coulehan JL. Chiropractic and the clinical art. *Soc Sci Med*. 1985;21(4):383-390.
76. Pellegrino ED. Toward a reconstruction of medical morality. *Am J Bioeth*. 2006;6(2):65-71.
77. Kahneman D. *Thinking, Fast and Slow*. Farrar, Straus, and Giroux; 2011.
78. Haidt J. *The Happiness Hypothesis*. Basic Books; 2006.
79. Haidt J. *The Righteous Mind: Why Good People are Divided by Politics and Religion*. Pantheon Books; 2012.
80. Heath C, Heath D. *Switch: How to Change Things When Change is Hard*. Broadway Books; 2010.
81. Akerlof GA, Shiller RJ. *Animal Spirits: How Human Psychology Drives the Economy, and Why it Matters for Global Capitalism*. Princeton University Press; 2009.
82. Mansell W. The perceptual control model of psychopathology. *Curr Opin Psychol*. 2021;41:15-20.
83. Powers WT. *Behavior: The Control of Perception*. 2nd Expanded ed. Benchmark; 2005.
84. Miller WR, Rollnick S. *Motivational Interviewing: Helping People Change and Grow*. 4th ed. The Guilford Press; 2023.
85. Weingarten E, Chen Q, McAdams M, et al. From primed concepts to action: a meta-analysis of the behavioral effects of incidentally presented words. *Psychol Bull*. 2016;142(5):472-497.
86. Lucas C. *Pharmacomastix: Or, the Office, Use, and Abuse of Apothecaries Explained*. S. Powell for Abraham Bradley; 1741. Accessed February 29, 2024. http://quod.lib.umich.edu/cgi/t/text/text-idx?c=ecco;idno=004838202.0001.000
87. Stange KC. The generalist approach. *Ann Fam Med*. 2009;7(3):198-203.
88. McWhinney IR. Family medicine in perspective. *N Engl J Med*. 1975;293(4):176-181.
89. Kroos K. Eclecticism as the foundation of meta-theoretical, mixed methods and interdisciplinary research in social sciences. *Integr Psychol Behav Sci*. 2012;46(1):20-31.
90. Pellegrino ED, Thomasma DC. *The Virtues in Medical Practice*. Oxford University Press; 1993.
91. Cosgrove L, Shaughnessy AF. Becoming a phronimos: evidence-based medicine, clinical decision making, and the role of practical wisdom in primary care. *J Am Board Fam Med*. 2023;36(4):531-536.
92. Epstein D. *Range: Why Generalists Triumph in a Specialized World*. Riverhead Books; 2019.

93. Armstrong D. Diagnosis and nosology in primary care. *Soc Sci Med*. 2011; 73(6):801-807.
94. Napel HT, van Boven K, Olagundoye OA, et al. Improving primary health care data with ICPC-3: from a medical to a person-centered perspective. *Ann Fam Med*. 2022;20(4):358-361.
95. van Boven K, Napel HT, eds. *ICPC-3 International Classification of Primary Care: User Manual and Classification*. 3rd ed. CRC Press; 2022.
96. Lynch JM, Dowrick C, Meredith P, et al. Transdisciplinary generalism: naming the epistemology and philosophy of the generalist. *J Eval Clin Pract*. 2021; 27(3):638-647.
97. Lynch JM, van Driel M, Meredith P, et al. The craft of generalism: clinical skills and attitudes for whole person care. *J Eval Clin Pract*. 2022;28(6):1187-1194.
98. Lynch JM. *A Whole Person Approach to Wellbeing: Building Sense of Safety*. Routledge; 2020.
99. Reeve J, Byng R. Realising the full potential of primary care: uniting the 'two faces' of generalism. *Br J Gen Pract*. 2017;67(660):292-293.
100. Reeve J, Beaulieu MD, Freeman T, et al. Revitalizing generalist practice: the Montreal statement. *Ann Fam Med*. 2018;16(4):371.
101. Gunn JM, Palmer VJ, Naccarella L, et al. The promise and pitfalls of generalism in achieving the Alma-Ata vision of health for all. *Med J Aust*. 2008; 189(2):110-112.
102. Council on Graduate Medical Education. *Advancing Primary Care*. U.S. Department of Health and Human Services, Public Health Service; 2010.
103. Stange KC, Miller WL, Etz RS. The role of primary care in improving population health. *Milbank Q*. 2023;101(S1):795-840.
104. Gray DJP, Sidaway-Lee K, White E, et al. Continuity of care with doctors—a matter of life and death? A systematic review of continuity of care and mortality. *BMJ Open*. 2018;8(6):e021161.
105. Etz RS, Zyzanski SJ, Gonzalez MM, et al. A new comprehensive measure of high-value aspects of primary care. *Ann Fam Med*. 2019;17(3):221-230.

SUPPLEMENT 2

Educational Resources

Introduction

This supplement is for those who are teachers of the generalist's craft and begins with a brief overview of how to use the *Field Guide* with different types of learners. I then share three GEMs, or generalist enhancement methods, you can use to help apprentices of the generalist's craft enhance and expand their observational skills and develop their appreciation for the interdependent and dynamic aspects of health. Instructions for three strategies for teaching the generalist's craft follow. The supplement concludes with two tools for assessing the craft.

Who you are—specifically, your preferred learning style—influences how you will best learn from using this *Field Guide*. The Kolb experiential learning cycle,[1] which underlies the guide's structure and organization, depicts what is required to master something new (see Figure S2.1).

What varies among individuals is where we prefer to start that learning: our learning style. I encourage everyone to begin with Module 2 to become acquainted with the language of the Clinical Hand and its three supporting tools. What you do next varies by learning style. Here's how.

Hands-on Learners: Some of us start by diving right into the clinical waters, to actively experiment and generate immediate concrete experiences and then pause to reflect on what happened. If that is you, take the *Field Guide* with you into your next clinical encounter and start with Module 3. After a few concrete experiences and reflections, step back and explore Module 4. Following a few more cycles, read Supplement 1 to learn the abstract concepts underlying what you are doing. If you are teaching a hands-on learner, recommend the above and help them connect what they are doing to the tools and suggestions in the *Field Guide*. Early observation is especially important to prevent misunderstandings and the development of inappropriate habits.

Observers: Others start by watching, by observing a few wizards of the generalist's craft, exploring what happened, and only then actively experimenting and trying it themselves, generating their own concrete experiences. If you

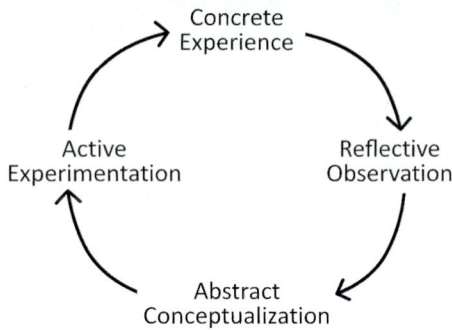

FIGURE S2.1. The Experiential Learning Cycle.

are one of those observational learners, begin by using the Observation Checklist at the end of this Supplement 2 to focus your observations. After watching several encounters, read Modules 3 and 4 before diving in and trying it yourself. Teachers of observers can encourage the above. You want to get them practicing sooner rather than later. Doing so by trying one unit from Module 3 at a time can be helpful.

Readers: Still others begin with reading and learning the abstract concepts. They want to understand before either observing or doing. If this is you, read Modules 3, 4, and Supplement 1. Move on to experimentation, either by observing others or trying it yourself. As a teacher, it is especially important to not allow your apprentice to linger too long with the reading.

Everyone should dip in and out of Module 1 to refresh their prerequisite thriving skills and ensure their self-care and wellness along the way.

GEMs: Generalist Enhancement Methods

GEMs are activities designed to help learners enhance and experience the embodiment of their senses of awareness as a means for awakening and expanding their fields of vision. They are methods that brighten the generalist perspective. GEMs are especially useful when done at the start of a generalist training program but are beneficial and entertaining at any time. And no, these don't fulfill any required professional competencies. That is part of the fun.

Camera Walk

Overview

When performing the generalist's craft, you must frequently and rapidly shift your focus back and forth between the particular details in front of you and the larger context informing and influencing the situation and concerns, all while remembering what you are learning. Quite a daunting task. The Camera Walk offers a way to practice that observational shifting while also enhancing your memory. You may be surprised at what you discover in places you thought you knew. That is the point of the activity.

Goals

After practicing the Camera Walk, you will improve the following:

- Your ability to shift fields of awareness
- Your observation and listening skills
- Your memory capacity for what is observed
- Your focus and attention

Participants and Their Roles

Teacher: Provides instructions, facilitates group sharing and discussion after the activity is completed.

Learner: Performs activity with a partner, describes "pictures" taken in the group setting.

Components of the Session (Session Takes 45-50 Minutes)

First: Share brief overview of the activity and then divide the group into pairs.
Second: Have each pairing perform the activity as follows:

- One person acts as the "camera," and the other serves as the "photographer."
- The "camera" keeps their eyes closed until given instructions by the photographer on how to take the picture. The "photographer" safely guides the "camera" to where they can take the desired picture and then positions the "camera" for the shot. The "photographer" instructs the "camera" on what picture to take, specifically, how long to keep their eyes open, whether to telephoto in for detail or to wide angle for the big picture or somewhere in between. The "camera" completes the instructions and places the picture observed into their memory.
- Each "camera" takes three pictures. These need to include at least one telephoto shot and one wide-angle image.
- The "camera" and "photographer" switch positions and repeat the above.

Third: Everyone gathers in a group, and each person describes the three pictures in their camera's memory. The "photographer" comments on how well the picture presented by the "camera" represented their intent. After everyone has shared their pictures, the group processes their experience, what they learned, and how it might relate to when they are seeing patients.

Fox Walking

Overview

Modern humans generally walk as if in a hurry, with our weight already committed forward before the next step hits the ground. When on uneven surfaces, such as walking in the woods, we need to frequently check on where our feet are landing to prevent stumbling. This makes it difficult to maintain observation of the surroundings. Fox walking offers an alternative way to walk that increases your awareness and observation of the world around you.[2]

Goals

After learning to Fox Walk, you will improve in the following:

- Slowing down
- Mindful awareness
- Observation and listening skills
- Familiarity with local habitat

Participants and Their Roles

Teacher: Demonstrates, instructs, supports learning.
Learner: Practices skill mastery.

Components of the Session (Session Takes 30 Minutes)

Share premise of activity: Forward foot placed on the ground before weight is committed forward results in a shorter stride and the ability to observe without watching the ground to check on your next step.

First: Learn the steps.

- Keeping weight on the back foot, begin to step forward with the lead foot.
- Forward foot lightly touches the ground using the entire outside edge of the foot including the heel, using the foot to feel what is on the ground.
- Slowly roll the foot inward until fully, but lightly, on the ground. Feel what is under the foot and adjust position if necessary.

- Shift weight from back foot to front foot.
- Repeat...

Second: Practice with backs straight and eyes off the ground.
Third: Practice until you do not need to think about it.

Sculpting Health

Overview

The dominant Western cultural worldview prioritizes the individual and a belief in individual autonomy. Our understanding of health often gets simplified and constricted within that perspective. The Sculpting Health activity reminds us that autonomy is an illusion in an interdependent world—that agency and communion are possible through recognizing and embracing connections and that health emerges from those relationships.

Goals

After completing the Sculpting Health activity, you will improve in the following:

- Embodied interdependent understanding of health
- Ability to work in a small group

Participants and Their Roles

Teacher: Provides instructions, facilitates group discussion after activity.
Learner: Creates and performs activity with others, shares experience and what is learned with the group.

Components of the Session (Session Takes 45-60 Minutes)

First: Share brief overview of activity, then divide larger group into groups of three to five people.
Second: Have each group perform the following activity:

- Huddle together and decide how, as a group, you will use your bodies to sculpt "health." Practice forming the sculpture in preparation for performing it before the larger group. Be prepared to describe how the sculpture enacts "health."

- Reconvene as a large group. Each small group then creates their sculpture of health for the others. Ask the viewers to describe what they see and how it depicts "health." Then ask the small group to share what it intended to describe.
- After all the groups are done sharing their sculpture, facilitate a large group discussion of the activity and how it helped better understand the many layers of meaning of "health."
- Note: The pull of individualism and autonomy is strong, and occasionally a group will elect to have each member of their small group sculpt their own health. Usually, asking them how the different versions of individual health relate to each other facilitates a shift toward recognizing the role of interdependence in creating health.

Teaching Strategies for Generalist's Craft

The three teaching strategies presented here will fit into most educational contexts. That said, the current high-volume, high-demand, and inadequately resourced environments of many generalist clinician educational settings can pose implementation challenges. At Lehigh Valley Health Network, we use two models to help us enhance the efficiency and effectiveness of the three teaching strategies.

The first is the Prepare, Orchestrate, Educate, Review (POwER) framework or model[3] that incorporates clinic planning to encourage more efficient teaching. In this model, the role of the teacher/supervisor/preceptor at a practice is to do the following:

1. Prepare: Review schedules, lead discussion with team (other faculty) to plan and assign learners.
2. Orchestrate: Anticipate needs, monitor flow, orchestrate team functioning, circulate throughout staffing session.
3. Educate: Use the One-Minute Precepting framework (see further).
4. Review: Intercept problems early, provide appropriate information, guide learners in defining, focusing, and reinforcing their own learning needs, and debrief team at the end of the session.

These activities require that the management team at the practice be well acquainted and educated on their involvement in the educational process and that the preceptor be well acquainted and educated on the operations and management of the practice.

The second model delineates the five-step microskills of One-Minute Precepting.[4,5] The five microskills are as follows:

1. Get a commitment: Learner makes a commitment to a diagnosis, workup, or therapeutic plan.
2. Probe for supporting evidence: Teacher helps the learner reflect upon the thought process used to make the commitment.
3. Teach general rules: Teacher provides teaching points from any gaps or mistakes in data, knowledge, or missed connections (may be skipped if the learner has performed well).
4. Reinforce what was done right: Teacher provides positive feedback.
5. Correct mistakes: Teacher provides corrective feedback.

The three teaching strategies that follow are intended to assist in both teaching the generalist's craft and evaluating learners in their progress. Enjoy!

Continuity Case Conference
Overview

Learning how to do continuity of care and appreciate its value is particularly difficult in current educational settings in primary medical care. Medical students are never around long enough, and matching patient needs to the sporadic availability of residents and interns is perplexing at best. Even more challenging is learning how to play out dramas, which can often take several years before conversion to a maintenance ceremony is possible. The Continuity Case Conference was developed to address these challenges.[6]

Goals

At the end of a Continuity Case Conference, the learner will be able to:

- Name and understand the many aspects of dramas.
- Identify the skills needed to improve their management and participation in dramas.
- Appreciate and articulate the value of continuity of care.

Participants and Their Roles

Organizer: Go over instructions with presenting learner at least 2 months in advance and provide support as learner prepares presentation; then facilitate the session.

Presenting Learner: Prepare the continuity case, present the case, write up the summary case report.

Others Present (students, residents, other faculty, clinic ensemble as available): Listen to case presentation, ask questions, and offer constructive comments in group discussion following case presentation.

Components of the Session (Session Takes 45-60 Minutes)

Optimally, the presenter is in their late second or early third year of training. The presenting learner selects a continuity case (at least five or more visits), which needs to be an ongoing drama in which the presenter feels stuck. The selection should occur at least 2 months prior to the session so there is enough time to organize the presentation. Sometimes, the drama selected began with residents who have already graduated and who may have presented an earlier part of the drama as a continuity case. It is especially valuable for the learner to gain access to that summary case report and review the older records.

The format for the session is as follows:

- Presenter presents a *timeline* of the drama and uses it to give a brief overview of the case, identifying core problems, encounter history, and the current dilemma.
- Presenter presents the details of the case, being sure to address the following (variation in content may vary depending on the case):
  - The *symptom/illness story*, tracking changing ideas, feelings, expectations, and effect on function and addressing the five limbs of the Naming and Caring Tree.
  - The *family story*, including a genogram and family life cycle information.
  - The *personal story* before the onset of the drama and how it has changed.
  - The role of *culture*, noting important beliefs and values and any patient and family explanatory models or illness prototypes.
  - The drama narrative *trajectory*, identifying the main conflicts, crisis points, and which "act" the drama appears to be in.
  - The *relationship* history, noting how it has changed, improved, or worsened. How has the presenter changed?
  - The *Finding Common Ground* history, tracking the changes to concerns, goals, and roles. Who else is involved in the drama?
  - The current situation, summarizing what has been learned while preparing the presentation.

- Organizer facilitates group input, questions, comments, suggestions.
- Presenter writes up summary case report, incorporating feedback from the session (due in 2 weeks).

Mega Clinic
Overview
Office sessions are a complex dynamic process requiring flexibility and the use of reflection in action. They also necessitate the ability to quickly shift among the different types of clinical encounters. The Mega Clinic was developed by Robin Pritham for his family medicine residency program in northern Maine and adapted at Lehigh Valley explicitly for teaching the generalist's craft.[7] In the Mega Clinic, a clinician tells a group about one of their recent clinic sessions. They talk about what happened and how they handled it. This is followed by comments from the preceptor and members of the clinical ensemble who participated in that session, then the Mega Clinic concludes with an open discussion.

Goals
At the conclusion of the Mega Clinic, the presenter will have gained insight into improving the following:

- Reflection in action and their ability to adapt
- Reflection on action
- Managing the dynamics of a half-day session (overall performance of session, time management, use of office system, types of clinical encounters)
- Appreciating the value and knowledge of their clinic ensemble

Participants and Their Roles
Presenter: Brings patient schedule from the session being presented; describes their session.

Moderator (usually faculty): Facilitates discussions after the presentation, protects the safety of the space.

Others (faculty, other learners, clinic ensemble): Listens to the presentation, shares comments and suggestions from their perspective in group dialogue.

Components of the Session (Session Takes 45-60 Minutes)
Moderator introduces the presenter and reviews the rules of engagement, which include no interruptions during the presentation.

Presentation of session with the following instructions:

- You will have 20 minutes to tell us about your office session.
- Share the big picture of the session, but include something about each patient and your feelings at the time.
- Highlight where things went well, where you had difficulty, what events impacted how the session went, and how you were reflecting in action and adjusting your actions.
- Identify the kinds of encounters you are describing.

Feedback by individuals: The preceptor for that session and the members of the clinician's clinical team respond to what they heard and share their perspectives on the session with facilitation by the moderator.

Open discussion: The moderator facilitates an open group discussion using the principles of reflection on action.

Paired Precepting

Overview

Precepting is a common means for teaching and monitoring learners in medical and nursing education and conventionally done one encounter at a time. The generalist's craft in primary care integrates multiple skills in an environment of competing demands and opportunities. These skills include clinical, management, and team-based ones. Paired Precepting was developed to address teaching and evaluating an apprentice of the generalist's craft as they navigate a half-day session in their clinic.

Goals

At the end of a Paired Precepting session, the apprentice clinician will have learned the following:

- Competence at implementing the generalist's craft in primary care, especially the ritual structure of the five fingers of direction on the Clinical Hand tool
- Strengths and challenges in managing time, the electronic health record, the clinic ensemble, and other contingencies that may arise
- Strengths and challenges related to clinical content knowledge, communication and relationship skills, and ability to connect to and facilitate care coordination within the community

Participants and Their Roles

Preceptor: Stay with learner throughout the half-day session, provide feedback throughout the half-day and in summary at the end of the session.

Learner: Focus on the work of the half-day, listen and respond to feedback from preceptor.

Components of the Session (Session Takes 3-4 Hours)

The half-day session proceeds as follows with improvisation expected as needs arise:

- Preceptor and learner meet at the beginning of the session, preferably a few minutes before the expected start time.
- Preceptor and learner review expectations and share any specific goals and expectations. For example, the learner may want a special focus on ability to negotiate and set the agenda or some advice on the care of a patient scheduled for the day.
- Preceptor follows the learner all through the half-day. They go into the exam room, are present for virtual visits, are there at any team huddles and all conversations with ensemble colleagues, and observe as the resident reviews and documents in the electronic health record. It is as if the preceptor were attached to the resident by a short cord.
- Preceptor shares feedback and asks questions as needed and/or as opportunities present while trying to minimize disruption. The same applies to the learner.
- Preceptor and learner debrief at the end of the half-day session for about 5 to 10 minutes. A written evaluation follows within the next week. The feedback includes the use of the core tools of the generalist's craft, clinical content and sensemaking, communication and relationship skills, care coordination, management of the clinic ensemble, the electronic health record, time management, and any other issues that surfaced.

Variations: The paired preceptor can also be a behavioral scientist, clinical pharmacist, social worker, communication specialist, or other who focuses on their particular areas of concern.

Assessment Tools

This section offers two assessment tools for evaluating the use of the generalist's craft in primary care. The first is a checklist developed by Bill Ventres, a wise practitioner of the craft with extensive cross-cultural experience. He developed a question list (Q-list) to help him assess his own mastery of the craft.[8] I share it in Table S2.1 for your use in doing the same.

The second is the observation tool used in the Lehigh Valley Family Medicine Residency Program to assess competence in the generalist's craft.

TABLE S2.1 Q-List for General Medical Practice

Domain of General Practice	Key Questions
Patient Presentation	What is my patient's presenting concern?
	Are other issues present?
	Are family members or significant others involved?
	Have other health care professionals been involved? Are they now?
Medicine	Do shared medical management goals exist?
	Do sufficient diagnostic data and treatment plans exist?
	Is my medical knowledge adequate for my role at the moment?
	Are other medical consultants involved?
History	Are other family members in my care?
	Are there important issues to consider from my patient's past hx.?
	Previous "rubs": How have I dealt with other issues with the patient?
	Are other team members involved in my patient's care?
	Have any significant milestones recently passed/are coming up?
Daily Reality	What is my patient's explanatory model?
	Are any of the following explicitly involved: Work? Family? Friends?
	What are my patient's spiritual beliefs?
	Do underlying contributing social stressors/drivers exist?
	What are my patient's strengths? Weaknesses?

Relational Issues:
- Patient Focus
  - Are any language issues involved?
  - Is my patient "health care" literate (verbally and written)?
  - What are my patient's needs re: power and authority?
  - Are particular patient ideologies/perspectives involved?
- Practitioner Focus
  - Do I understand my patient?
  - Am I responsive to my patient's expressed needs?
  - Am I communicating at an appropriate level?
  - Am I aware of power dynamics in my communication?
  - Have I examined my personal ideologies/perspectives re: my patient?
- Trust
  - Do I trust and respect my patient?
  - Does my patient trust, respect, and have faith in me?

Learning
- What are my patient's goals of management or resolution?
- What is meaningful in my patient's life re: the presenting concern?
- Am I really interested in this patient?
- What do I need to learn from this particular patient?

Care of the Patient
- Have I explored the dynamics of the biopsychosocial process?
- Have I uncovered previously unexposed issues of pertinence?
- How can I enrich my ability to care for the patient?
- Who else can help in the care of the patient?

Adapted from Ventres WB. The Q-List manifesto: how to get things right in generalist medical practice. *Fam Syst Health*. 2015;33(1):5-13.

Here is the latest version of the Clinical Hand Direct Observation Tool

Clinical Hand Direct Observation Tool

Ground Rules and Goals

Quietly observe clinical encounter(s). Note behaviors and interactions that correspond to various parts of the Clinical Hand and other tools by checking what you observe in the key points provided. Note specific interactions, words, etc., that you thought were examples of utilizing tools in the Notable Observations columns.

Date of Observation, Observer, and Physician/NP/PA Observed:	Faculty: Date:
Number and Types of Patient Visits	Routine Ceremony: Maintenance Transition Drama

Key Points	**Connect**	Notable Observations
Prepares *Welcomes* *Comforts* *Develops Rapport* *Orients to EHR*		

Key Points	**Set Agenda**	Notable Observations
Elicit Agenda *Identifies chief concern* *Elicits other concerns* *Shares own goals* *Identifies actual reason for connecting* **Prioritizing** *Recognizes encounter type* *Negotiates agenda*		

Key Points	**Clinical Discovery**	Notable Observations

Tracks illness and sickness experience and cues
Tracks disease experience and cues
Obtains relevant context
Weaving of foraging and hypothesis evaluation
Builds story and swings on tree limbs
Opens family window
Communication Skills
Active listening
Weaving of open-ended and closed questions

Key Points	**Hand Over**	Notable Observations

Common Ground
Presents findings and treatment options clearly and in pt.'s language and learning style
Uses Round Table of Evidence
Share Power
Elicits feedback and seeks clarification
Patient included in treatment planning process
Confirms pt.'s understanding of next steps
Matches care burden to patient capacity
Debriefs what's in EHR

Key Points	**Safety Net**	Notable Observations

Prognosis review with self
Precepting
Presents an organized story
Asks key questions
Listens openly
Remains the clinician

Key Points	**Housekeep**	Notable Observations
Documentation check Performs self-review of visit Checks in with staff in supportive ways Mindful hand washing—attends to emotions and baggage between visits		

Key Points	**BATHE**	Notable Observations
Background **A**ffect **T**roubles **H**andle **E**mpathy		

Key Points	**Naming and Caring Tree**	Notable Observations
Emotional Limb (threat, expressions, loss) Physical Limb (anatomy and physiology) Cognitive Limb (illness stories, self-image, explanatory models, attributions) Social Limb (troubles, ties, traditions) Spiritual Limb (soul stories)		

Key Points	**Goals for Visit**	Notable Observations
Addresses actual reason for connecting Patient has engaging plan Addresses a related, resistant health issue		

Key Points	**Build Relationship**	Notable Observations
Practices open and honest communication Demonstrates respect		

REFERENCES

1. Kolb DA. *Experiential Learning: Experience as the Source of Learning and Development.* 2nd ed. Pearson Education; 2015.
2. Brown T Jr, Brown J. *Tom Brown's Field Guide to Nature and Survival for Children.* Berkley Books; 1989.

3. Lillich DW, Mace K, Goodell M, et al. Active precepting in the residency clinic: a pilot study of a new model. *Fam Med.* 2005;37(3):205-210.
4. Neher JO, Gordon KC, Meyer B, et al. A five-step "microskills" model of clinical teaching. *J Am Board Fam Pract.* 1992;5(4):419-424.
5. Furney SL, Orsini AN, Orsetti KE, et al. Teaching the one-minute preceptor. *J Gen Intern Med.* 2001;16(9):620-624.
6. Sternlieb JL. Teaching the value of continuity of care: a case conference on long-term healing relationships. *Fam Syst Health.* 2012;30(4):302-307.
7. Sternlieb JL. Teaching housekeeping: learning to manage the emotional impact of patient care. *Fam Syst Health.* 2008;26(3):356-364.
8. Ventres WB. The Q-List manifesto: how to get things right in generalist medical practice. *Fam Syst Health.* 2015;33(1):5-13.

Glossary of Mnemonics

General Mnemonics

BATHE—Technique when the patient is in distress
    B—Background
    A—Affect
    T—Troubles
    H—Handles
    E—Empathy

DOE—Disease-Oriented Evidence

FICA—Spiritual assessment tool
    F—Faith
    I—Importance
    C—Community
    A—Address

FIFE—Exploring the illness experience
    F—Feelings
    I—Ideas
    F—Function
    E—Expectations

LATE—How to do a transition ceremony
    L—Listen to the story
    A—Address fear
    T—Touch the trouble
    E—Express hope and enact a plan

LETS HEAR—Eliciting an explanatory model
    L—Label
    E—Etiology
    T—Time
    S—Severity

H—History (natural)
E—Effects
A—Affects
R—Rx (treatment)

MENCH—Multiple stories of the generalist's craft
M—Mindful stories (clinician)
E—Evidentiary stories
N—Narrative stories (patient and family)
C—Centered stories (context and place)
H—Health care stories

POEM—Patient-Oriented Evidence that Matters

POISED—How to use the electronic health record
P—Prepare
O—Orient
I—Information gather
S—Share
E—Educate
D—Debrief

POwER—Teaching model for clinic setting
P—Prepare
O—Orchestrate
w
E—Educate
R—Review

SCREEM—Resources
S—Social
C—Cultural
R—Religious
E—Educational
E—Economic
M—Medical

STEPS—Tool for evaluating pharmacotherapeutics
S—Safety
T—Tolerability

E—Effectiveness
P—Price
S—Simplicity

Diagnostic Mnemonics

ANCIENT DIVA—Physical diagnostic categories
    A—Anatomy
    N—Neoplasm
    C—Congenital/Genetic
    I—Infectious
    E—Endocrine/Metabolic
    N—Nutritional
    T—Trauma
    D—Degenerative
    I—Inflammatory
    V—Vascular
    A—Allergic/Autoimmune

ISEA—Cognitive diagnostic categories
    I—Illness prototypes
    S—Self-image
    E—Explanatory models
    A—Attributions

PAW SCAB—Habitat diagnostic categories
    P—Plants
    A—Animals
    W—Water
    S—Soil
    C—Climate
    A—Air
    B—Buildings

SAVE—Spiritual diagnostic categories
    S—Soul story
    A—Awakened soul
    V—Visited soul
    E—Escaped soul

TEL—Emotional diagnostic categories
- T—Threat (anxiety disorders)
- E—Expression (addiction, somatoform, complex pain disorders)
- L—Loss (affective disorders)

TTTS—Social diagnostic categories
- T—Troubles
- T—Ties
- T—Traditions
- S—SCREEM resources

Index

Note: Page numbers followed by *f* indicate figures; those followed by *t* indicate tables.

A

Abstract conceptualization, 159
Active experimentation, 159
Active listening, 42, 56, 100, 101*t*, 104, 123
Actual reason for connecting (ARC), 44, 80–82, 83*t*, 86, 88, 91, 96, 127, 152, 161, 181
    new information about, 93
    patient's, 83
    Pedro's, 164
Adverse childhood experiences, 239
Adverse community environments, 239–240
Affinity, 110, 111*t*
Anatomy, Neoplasm, Congenital/Genetic, Infectious, Endocrine/Metabolic, Nutritional, Trauma, Degenerative, Inflammatory, Vascular, Allergic/Autoimmune (ANCIENT DIVA), 130, 291
Anchoring, 212
    heuristic, 124
    social, 150
ANCIENT DIVA. *See* Anatomy, Neoplasm, Congenital/Genetic, Infectious, Endocrine/Metabolic, Nutritional, Trauma, Degenerative, Inflammatory, Vascular, Allergic/Autoimmune (ANCIENT DIVA)
Ancient forest standard, 142
Angel limb. *See* Spiritual limb
Anthropology, 6
Antifragility, 136, 187, 243–244, 249
Aphorisms, 4, 13, 225–226
ARC. *See* Actual reason for connecting (ARC)
Assessment tools, 281–283
Associational heuristic, 124
Associations, 124, 212
Attending. *See* Mindfulness and attending
Attending Imagery Technique, 27, 28*t*, 29*f*
Attentive observation, 26
Availability, 193, 212
    rule of thumb, 124
    up-to-date evidence databases, 1

B

Background, Affect, Troubles, Handle, and Empathy (BATHE), 19, 30, 50, 289
    features, 32*t*
    on fingernails, 32*f*
Balint group, 28, 184, 195
BATHE. *See* Background, Affect, Troubles, Handle, and Empathy (BATHE)
Beginner's mind, 26–27
Behavior rules of thumb, 209*t*
Behavioral inheritance, 205, 206*t*
Biases, 212, 213–215*t*
Bioculture, 136, 204, 207–208*t*
Bioenergy, 135
Biomedical treatment, 93, 95*t*, 129
Biophilia hypothesis, 209
Bioregion, 202
    features of, 203*t*
    with health care services, 51
Bureaucratic fulfillment, 93, 95*t*

C

Calgary-Cambridge model, 8
Camera Walk, 272–274
Capacity-to-burden ratio, 161, 169

CARE approach, 8
Celebrate, 83, 172
Ceremonies, 13, 49, 84, 85*t*
    decaying maintenance, 92
    growing maintenance, 92
    heroic transition, 90
    labeling transition, 90
    life cycle maintenance, 92
    maintenance, 84, 90–91, 91*t*, 92*t*, 182–184, 183*t*, 184*t*
    religious, 35
    stuck maintenance, 92
    transition, 89, 89–90*t*, 178, 191, 193
Chaos, 41, 88, 175, 178, 191, 192
    domain, 177*t*, 178
    narratives, 87, 189, 216
Clinical circumstances, 144*t*
Clinical discovery, 48, 54, 69, 80, 93, 98, 103, 121
    diagnostic work of, 56
    and evaluation, 119
    expanding field of shared understanding, 122*f*
    recognition processes, 125*t*
    and sensemaking, 121*f*
    strategies and related tactics, 123*f*
    touching skills, 119–121
Clinical encounter, 1, 12–13, 19, 30, 32, 47, 49–51, 54, 56, 59, 175, 185, 193, 279
    achieving situational awareness using Ecological Clinical Map, 71, 72*f*
    attending and Grip of Power, 74–75, 76*t*
    Cynefin framework, 175, 176*f*
    journey of, 67, 68*f*, 71, 80, 85*t*
    orientation, 71, 80
    prepare and open hand, 72–74, 73*t*, 74*f*
    ritual structure of, 48
    routines, 179–181
    wrist lines of guidance, 81
        Guiding Pulses, 84–92
        Guiding Wrist, 81–84
Clinical Hand add-ons, 204
    Swinging Cultural Ape, 204–210
Clinical Hand Direct Observation tool, 284
    ground rules and goals, 284–286
Clinical Hand tool, 8, 47–51, 47*t*, 48*f*, 67, 68*f*, 81*f*, 135, 153, 159
    BATHE letters on nails of, 31
    of generalist craft, 6–8
    highlights, 49*t*
Clinical jazz, 11, 39, 69, 148, 183, 195
    features of clinical jazz improvisation, 60, 60–61*t*
    generalist relational, 14
    of generalist's craft, 1
Clinical reality, 2, 3*t*
Clinicians, 4, 12, 14, 54, 56, 76, 87, 90, 122, 136, 164, 190, 262
    experienced, 5
    generalist, 6, 39, 88, 129, 147
    medical routines to, 89
    new "understudy", 186
    patterns for, 111
    personal, 185
    primary care, 42, 186
    in training, 170
Clues, 102, 120, 159, 189, 212, 213–215*t*
Cognitive limb, 21, 129, 131
Cognitive naming and caring, 131, 132*t*
Cognitive self-care, 20*t*
Collaborative Deliberation framework, 8
Community capacities, 144*t*
Community-oriented primary care, 200
    features of, 200, 202*t*
Complex domain, 177*t*, 178
Complexity theory, 40
    conceptual history and insights from, 242
    health in, 243–245
    implications of, 245
Complicated domain, 176*t*, 178

Concerns, 161
  health, 206
  patient's, 81, 99
  prioritized, 84
Concrete experience, 159, 271
Connect Finger, 71, 71f
Connect guidepost, 69, 74, 75–79
  Path to Connect, 75–79
Consultation Model (Pendleton), 8
Contact access, Continuity, Comprehensiveness, and Coordination (four Cs of primary medical care), 108, 232, 233t
Contextualizing care, 149
Continuity, 107–108, 110, 111t, 186
  of care, 185, 232
  case conference, 277–279
Continuum of Decision-Making, 160, 160f
Conventional physician-centeredness, 200
Craft, 5, 191. *See also* Generalist's Craft
  of generalist primary medical care, 226
  learning and mastering, 1–4
  origins of, 5–6
  purpose, 4–5
Critical curiosity, 26
Cultural change, 206
Cultural healing traditions, 134–135
Cultural traditions, 6, 105
Culture, 3, 9, 26, 53, 87, 104, 113, 129, 136, 205, 210, 242, 278
  human biology wired for, 199
  importance of, 50
Cynefin framework, 175, 176f
  domains of, 176–177t

D

Decaying maintenance ceremonies, 92, 92t
Decision-making, 149, 160, 209
Denial, 131, 218, 238
  of disease, 220
  faces of, 219t
  of health, 220
  patient, 218–220
Developmental trauma, 229, 238–241, 254
  impact of, 10
  people with, 131
  sources, 239
Diagnostic mnemonics, 130, 291–292
Diagnostic strategy, 123
Direct reciprocity, 206t
Discipline, 21, 29, 46, 69, 123, 172, 179, 256
Disease-Oriented Evidence (DOE), 58, 147, 147t, 289
Disease story, 54, 104–105
Distal context, 54, 109–110, 183, 188, 190
Diversity, 6, 21, 110, 136, 209
DOE. *See* Disease-Oriented Evidence (DOE)
Dramas, 13, 49, 84, 85t, 87, 185–190, 216
  breakthrough tactics for, 190t
  facilitators of effective, 186t
  family questions in, 189t
  features of, 88t
  illness trajectory, 187f
  mastering, 188t

E

Eclectic, 256–257
Ecological Clinical Map, 13, 47, 47t, 51–54, 75
  achieving situational awareness using, 71, 72f
  clinic, community, and healing landscapes, 199–204
  highlights, 52–53t
  patient, 196–199
  tool, 52f
Ecological identity, 113, 203, 203t

Ecology of medical care, 233–234
Educational resources, 13, 271
    assessment tools, 281–283
    Clinical Hand Direct Observation tool, 284
        ground rules and goals, 284–286
    GEMs, 272–276
        Camera Walk, 272–274
        Fox Walking, 274–275
        Sculpting Health, 275–276
    teaching strategies for generalist's craft, 276–281
EHR. *See* Electronic health record (EHR)
Electronic health record (EHR), 12, 72, 76, 280–281
    POISED mnemonic for using, 78*t*
Electronic medical record, 12
Elephant and the Rider of Changing Behavior, The, 40, 40*t*, 44–46, 45*f*, 253–254, 253*f*
Elicit Agenda, 94*t*
Emergence, 136, 200, 242, 243*t*, 252
Emotional intelligence, 24, 25*t*, 199
Emotional limb, 21, 128–129
Emotional naming and caring, 130, 131*t*
Emotional self-care, 20*t*
Emplotment, 217
Enactment, 151
Endosymbiosis, 205, 206*t*
Epigenetics, 205, 206*t*, 239
Evidence, 9, 43, 56–57, 59, 140, 153, 205, 220, 229, 262
    types and sources of, 144–145*t*
    up-to-date evidence databases, 1
Evidence-informing, 120
Evolution
    bioculture and evolution matter to clinicians, 207–208*t*
    drivers of life story, 205*f*
    mechanisms of heritable change and variation, 206*t*

Experiential learning cycle (Kolb), 159, 271, 272*f*
Expertise, 10–11, 43, 141, 144*t*
Explanatory model, 105, 106*t*
Expressive eyes, 94, 101, 102*f*
Eye juggling, 19, 29–30, 30*f*, 31*t*, 88, 150
Eye of context, 29
Eye of self, 29
Eye on the patient, 29

F

Faces of patients, 197, 197*f*
    characteristics, 198*t*
Faces of safeguarding and denial, 219*t*
Faith, Importance, Community, Address (FICA), 135, 289
Family, 110, 111*t*
    APGAR, 112, 113*t*
    circle, 111
    life cycle, 111, 112*f*
Family medicine, 1–2, 200
    clinical content, 5
    educator, 7
    generalist's craft to, 46
    LVHN, 13
    residencies, 28–29
Feelings, Ideas, Function, Expectations (FIFE), 105, 105*t*, 289
FICA. *See* Faith, Importance, Community, Address (FICA)
Field Guide, 1–2, 4–5, 14, 219, 260, 265, 271
    attribution of single authorship, 6
    purposes, 257
    in River of Health metaphor, 247
    strategies in, 69
    tools and curriculum, 8
Field Guide for the Generalist's Craft, 4–5, 10, 12–13
FIFE. *See* Feelings, Ideas, Function, Expectations (FIFE)

Index   297

Finding Common Ground
   conceptual strategies for, 158–161, 158f
   history, 278
   work of, 151
Fingers of Direction, 67, 69, 70f
Five Fingers of Direction, 48, 49t, 59, 99, 280
Five-limb processing and encoding, 235
Folk Model (Helman), 8
Four Areas framework (Stott and Davis), 8
Four-Circle Curriculum, 9f
Four Habits model, 8
Fox Walking, 274–275
Frequent attenders, 238
Frequent symptom reporters. *See* Frequent attenders

G
GEMs. *See* Generalist enhancement methods (GEMs)
general health advice, 93, 95t
General practitioners, 3, 220
   examples of current tensions and pressures facing, 3t
   international, 260
Generalism, 24, 122, 142–143, 230, 254, 262–264
   features and principles of, 264
   generalist ways, 254–256, 255t
   jack-of-all-trades, polymath, eclectic, and phronimos, 256–257
   Montreal statement on Generalist Practice, 260, 260–261t
   principles of, 257–260
   simple rules, 56, 265
Generalist enhancement methods (GEMs), 13, 271, 272
   Camera Walk, 272–274
   Fox Walking, 274–275
   Sculpting Health, 275–276

Generalist Wheel of Inquiry, 141–142, 141f, 259, 259f
Generalists, 42–44, 143, 195, 256
   additional evidence questions for, 143t
   medical, 242, 245
   practice, 1
   relational clinical jazz, 14
   ways, 254–256, 255t
Generalist's craft, 1–2, 7, 229
   artisans of, 122
   clinical hand and supporting tools of, 47, 47t
      Clinical Hand tool, 48–51
      Ecological Clinical Map tool, 51–54
      Relationship-Centered Clinical Method tool, 54–56
      Round Table of Evidence tool, 56–59
   Clinical Hand tool of, 6–8
   generalism, 254–264
      eclectic, 256–257
      generalist ways, 254–256
      jack-of-all-trades, 256–257
      Montreal Statement on Generalist Practice, 260–261
      phronimos, 256–257
      polymath, 256–257
      principles, 257–260
   health and healing, 241–252
   high-value primary medical care, 262–264
   human behavior, 252–254
   metaphors of, 39–46, 40t
   of primary care healing, 4
   primary medical care, 230–241
      connects with, 239t
      developmental trauma and trauma-informed care, 238–241
      ecology of medical care, 233–234
      four functions of, 232t

Generalist's craft (*continued*)
    frequent attenders and power laws, 238
    functions, facilitators, and principles, 231–233
    health, symptoms, and illness behavior, 234–237
    primary health care, 230–231
    symptom awareness process, 235*f*
    principles informing design and selection of tools of, 11*t*
    principles of, 258*t*
    story and, 108*t*
    teaching strategies for, 276–281
        Continuity Case Conference, 277–279
        Mega Clinic, 279–280
        Paired Precepting, 280–281
Genes, 149, 199, 205
Genetics, 205, 206*t*
Genogram, 111, 190
Goal-oriented care, 82, 161–163
Goals, 42, 46, 49, 56, 67, 273, 277, 280
    of care, 107, 158, 161–163
    of encounter, 81–84
    questions to guide tailoring care plan, 163*t*
    types, 162*t*
    values history, 162*t*
Gold standard, 142
Good Generalist Craft, outcomes of, 10*t*
Grip of Power, 74–75, 75*f*, 76*t*
Group selection, 206*t*
Growing maintenance ceremonies, 92, 92*t*
Guiding Pulses, 84, 84*f*
Guiding Wrist, 81–84, 82*f*

H
Habitat, 11, 19, 49, 110, 129, 135, 249
    features, 144*t*
    naming and caring, 135, 135*t*
    self-care, 20*t*
Habits of mind, 26
Hand Over Finger, 98, 98*f*
Hand Over guidepost, 78, 98–100, 167, 167*t*
Hands-on Learners, 271
Hands-on oral tradition, 11
Harm, 74, 145, 158–159, 191
Healer, 10, 12, 44
    generalist, 27, 81, 121, 129, 175, 225, 241, 254
    healer–patient relationship, 111
    primary care, 50–51, 54
Healing, 2, 10, 200, 241, 257
    common factors, 251*t*
    cultural healing traditions, 134–135
    generalist's craft of, 5, 11, 40, 67
    landscape, 200
    multilayered symbols, 34
    relationships, 5, 250–252
    significant aspects of healing relationships, 251*t*
    Spiral of Healing, 252, 252*f*
    symbols, 136
    three ways for, 249*t*
Health, 225, 241
    in complexity theory, 243–245
    as concept, 242–243
    definitional features of, 246*t*
    drivers of, 247, 248*t*
    maintenance visits, 162
    as membership, 245–247
    properties of complex adaptive systems, 243–244*t*
    River of Health, 247, 247*f*
    story, 212–217
health-seeking process, 234, 234*f*
"Heartsink" patients. *See* Frequent attenders
Helicobacter pylori, 209–210
Heroic transition ceremonies, 90
Heuristics, 44, 124, 126, 212, 213–215*t*, 253

High-value primary medical care, 262–264, 262*t*
  equation for, 262
  features of, 263*t*
Horizontal integration, 231
Housekeep Finger, 171, 171*f*
Housekeep guidepost, 69, 171–173
  indicators of completing, 173*t*
  tools for, 172*t*
Human behavior
  challenges of changing, 10, 252–254
  resistant, 44
Human limb. *See* Cognitive limb
Hypotheses, 56, 84, 124, 126
  generating and evaluating, 127
  working, 90, 123, 126

I

"I" perspective, 57–58, 142
ICD. *See* International Classification of Diseases (ICD)
ICPC. *See* International Classification of Primary Care (ICPC)
Illness prototypes, 105, 106*t*, 124, 132
Illness prototypes, Self-image, Explanatory models, Attributions (ISEA), 291
Illness story, 104–105, 278
Improvisational jazz, 14, 59
Indirect reciprocity, 206*t*
Induction, 122
Information evaluation, four questions for, 145*t*
Information mastery, 142, 147–148
  minitools of, 58
  publications and workshops on, 8
Inner chatter, 21–24, 26, 28, 30, 94, 104, 132
Integrated care, 257
Integrated self, 217
Interdependence, 21, 44, 71, 114, 136, 206, 209, 245–246

International Classification of Diseases (ICD), 104, 257
International Classification of Primary Care (ICPC), 257
Interpretive care, 257
Intimacy, 6, 110, 111*t*, 217
ISEA. *See* Illness prototypes, Self-image, Explanatory models, Attributions (ISEA)
"It" perspective, 58
"It's" perspective, 58

J

Jack-of-all-trades, 255–257
Jazz, 59
  clinical, 11, 39, 69, 148, 183, 195
  improvisational, 14, 59
Johari window, 122

K

Kairos time, 34
Kin-based groups, 4
Kin selection, 206*t*
Knowledge in action, 195

L

Label, Etiology, Time, Severity, History, Effects, Affects, Rx (LETS HEAR), 289–290
Labeling transition ceremonies, 90
Language, 11–12, 39, 99, 123, 256
  body, 86
  selective pressures for, 204
  symbolic, 199
LATE. *See* Listen, Address the fear, Touch the trouble, and Express hope (LATE)
Lehigh Valley Health Network (LVHN), 7–10
Life cycle maintenance ceremonies, 92, 92*t*

Listen, Address the fear, Touch the trouble, and Express hope (LATE), 193, 289
Listening skills, 100–103
Livelihood self-care, 20*t*
Livelihoods identity, 114, 114*t*
A LOT Moments, 94, 95*f*, 101
LVHN. *See* Lehigh Valley Health Network (LVHN)

M

Maintenance ceremonies, 84, 90–91, 182–184. *See also* Transition ceremonies
  features of, 91*t*
  mastering, 184*t*
  remembering the family in, 183*t*
  types of, 92*t*
Malady experience, 104, 107
Masquerades, 126
Meaning response, 249–250
Medical Information, 93, 95*t*
Medicare annual wellness exams, 162
Medicine of neighbors, 182
Mega Clinic, 279–280
MENCH. *See* Mindful, Evidentiary, Narrative, Centered, Health care (MENCH)
Meta-models, 102, 103*t*
Metaphors, 13, 39
  of generalist's craft, 39–46, 40*t*
    The Elephant and the Rider of Changing Behavior, 44–46
    River of Health, 40–41
    Spiral of Healing, 41–42
    Windmill Sails of Generalism, 42–44
Migration, 206
Mindful, Evidentiary, Narrative, Centered, Health care (MENCH), 217, 217*t*, 290
Mindful handwashing, 172, 173*t*
Mindful practice, 24, 26–28, 27*t*

Mindfulness and attending, 19, 23
  clinical tools for, 27–29
  emotional and social intelligence, 24, 25*t*
  mindful practice and mindfulness meditation, 26–27
Mindfulness meditation, 24, 26–27, 26*t*
Mindlines, 220–221, 220–221*t*
Mnemonics, 287–289
Montreal statement on Generalist Practice, 260, 260–261*t*

N

Naming and Caring Tree, 49, 127, 128*f*, 135, 151
  naming or diagnostic limbs, 189
  SCREEM resources on social limb of, 161
Natural cooperation, 205, 206*t*
Nervous system, 205
Network reciprocity, 206*t*
Numbers, 58, 142, 145, 159, 249
Nurse practitioners, 12, 230

O

Observation skills, 100–103, 100*t*
Observers, 271–272
Obvious domain, 176*t*
"One Health" concept, 246
Online self-presentations, 114
Optimal healing environments, 200, 201*t*
Oral traditions, 11–12
Ottawa Ankle Rules, 82

P

Paired precepting, 280–281
Palm of Hope, 49, 49*t*, 127–137, 128*f*
Pareto distribution, 238
Partners in health, 225
Path to Connect, 75–79, 77*t*

Patient capacities, 144*t*
Patient-Centered Interviewing approach (Robert Smith), 8
Patient denial, 218–220
Patient expectations, 3*t*, 169, 185
Patient-Oriented Evidence that Matters (POEMs), 58, 147, 147*t*, 290
Patient requests, 93, 95*t*
Patient's stories, 54, 56, 103, 212
    exploring, 104–107
    weaving among the stories, 103*f*
PAW SCAB. *See* Plants, Animals, Water, Soil, Climate, Air, Buildings (PAW SCAB)
Payoff, 126
PCPCM. *See* Person-Centered *Primary Care Measure* (PCPCM)
Person-Centered Primary Care Measure (PCPCM), 262, 264*t*
Person face, 199
Personal expectations, 2, 3*t*
Personalizing, 126, 149, 161–163
Phronimos, 256–257
Physical limb, 19, 128, 130
Physical Naming and Caring, 130, 130*t*
Physical self-care, 20*t*
Physicians, 3, 12, 230, 253
    family, 87, 217
    primary care, 182
    services of, 230
Placebo effect, 250
Placebo response, 130, 250
Plants, Animals, Water, Soil, Climate, Air, Buildings (PAW SCAB), 135, 291
POEMs. *See* Patient-Oriented Evidence that Matters (POEMs)
POISED. *See* Prepare, Orient, Information Gather, Share, Educate, Debrief (POISED)
Polymath, 256–257
Positive criticism, 160, 160*t*
Post-it Notes[*], 76
Potential harms, 209

Power, 5, 54, 74–75, 76*t*, 85, 90, 98–99, 107, 108*t*, 115, 119, 129, 134, 136, 145, 158, 178, 250
Power laws, 238
Practice/health system expectations, 3*t*
Practitioners, 1, 5, 12, 257
    general, 3, 6
    of generalist's craft, 122
    nurse, 12, 230
Precautionary principle, 209
Precepting, 170, 280
Precise treatment, 181, 181*t*
Prepare, Orchestrate, Educate, Review (POwER) framework, 276
Prepare, Orient, Information Gather, Share, Educate, Debrief (POISED), 77, 78*t*, 290
Primary care healers, 3–4, 6, 23, 41
Primary health care, 6, 107, 230
    domains and context of, 231*f*
Primary medical care, 1, 4, 10, 34, 48, 51, 230
    connects with, 239*t*
    developmental trauma and trauma-informed care, 238–241
    ecology of medical care, 233–234
    four functions of, 232*t*
    frequent attenders and power laws, 238
    functions, facilitators, and principles, 231–233
    health, symptoms, and illness behavior, 234–237
    primary health care, 230–231
    symptom awareness process, 235*f*
Principled negotiation, 160, 160*t*
Prioritize Agenda, 94*t*
Prioritizing, 44, 73, 93, 94*t*, 96, 126, 163, 260, 262
Probability, 90, 126
Proximal context, 109–110
Psychosocial assistance, 93, 95*t*
Psychotherapy, 250
Public health, 143, 150, 230

Q

Q-list. *See* Question list (Q-list)
Qualitative studies, questions for evaluating, 145, 146t
Quantitative studies, questions for evaluating, 145, 146t
Quest narratives, 189, 216
Question list (Q-list), 281, 282–283t

R

Randomized clinical trials (RCTs), 250
RCTs. *See* Randomized clinical trials (RCTs)
Readers, 272
Reason for visit (RFV), 238
Reciprocity, 110, 111t
Recognize, 21–22, 24, 39, 43, 72, 115, 137, 156, 241t
Red flags, 126, 153, 210
Reflection in action, 195, 279
Reflection on action, 195, 279–280
Reflective observation, 159
Reflective pause, 46–47, 109–116, 137
Reflective practice model, 195, 196t
Relationship-building, 81, 87, 120
Relationship-Centered Clinical Method, 7, 13, 47, 47t, 54–56, 55f, 98
  add-ons, 210
  health story, 212–217
  heuristics, clues, and biases, 212
  highlights, 57t
  patient denial, 218–220
  tool, 7, 58f
  use of, 99
  whole person, 210–211
Relationship: Establishment, Development, Engagement (REDE) model, 8
Representative rule of thumb, 124
Representativeness, 212
Research evidence, 141, 145t
  residency curriculum design, 10
Resilience, 136, 187, 243–244, 249
Restitution narratives, 87, 212, 216
RFV. *See* Reason for visit (RFV)
Ritual, 7, 19, 33, 33t, 136, 192–193
  components, 35t
  functions, 36t
  symbols, 136
River of Health, 13, 39, 40–41, 40t, 41f, 247, 247f
Robustness, 136, 187, 243–244
Roles, 7, 56, 127, 134, 161, 164–166, 164t
  for generalist healer, 129
  Pedro's explanatory story and engaging plan, 165–166t
  social, 104
Round Table of Evidence, 8, 13, 47, 47t, 56–59, 59t, 140–146, 140f
  add-ons, 220–221
  tool, 142
Routines, 13, 49, 84, 85t, 87, 179–181
  features of, 86t
  mastering, 181t
  precise treatment, 181t
  remembering family in, 180t
  ritualized, 4
Rules of thumb. *See* Heuristics

S

Safeguarding, 131, 218, 219t, 238
Safety Net Finger, 169, 169f
Safety Net guidepost, 169–171, 170t
Safety, Tolerance, Efficacy, Price, Simplicity (STEPS) approach, 58, 148, 148t, 290–291
Sanctioning, 86, 88
SAVE. *See* Soul story, Awakened soul, Visited soul, Escaped soul (SAVE)
SCREEM resources. *See* Social, cultural, religious, educational, economic, and medical (SCREEM resources)
Sculpting Health, 275–276
Self-care, 19–23, 20t

Self-organization processes, 205
Sensemaking, 149–156, 220–221
   process for Pedro's clinical encounter, 154–155t
   process in clinical encounter, 151t
   sensible scales, 149, 150f
Sensible scales, 149, 150f
Set Agenda
   Finger, 80, 80f
   Guidepost, 78, 92–96
   indicators of completing, 96t
Shared principles of primary medical care, 233, 233t
Shinrinyoku (forest bathing), 135
Short-term goals, 162
Sickness story, 105, 107t
Sick role, 36, 83, 104
Six Phases model (Byrne and Long), 8
Social anchoring, 150
Social, cultural, religious, educational, economic, and medical (SCREEM resources), 133–134, 133t, 290
Social intelligence, 24, 25t
Social limb, 21, 129, 132, 161
Social Naming and Caring, 132, 132t
Social self-care, 20t
Social/ecological/political issues, 3t
Society, 205
Soul story, Awakened soul, Visited soul, Escaped soul (SAVE), 291
Specialism, 245, 255
Specialists, simple rules of, 42–43, 43t
Speech cues, 101, 103t
Spiral of Healing, 13, 39, 40t, 41–42, 42f, 252, 252f
Spiritual limb, 21, 129, 134
Spiritual Naming and Caring, 134, 134t
Spiritual self-care, 20t
Spirituality, 134–135, 199
Stacey matrix, 40
Statistics, 145
Stories, 4, 6, 107–108, 217
   and generalist craft, 108t
   malady, 54
   tools, 216t
Stress, 35, 124, 245
Stuck maintenance ceremonies, 92, 92t
Swinging Cultural Ape, 49t, 50, 204, 204f
Swinging on the Tree, 99, 127–137, 153
Symbolic inheritance, 205, 206t
Symbols, 34, 39
Symptom formation process, 235, 236t

T

Teaching strategies for generalist's craft, 276
   continuity case conference, 277–279
   Mega Clinic, 279–280
   paired precepting, 280–281
Techno-consumer, 196, 198–199
TEL. *See* Threat, Expression, Loss (TEL)
Therapeutic listening, 93, 95t
"Think aloud" strategy, 99, 159
Threat, Expression, Loss (TEL), 292
Three Function model, 8
Thriving skills, 19
   BATHE technique, 30–33
   creative hero(ine), tools of, 23t
   eye juggling, 29–30, 30f
   mindfulness and attending, 23–29
      clinical tools for, 27–29
      emotional and social intelligence, 24, 25t
      mindful practice and mindfulness meditation, 26–27
   ritual, 33–36
   self-care, 19–23
   wellness, importance of, 19–23
Tools, 59–61, 60f
   of Generalist's Craft, 10–11
   of Turtle Craft, 7
Touching skills, 119–121
   examining patients, 120t
   preparation for, 120t

Transition ceremonies, 84–85, 89, 191–193. *See also* Maintenance ceremonies
  aims for, 192*t*
  features of, 89*t*
  mastering, 193*t*
  types of, 90*t*
Trauma-informed approach, key principles of, 240*t*
Trauma-informed care, 56, 238–241
Trauma-informed primary medical care at practice level, 241*t*
Trouble tool, 49*t*, 50
Troubles, ties, and traditions (three Ts), 132
Troubles, Ties, Traditions, SCREEM resources (TTTS), 292
Trust-inducing, 120
TTTS. *See* Troubles, Ties, Traditions, SCREEM resources (TTTS)
Turtle Craft tools, 8–10

U

Useful information, questions to identify, 148*t*
Usefulness equation, 147

V

Values and preferences, 144*t*
Values history, 162*t*
Vertical integration, 231

W

Way of Being, 255, 255*t*
Way of Belonging, 255, 255*t*
Way of Doing, 255, 255*t*
Way of Knowing, 255, 255*t*
Way of Perceiving, 255, 255*t*
"We" perspective, 58, 142
Wellness, importance of, 19–23
WHO. *See* World Health Organization (WHO)
"Whole Health" concept, 246
Whole person
  change, six stages of, 116*t*
  in context, 107, 210–211, 211*t*
  life story, 115*t*
  story and generalist craft, 108*t*
  understanding, 109*f*, 110*t*
  wheel of readiness to change, 117*f*
Windmill Sails of Generalism, 39–40, 40*t*, 42–44, 43*f*, 143, 259, 259*f*
Wisdom, 225–226
Work relative value units (wRVUs), 2, 74
World Health Organization (WHO), 230
Wrist Lines of Guidance, 49, 49*t*, 81
  Guiding Pulses, 84–92
  Guiding Wrist, 81–84
wRVUs. *See* Work relative value units (wRVUs)